Fungal Infection: Diagnosis and Management

Fungal Infection: Diagnosis and Management

Editor: Sanda Warne

AMERICAN
MEDICAL PUBLISHERS
www.americanmedicalpublishers.com

AMERICAN
MEDICAL PUBLISHERS
www.americanmedicalpublishers.com

Cataloging-in-Publication Data

Fungal infection : diagnosis and management / edited by Sanda Warne.
p. cm.
Includes bibliographical references and index.
ISBN 978-1-63927-672-1
1. Mycoses. 2. Mycoses--Diagnosis. 3. Mycoses--Prevention.
4. Mycoses--Treatment. 5. Medical mycology. I. Warne, Sanda.
RC117 .F86 2023
616.969--dc23

American Medical Publishers,
41 Flatbush Avenue,
1st Floor, New York,
NY 11217, USA

ISBN 978-1-63927-672-1 (Hardback)

Contents

Preface

This book aims to highlight the current researches and provides a platform to further the scope of innovations in this area. This book is a product of the combined efforts of many researchers and scientists, after going through thorough studies and analysis from different parts of the world. The objective of this book is to provide the readers with the latest information of the field.

Fungal infection is referred to as a disease caused by fungi, which are microorganisms identified by chitin, a substance present in their cell walls. Some common types of fungal infections are ringworm infection, yeast infection, athlete's foot infection and onychomycosis. The risk of developing fungal infection is dependent upon environmental factors along with the processes happening inside the body, such as humidity and dampness, poor circulation of blood, menopause in women, skin or nail injury, and suppressed immune system. These infections can spread from one person to another. To prevent the spread of fungal infections, it is essential to maintain good hygiene. Preventive measures like washing hands often, keeping skin dry and clean, not using other people's personal care products, etc. can help in avoiding fungal infections. The topics included in this book on the diagnosis and management of fungal infections is of utmost significance and bound to provide incredible insights to readers. It is appropriate for students seeking detailed information in this area as well as for experts.

I would like to express my sincere thanks to the authors for their dedicated efforts in the completion of this book. I acknowledge the efforts of the publisher for providing constant support. Lastly, I would like to thank my family for their support in all academic endeavors.

Editor

1

The Burden of Fungal Infections in Ethiopia

Tafese B. Tufa [1,2,*] **and David W. Denning** [3,4]

1 Asella Teaching and Referral Hospital, College of Health Sciences, Arsi University, P.O. Box 04, Asella, Ethiopia
2 Hirsch Institute of Tropical Medicine (HITM), Heinrich-Heine University, P.O. Box 04, Asella, Ethiopia
3 The National Aspergillosis Centre, Wythenshawe Hospital, Manchester M23 9LT, UK
4 The University of Manchester and Manchester Academic Health Science Centre, Manchester M13 9PL, UK; ddenning@manchester.ac.uk
* Correspondence: tafeseb.tufa@yahoo.com

Abstract: The burden of severe fungal infections (FIs) is not well addressed in Ethiopia. We have estimated the burden of FIs from multiple demographic sources and by searching articles from PubMed. Opportunistic FIs were estimated using modelling and 2017 national HIV data. The burdens of chronic pulmonary aspergillosis (CPA) and allergic bronchopulmonary aspergillosis (ABPA) were estimated by using the prevalence of asthma, chronic obstructive pulmonary disease, and annual the incidence of tuberculosis. Of the 105,000,000 estimated Ethiopian population, 610,000 are thought to have HIV infection. Our estimation of HIV-related FIs were: 9900 cryptococcal meningitis (CM), 12,700 *Pneumocystis jirovecii* pneumonia (PCP), 76,300 oral and 56,000 oesophageal candidiasis cases. A remarkable 7,051,700 4–14-year-olds probably have tinea capitis and 1,469,000 women probably have recurrent *Candida* vaginitis. There were 15,200 estimated CPA cases (prevalence) and 11,500 invasive aspergillosis (IA) cases (incidence). Data are scant, but we estimated 5300 candidaemia and 800 Candida peritonitis cases. In conclusion, approximately 8% of Ethiopians suffer from FIs annually, mostly schoolchildren with tinea capitis. IA, CM and PCP are the major causes of fungal deaths. The absence of CD4 count is challenging the identification of HIV patients at risk of opportunistic FIs. There is a pressing need to improve FI diagnosis, probably including national surveillance.

Keywords: invasive fungal infections; tinea capitis; epidemiology; Ethiopia

---

1. Introduction

Pathogenic, opportunistic and allergenic fungi cause a very wide range of diseases from simple superficial mycosis to complex disseminated endemic or opportunistic mycosis [1]. Unlike superficial or cutaneous mycosis, disseminated fungal infections (FIs) are life threatening if not appropriately treated. In resource-limited settings (RLSs), invasive FIs remain understudied and underdiagnosed despite their high mortality rates when compared with other infectious diseases [1,2].

The number of immunosuppressed individuals who are at risk of developing opportunistic mycosis is increasing due to HIV/AIDS even though the rate is reduced because of antiretroviral therapy (ART), the expansion of intensive care units (ICUs), chronic diseases, malignancies and sophisticated procedures such as stem cell or organ transplantation [3]. The most common opportunistic FIs are cryptococcal meningitis (CM), Pneumocystis jirovecii pneumonia (PCP), invasive candidiasis and disseminated aspergillosis [4]. Diagnosis and management of these opportunistic mycosis in RLSs is challenging as standard diagnostic methods and essential antifungal medicines are often absent [5].

Many populations are sensitive (allergic) to fungi and develop severe asthma or exacerbation of pre-existing respiratory diseases [6]. Anyone in the general population may develop dermatophytoses and vaginal candidiasis is common in women [1]. Although less attention is given to the management of dermatophytoses, the prevalence of atypical dermatophytoses is increasing and has become an emerging public health problem, with the new development of extensive terbinafine resistance [7]. Antifungal resistance in Trichophyton spp. is due to two amino acid substitutions or point mutations [8]. As studies from India indicate, the predominant causative organism of dermatophytoses has shifted from T. rubrum to T. mentagrophytes [9–11]. The two main causative agents of dermatophytoses survive on towels for <12 weeks for T. rubrum but >25 weeks for T. mentagrophytes [12]. This change may be responsible for the widespread and inflammatory lesions associated with T. mentagrophytes and transmitted by sharing fomites.

Across the world, over one billion people of all ages suffer from FIs annually [13], accounting for over 1.6 million deaths and contributing to the poor and fatal outcome of many more diseases [14]. This figure is three-fold higher than the annual deaths from malaria and comparable to the number of tuberculosis deaths per year [2].

Even though invasive FIs are life threatening, they do not receive sufficient attention from many global health organizations or governments. Particularly in sub-Saharan African countries, data on the incidence and prevalence of these infections are lacking and limited diagnostic facilities, few evidence-based case management protocols and the unavailability of appropriate antifungal medications and specialists in the field amplify the problems [1,2]. This situation results in high and preventable case mortality and morbidity.

Robust estimates of fungal disease incidence and prevalence are lacking in Ethiopia [2]. In the absence of either population- or hospital-based surveys as source epidemiological data, we sought to provide estimates by modelling using available data on FIs in Ethiopia and assumptions drawn from published literature. This estimation of FIs in Ethiopia will allow a baseline estimate for future studies and serve as a reference for policy makers.

2. Materials and Methods

Data Sources

For the estimation of the serious FI burden in Ethiopia, we used the 2017 estimated Ethiopian total population for the general healthy population. We used different risk groups including people living with HIV/AIDS (PLWHA), patients with asthma, chronic obstructive pulmonary disease (COPD), cancer, pulmonary tuberculosis and postsurgical patients, and those admitted to ICUs to estimate specific infections. To estimate tinea capitis prevalence, we determined the number of children in the high-risk age group (3–14 years old) from the Ethiopia National Education [15] and Education for All National Review Report [16]. Data on PLWHA numbers were obtained from the HIV/AIDS [17] 2017 Global report [18]. Data about tuberculosis annual incidence in Ethiopia were obtained from the 2017 World Health Organization (WHO) tuberculosis report [19]. We also used data from published reports to identify the most accurate numerators and denominators for each FI as described below.

We searched published articles from PubMed related to FIs in Ethiopia and used the prevalence and/or incidence rates of FIs for our estimations. Where published data was missing, we used unpublished data from government institutions of regional or national reports. In the absence of local data from the country, published data were used from neighbouring countries. In our modelling, different populations are included as risk groups for particular FIs as risks vary. Therefore, systematic reviews and meta-analysis were not applicable to compare the heterogeneity. A narrative approach was taken to report the findings of the studies included. Our estimates are based only on well-defined risk populations, which might be the lowest incidence rates of FIs and rounded to the nearest 100 to be less precise.

3. Results

3.1. Country Profile

In 2017, the Ethiopian total population was estimated to be 105 million, with 51.3% being female (Table 1). Of the general population, 41% were younger than 15 years and only 5% of Ethiopians are over age 60 years [20]. The gross domestic product per capita was USD 768 in 2017. According to the WHO 2017 report, 610,000 Ethiopians were estimated to be HIV-infected, with 170,000 of them not receiving antiretroviral (ARVs), and of those on ARVs, less than 50% had HIV viral load suppression [17,21]. New AIDS cases and AIDS-related deaths have been decreasing sharply since 2011, with a fall from 32,000 to 15,000 deaths in 2017 [17,21]. Of all PLWHA in 2017, 50% were receiving ART. Approximately 184,500 adult HIV-positive patients had CD4 counts <200 cells/μL and we estimated that 50% of them were severely immunosuppressed and therefore at a higher risk of opportunistic FIs (Table 1).

Table 1. Country's profile, populations and rates required to calculate the burden of fungal infections.

Demographic data	Total population = 105,000,000 of children (<15 years) = 41% Total number of adults = 60,180,000 Adult women = 31,293,600 % women over 60 = 5% % women 15–50 = 24,482,600	Source: WHO Tuberculosis (TB) stats 2011 [21]; http://aidsinfo.unaids.org/
	Children age 4–14 years = 21,832,000	Source: Education for All 2015 national review report [16]
HIV/AIDS	Current total HIV/AIDS in 2017 = 610,000 Proportion of diagnosed cases on ARVs = 440,000 Annual new AIDS cases (at risk of OIs) = 169.5	Source: https://www.unaids.org/en/resources/documents/2018/unaids-data-2018
	Proportion of AIDS patients presenting with *Pneumocystis jirovecii* pneumonia (PCP) = 30%	Source: Aderaye, G. et al. (2008)
	Proportion of AIDS patients presenting with cryptococcal meningitis = 12% = 44,400	Source: Awoke D. et al. (2018)
	AIDS-related deaths in 2017 = 15,000	http://www.who.int/hiv/pub/progressreport2011
Tuberculosis	Pulmonary tuberculosis annual incidence Total = 105,200	Source: WHO Global Tuberculosis report 2016 [22]
Adults with asthma	Prevalence of asthma in adults = 2.0% Asthma prevalence in adults = 1,239,000	Source: To et al. [23]
COPD	COPD prevalence (all GOLD stages) = 7.8% and 10% admitted to hospital annually	Source: Musafiri et al. [24]
Patients with leukaemia	AML population = 3000	Source: Globocan (2018)
Lung cancer	Estimation of lung cancer = 2000	Source: Globocan (2018)
All cancer sites	otal cancer incidence = 67,600	Source: Globocan (2018)
Number of critical care patients	Estimated number of critical care beds = 1500 (5% of hospital beds in Ethiopian) Hospital beds (per 1000 people) in Ethiopia = 0.7	Source: World Bank, country Indicator: Number of hospital beds

COPD, chronic obstructive pulmonary disease; GOLD, Global initiative for Obstructive Lung Disease; ARV, antiretroviral; AML, acute myeloid leukaemia.

Table 2. Incidence and prevalence rates previously reported used to estimate the burden of fungal infections.

Diseases	Population	Prevalence	Reference
Cryptococcal Infection	Cryptococcal antigen (CrAg)–positive HIV-infected persons <150 CD4 cells/μL	6.2%	Beyene et al. [25]
	Cryptococcal antigenemia among HIV-infected patients receiving antiretroviral therapy in Ethiopia	8.4%	Alemu et al. [26]
	Cryptococcal disease among hospitalized HIV–infected adults in Ethiopia	9.1%	Mamuye et al. [27]
	Cryptococcal antigenemia ART-naïve and experienced HIV-infected persons	10.2%	Beyene et al. [28]
	Cryptococcal antigenemia among HIV-infected patients at a referral hospital	11.7%	Derbie et al. [29]
PCP	Pulmonary infections in TB smear-negative HIV-positive patients with atypical chest X-ray in Ethiopia	29.7%	Aderaye et al. [30]
	HIV-positive patients with suspected pulmonary tuberculosis in Ethiopia	10.9%	Aderaye et al. [31]
Oral candidiasis	PLWHA ART-naive with CD4 <200 cells per μL	90%	Fabian et al. [32]
Oesophageal candidiasis	AIDS patients in Denmark. In total, 20% of patients with HIV not on ARVs and 5% of those on ARVs	20% ART-naive and 5% of those on ART	Smith and Orholm [33]
ABPA	Adult asthmatics	2.5%	Denning et al. [34]
CPA	Chronic pulmonary aspergillosis commonly complicates treated pulmonary tuberculosis with residual cavitation	6.5% annually in those with tuberculosis cavity and 0.2% with no cavities, assumed to be 67% of all TB-related CPA	Page et al. [35]
SAFS	Severe asthmatics (adults). In total, 10% of asthmatics have severe asthma	33%	Denning et al. [34]
rVVC	Adult women	6%	Sobel et al. [36] Foxman et al. [37]
Tinea capitis	School-age children	32.3%	Hibstu et al. [38]
	Children	29%	Figueroa et al. [39]
	Children from grade 1 to grade 4	27.4%	Murgia et al. [40]
	Primary school children in rural areas	24.6%	Leiva-Salinas et al. [41]

CrAg, cryptococcal antigen; PLWHA, people living with HIV/AIDS; ART, antiretroviral therapy; ABPA, allergic bronchopulmonary aspergillosis; CPA, chronic pulmonary aspergillosis; SAFS, severe asthma with fungal sensitisation; rVVC, recurrent vulvovaginal candidiasis; IQR, interquartile range; TB, Tuberculosis; PCP, *Pneumocystis jirovecii* pneumonia.

3.2. *Cryptococcal Meningitis*

CM is among the leading causes of mortality among adult HIV/AIDS patients in sub-Saharan Africa [42,43]. Early screening with cryptococcal antigen (CrAg) among the target population or advanced HIV-infected patients and giving pre-emptive treatment can prevent the development of CM and associated mortality. The prevalence of cryptococcal antigenaemia ranges from 6% to 11.7% among low CD4 T-cell count or among HIV/AIDS patients [25–29] (Table 2). We estimated the annual burden of CM by applying the 11.7% rate of cryptococcal antigenaemia among the 169,500 HIV patients thought to be at risk and calculated 9900 cases of cryptococcosis (9.4 cases per 100,000 person-years) (Table 3). If left untreated, all cryptococcal antigenaemia patients will develop CM [44]. We have not attempted to estimate non-HIV-related cases of CM.

Table 3. The estimated annual case load of serious fungal infections in Ethiopia.

Fungal Infection	Predominant Groups at Risk	Rate Per 100,000	Estimated Number of Cases
Cryptococcosis	AIDS	9.4	9900
PCP	AIDS	12.1	12,700
IA	Haematological Malignancy, lung cancer, 4% of AIDS deaths and 1.3% of COPD admissions to hospital	10.9	11,500
CPA	Tuberculosis patients and other respiratory disorders	14.5	15,200
ABPA	Adult asthma patients	28.6	30,100 *
SAFS	Adult asthma patients	38.9	40,900 *
Candidaemia	Hospitalised patients	5.0	5300
Candida peritonitis	Post-surgical patients	0.8	800
Oral candidiasis	HIV patients	72.7	76,300
Oesophageal candidiasis	HIV infection	53.2	55,900
Recurrent vaginal candidiasis	Adult women	1399	1,469,100
Tinea capitis	4–14-year-old children with poor hygiene	6716.0	7,051,700
Total burden estimated			8,738,300

ABPA, allergic bronchopulmonary aspergillosis; IA, invasive aspergillosis; SAFS, severe asthma with fungal sensitisation; CPA, chronic pulmonary aspergillosis; COPD, chronic obstructive pulmonary disease. * Duplication between ABPA and SAFS is likely as both are sensitised to *Aspergillus*.

3.3. *Pneumocystis jirovecii Pneumonia*

PCP is among the more common life-threatening opportunistic mycoses and may be mistaken as bacterial pneumonia due to a lack of standard diagnosis and management (including high-dose corticosteroids) in RLSs [45]. Early rapid diagnosis and treatment drive survival has outcomes of >70% in Africa and up to 90% in developed countries [45].

In Ethiopia, all patients with advanced immunosuppression (CD4 count less than 200 cells/µL) due to HIV are recommended to receive co-trimoxazole prophylaxis for prevention of PCP. The maximum prevalence of PCP diagnosed by nested PCR was 30% irrespective of ART status or co-trimoxazole prophylaxis [46] (Table 2). We used 7.5% as the minimum prevalence (or $\frac{1}{4}$ of the maximum prevalence) to avoid over the estimation of PCP cases due to oversensitive nested PCR or *Pneumocystis jirovecii* colonization (Table 2).

We therefore estimated an incidence of 12,700 cases of PCP in 2017 (12.1 cases per 100,000 person-years) assuming that 15% of all 169,500 adults are at risk over 2 years (Table 3). Due to lack of data, we could not make a reliable estimate of the incidence of PCP in children among those infected with HIV, or infections in non-HIV-infected adults.

3.4. *Oral Candidiasis*

Approximately 50% newly HIV diagnosed patients with low CD4 T-cell count commonly show oral candidiasis as an initial presentation of symptomatic HIV-infected patients [47,48]. Over the course of a year, this rate rises to ~90% of PLWHA not taking ART [32,49] (Table 2).

We estimated oral candidiasis to affect 76,300 Ethiopian at a rate of 72.6 per 100,000 person-years (Table 3). This burden was estimated by assuming that 90% of the patients at risk with advanced HIV (169,500 cases) will develop oral candidiasis over 2 years (Table 1).

3.5. *Oesophageal Candidiasis*

Oesophageal candidiasis is a common AIDS-defining illness occurring in those with advanced HIV, thus commonly among ART-naïve patients or ART-defaulters.

Oesophageal candidiasis cases were estimated to be 55,900 at a rate of 53.3 per 100,000 person-years (Table 3) under the assumptions that 20% of AIDS patients at risk, and 0.5% of those on ART develop oesophageal candidiasis [33] (Table 2).

3.6. *Allergic Fungal Respiratory Diseases*

Allergic bronchopulmonary aspergillosis (ABPA) is an occasional complication of asthma and cystic fibrosis (CF). Chronic *Aspergillus fumigatus* airways infection is a feature of chronic pulmonary aspergillosis (CPA) [50,51]. One study from South Africa reported a 2.5% prevalence of ABPA among adults with asthma presenting to secondary care [34] (Table 2).

We used data collected as part of the World Heath Survey (2002–2003) for Ethiopia on the prevalence of adult asthma (2.0%) to estimate the prevalence of fungal asthma in adults in Ethiopia (23) (Table 1). There are no reliable published data for CF prevalence.

Assuming a 2% adult asthma prevalence [23] (1,203,600 adults) (Table 1) and the estimated 2.5% ABPA prevalence among asthmatic adults (Table 2) [34], 30,100 adults were estimated to have ABPA in 2011 (Table 3). We only used asthma prevalence among adults, as asthma is more common in children and ABPA is less common. [34,52]. CPA is exclusively an adult disease.

We also estimated the burden of severe asthma with fungal sensitisation (SAFS) in Ethiopia from the adult asthmatic population. Among these adult asthmatics, approximately 10% will suffer from severe asthma. Of these, 33% have been reported to be sensitized to *Aspergillus* or another mould [34] (Table 2). We calculated from these assumptions that SAFS affects 40,900 Ethiopians—a prevalence of 38.9 cases per 100,000 person-years (Table 3).

3.7. *Chronic Pulmonary Aspergillosis (CPA)*

CPA is a long-term sequel of several lung conditions, often following treated pulmonary tuberculosis [51,53]. In RLSs and in tuberculosis-endemic areas such as Ethiopia, a lack of diagnosis of *A. fumigatus* causing CPA probably leads to underdiagnoses and mismanagement. Such patients are mostly treated as cases of sputum smear-negative (and Xpert®negative) tuberculosis [54]. CPA presents with several different radiological features including simple aspergilloma, chronic cavitary pulmonary aspergillosis and chronic fibrosing pulmonary aspergillosis [53].

We calculated the annual incidence and prevalence of CPA using tuberculosis annual incidence and by applying the model described by Denning et al. from 2011 [53] (Table 2). In 2016, tuberculosis was reported in 182,000 individuals—of which, it is assumed that 68% are pulmonary and 85% survived, leaving 105,200 [22] (Table 1). According to Page et al. in a prospective study in Uganda, the annual rate of CPA was 6.5% among those with a cavity in the 2–7 years after completing therapy for pulmonary tuberculosis and 0.2% in those without visible cavities [35] (Table 2). This translates to 2200 cases annually and, assuming 10% mortality, the CPA prevalence after TB is estimated at 8100 cases. This estimate omits two other elements: those who were misdiagnosed as having TB and in fact had CPA and did not survive long enough to be assessed in the Uganda study and those with other underlying diseases such as COPD, pneumothorax and other pulmonary disorders. We have assumed that post-TB CPA is 67% of the total and that pulmonary tuberculosis is responsible for 80% of all CPA cases in Ethiopia. Overall, we estimated 15,200 cases of CPA at a rate of 14.5 cases per 100,000 persons per years (Table 3).

3.8. *Invasive Aspergillosis (IA)*

We estimated 700 cases of IA in 2011—an annual incidence of 0.65 per 100,000 person-years. We calculated this from the most immunosuppressed patients with leukaemia, assuming that 10% of patients with acute myeloid leukaemia will develop IA [53,55], and that there is an equal number of people with IA complicating all other leukaemias and lymphoma patients. We also assumed that 2.6% of lung cancer patients will develop IA [56] and that 4% of AIDS deaths are attributable to IA [44]. There are an estimated 7.8 people over 40 years of age with COPD and approximately 10% are admitted to hospital each year. Assuming 1.3% develop IA [57], we anticipate an annual IA incidence of 10,200 in COPD patients. Overall, we estimated 11,500 IA cases at a rate of 10.92 cases per 100,000 person-years (Table 3).

3.9. *Candida Infections*

Recurrent vulvovaginal candidiasis (rVVC) is defined as four or more episodes per year [36]. rVVC is usually caused by *Candida albicans*. *Candida glabrata*, which is fluconazole resistant, and other species are implicated less often. The absence of rapid, simple, and inexpensive diagnostic tests continues to result in both over- and underdiagnoses of vulvovaginal candidiasis at the same time. It is thought that approximately 70% of women suffer from vulvovaginal candidiasis at least once in their lives, more often during pregnancy [36].

Recurrent attacks of vulvovaginal candidiasis have been estimated to affect 5–10% of women annually [58,59], primarily based on data from Foxman et al [36,37] (Table 2). Estimates of rVVC are intrinsically difficult to conduct to reliably estimate the incidence and prevalence of rVVC among women [59].There are no reports of rVVC from East Africa, but a study in Tunisia found a similar prevalence of 6.1% [60].

We estimated rVVC among adult women aged 15–50 years, assuming that 6% are affected. Recurrent VVC is not common in post-menopausal women in the absence of hormone replacement therapy. Out of a total of 24,482,600 women aged 15–50 years, approximately 1,469,100 women could be affected by rVVC in 2017 at a rate of 1399 women per 100,000 person-years (Table 3). We made no allowance for HIV infection.

The incidence of candidaemia and candida peritonitis were estimated by considering cancer patients, postsurgical patients and patients admitted to ICU wards as high risk for candidaemia case development (Table 1). We estimated that candidaemia affects 5300 women, with an annual incidence of 5 per 100,000 person-year, and that there are 800 episodes of *Candida* peritonitis (intra-abdominal candidiasis), with 0.75 per 100,000 person-years, respectively (Table 3). We calculated the annual incidence of *Candida* peritonitis using the assumption that if candidaemia occurs at a population rate of 5 cases/100,000, one-third are in ICU wards or an equivalent ward and so there will be one patient with *Candida* peritonitis for every two patients with candidaemia in ICUs [53]. It is not easy to confirm this estimate of candidaemia in Ethiopia, as blood cultures are infrequently performed even though we have been observing cases during daily clinical practice.

3.10. *Other Fungal Infections*

A recent publication indicates that tinea capitis affects 32.3% of primary school children in Ethiopia [38] (Table 2). According to the Education for All 2015 report, there are 21,832,000 nursery school- and primary school-aged children in Ethiopia [16] (Table 1). We estimated from these reports that 7,051,700 school children suffer from tinea capitis each year at a rate of 6716 per 100,000 person-years (Table 3).

There was only one African histoplasmosis case reported from Ethiopia [61].

3.11. *Estimate of Fungal Infections-Associated Mortality in Ethiopia*

Opportunistic invasive FIs such as cryptococcosis, IA and PCP are the principal cause of mortality among people living with HIV in Ethiopia. According to our estimations, they contribute to 20,500 to 34,600 Ethiopian deaths annually. In Ethiopia, CM has been reported to have a 100% fatality rate within a year if not treated with an appropriate antifungal and up to a 68% case fatality rate when treated with high-dose fluconazole monotherapy [25,43]. In 2017, we estimated that out of the total 9900 CM cases, the minimum and maximum CM case mortality would be between 6700 and 9900 (Figure 1).

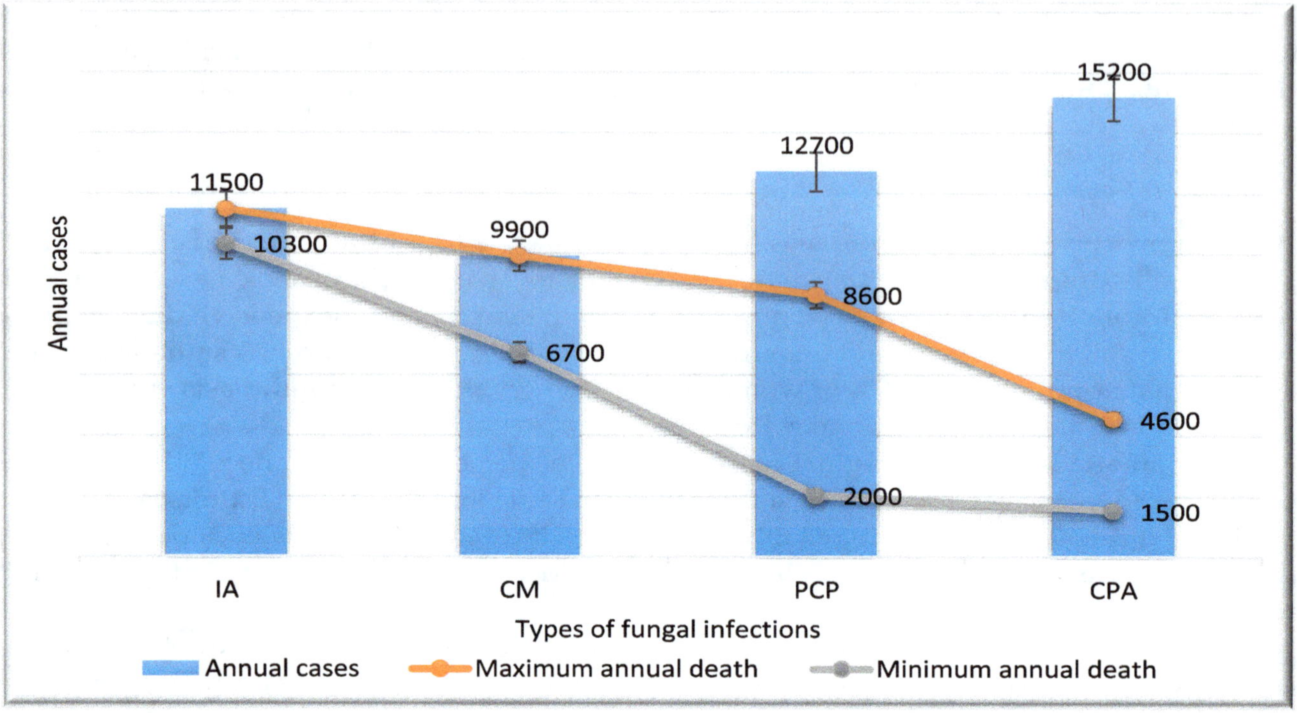

Figure 1. Annual estimates of the number of cases and deaths associated with the most relevant fungal infections in Ethiopia. IA, Invasive aspergillosis; CM, cryptococcal meningitis; PCP, *Pneumocystis jirovecii* pneumonia; CPA, chronic pulmonary aspergillosis.

Available evidence data demonstrate that IA has a case fatality of 90% in leukaemia patients if diagnosed late [62] and if left untreated, it has a case fatality of 100% [63]. We estimated AI could contribute to 10,300 to 11,500 deaths annually in the country.

The case fatality rate of PCP ranges from 16% to 68% in Africa [45]. We used this case fatality to estimate PCP-related annual death in Ethiopia. Out of the total 12,700 PCP cases estimated in Ethiopia, between 2000 and 8600 deaths could occur annually in the country. Denning et al. (2013) reported that the annual CPA fatality rate ranges from 10% to 30% [34] and we calculated that CPA is responsible for 1500 to 4600 deaths annually. In Ethiopia, AIDS remains the leading cause of premature death and years of life lost. Both CM and PCP make major contributions to these many early deaths.

We estimated that over 3600 candidaemia [64] and *Candida* peritonitis patients probability died in the country by using a 60% candidaemia case fatality rate from a report in South Africa [61]. Tinea capitis, ABPA, and recurrent vaginitis are not common causes of death. According to the report in 2013, approximately half a million people died due to severe asthma in the world [65]. However, according to the recent estimated data, the prevalence of fungal asthma was estimated to be 4% and could contribute to 62,544 deaths in Africa alone [66], but it is unclear how many deaths occur in Ethiopia.

4. Discussion

This is the first attempt to estimate the burden of FIs in Ethiopia. Overall, approximately 8% of Ethiopians suffer from serious FIs yearly, including the non-lethal but highly problematic tinea capitis and rVVC. More data are available on the HIV population and tinea capitis than on other groups of patients in Ethiopia. HIV fungal opportunistic infections contribute to 2% of the total FIs and significantly to the number of deaths due to FIs in the country.

IA, CM, PCP, and CPA are the major causes of mycoses-related deaths, though to contribute 33%, 29%, 25%, and 13% of FI deaths, respectively. This is similar to mycoses-related mortality in East

African countries [67,68]. Our estimates indicate that most FIs in the country affect PLWHA. This could be because of a host immunity defect due to HIV infections and more data are available on the HIV population in Ethiopia than on other groups of patients with immunosuppressive conditions.

The current Ethiopian national guidelines recommend ART initiation irrespective of CD4 T-cell count following the latest WHO "treat all" guidelines [69]. Currently in the country, there are no CD4 T-cell count test services available in governmental hospitals. Thus, the identification of target populations at greatest risk for opportunistic infections in need of co-trimoxazole and fluconazole prophylaxis is often not possible. The other big problem is the absence of CD4 T-cell testing services in the country, and so screening for cryptococcal infection among HIV advanced patients is not performed. The WHO recommends CrAg screening in HIV-infected patients with a low CD4 T-cell count (<100 cells/μL) prior to ART initiation to prevent CM development and cryptococcal infections associated with immune reconstitution inflammatory syndrome [51]. Delayed ART initiation by 4–6 weeks for CM patients has survival benefits [70]. In a country such as Ethiopia, where CM and PCP are highly prevalent, the viral load alone is not enough to monitor HIV advanced patients.

We estimated 12,700 annual cases of PCP from a study which diagnosed PCP using bronchoalveolar lavage and the nested PCR method among HIV-positive patients with suspected pulmonary tuberculosis. In our study, almost half of the patients were on ART and co-trimoxazole. So, our estimation may be higher than expected as our denominator did not include patients on co-trimoxazole prophylaxis.

In Ethiopian HIV clinics, PCP is diagnosed clinically as the presence of cough and low oxygen saturation. Even though Toluidine Blue O and Giemsa staining have an acceptable sensitivity and high specificity both in expectorated sputum and bronchoalveolar lavage (BAL) samples for the diagnosis of PCP, these recommended diagnostic methods using induced sputum and BAL are not technically feasible and affordable in Ethiopia [35].

The updated HIV treatment guidelines in Ethiopia recommend co-trimoxazole prophylaxis initiation among all HIV patients who had CD4 <200 cells per μL [71]. Patients with advanced HIV-disease receive drugs such as co-trimoxazole and fluconazole free of charge unless there is a drug stock out. Co-trimoxazole is a broad-spectrum antibiotic used as a prophylaxis for severe immunocompromised patients in order to prevent PCP, toxoplasmosis, malaria and respiratory and enteric infections.

Ethiopia is not an endemic area for systemic mycosis infections such as histoplasmosis, paracoccidioidomycosis or blastomycosis and non-tuberculous mycobacterial infections may be indistinguishable from pulmonary tuberculosis. This is especially the case in a tuberculosis-endemic area such as Ethiopia. The proportion of smear-positive pulmonary, smear-negative pulmonary and extra pulmonary tuberculosis were 20%, 34% and 46%, respectively [72]. Some of the above described fungal respiratory infections may have been misdiagnosed and treated as smear-negative tuberculosis cases.

We estimated 15,200 cases of CPA in 2017 among patients who recovered from TB. This large case load of affected people should be incorporated into national tuberculosis treatment guidelines in Ethiopia. To diagnose CPA, an ELISA for *Aspergillus* IgG antibodies or a lateral flow assay is needed [73]. Although widely available in developed countries, in RLSs, they are not usually available, as in Ethiopia. As a result, patients are typically treated with months of anti-tuberculosis medication even with no acid-fast bacillus seen [54]. A new rapid point of care, the *Aspergillus* IgG antibody test may facilitate a change in practice [74].

Our estimate of asthma prevalence in adults (2%) is likely to be a significant underestimate as a systematic review found that 16.3% of Ethiopians had had asthma at some point [75] and these higher prevalence rates are consistent with many other African countries [23]. Clearly, epidemiological data on asthma prevalence and fungal sensitization rates in Ethiopia are required.

We estimated 7,051,700 tinea capitis cases (6716 per 100,000) among children aged between 3 and 15 years in Ethiopia annually. Tinea capitis accounted for the highest prevalence of FIs in the country. This could be due to poor individual and environmental sanitation, limited health facilities, the shortage of water supply at school or home for children, poor handwashing behaviour, strong and close contact with animals, highly populated one-room schools and the tropical region with high humidity [76–78].

Candidaemia is a leading cause of nosocomial bloodstream infection across the world [79]. The annual mortality of invasive candidiasis in Ethiopia could be over 3600 due to the unavailability of appropriate diagnosis and antifungals. Immunocompromised patients such as those with haematological malignancy and those in ICUs are at high risk of developing candidaemia and *Candida* peritonitis. Data to support our estimate of the number of invasive candidiasis cases are lacking in Ethiopia. For instance, it is difficult to obtain the exact number of ICU beds in Ethiopia. Therefore, we assumed that up to 5% of all hospital beds in Ethiopia serve as ICU beds. From personal communications, we found that only teaching and referral hospitals have ICU services in Ethiopia. In general, we may underestimate the invasive candidiasis, since we did not consider other risk factors such as prolonged antibiotic therapy and low infection prevention practices in the country.

Our study has several limitations. Despite an exhaustive search, we could not obtain enough data, particularly for the incidence of invasive FIs and associated mortality in the country. So, we used data from other neighbouring countries. We also could not obtain data on how many people from Ethiopia used immunosuppresses agents due to organ transplantations and autoimmune diseases. To our knowledge, there is no official or unofficial registry of patients who have had an organ transplant or those who have had surgeryin the country. We assumed that the lack of data about the risk groups for specific FIs might have resulted in the overestimation or underestimation of the number of some invasive FIs.

In general, our estimates probably have wide confidence limits, due to the modelling style we used and the lack of evidence data for some invasive FI risk groups from Ethiopia. Despite these shortcomings, the burden of FIs in Ethiopia was addressed for the first time. Policy makers and stockholders may use these results for programmes and interventions in order to improve the diagnosis and management of FIs in the country.

5. Conclusions

To our knowledge, this is the first review report on the burden of FIs in Ethiopia. We estimated that fungi could infect approximately 8% of people in Ethiopia every year. However, the actual number of FIs in the country may be higher than our estimates, since we only used HIV infection to determine the immunosuppressed population and some other immunocompromised populations were not considered. Our estimates could be used as basis for future epidemiological studies and national FI surveillance for Ethiopia. In this study, we addressed the neglected fungal diseases in the country, which was a major public concern. Our estimates clearly point to the need for national FI surveillance, improving the mycology laboratory and point-of-care diagnostics, and accessibility to optimum antifungal drugs. The CD4 T-cell count test services should be available for opportunistic FI management and prevention for HIV late presenters. We recommend creating awareness for FIs and supporting mycosis research in the country. Upgrading the diagnosis and management of FIs is urgently needed to reduce their high mortality and morbidity in Ethiopia.

Author Contributions: Conceptualization, D.W.D. and T.B.T. methodology, D.W.D. and T.B.T.; software D.W.D. and T.B.T.; validation D.W.D. and T.B.T.; formal analysis, D.W.D. and T.B.T.; investigation, D.W.D., and T.B.T.; resources, D.W.D.; data curation, D.W.D. and T.B.T.; writing—original draft preparation, D.W.D. and T.B.T.; writing—review and editing, D.W.D. and T.B.T.; visualization, D.W.D. and T.B.T.; supervision, D.W.D.

Acknowledgments: The authors are grateful to all authors and institutes who provided raw and unpublished data on their previous works necessary for estimating the burden of fungal infections in Ethiopia.

References

1. Brown, G.D.; Denning, D.W.; Levitz, S.M. Tackling Human Fungal Infections. *Science* **2012**, *336*, 647. [CrossRef] [PubMed]
2. Bongomin, F.; Gago, S.; Oladele, R.O.; Denning, D.W. Global and Multi-National Prevalence of Fungal Diseases-Estimate Precision. *J. Fungi* **2017**, *3*, 57. [CrossRef] [PubMed]
3. Visentin, A.; Gurrieri, C.; Imbergamo, S.; Lessi, F.; Di Maggio, S.A.; Frezzato, F.; Adami, F.; Zambello, R.; Raumer, F.; Piazza, F.; et al. Epidemiology and Risk Factors of Invasive Fungal Infections Among 795 Patients with Chronic Lymphocytic Leukemia from the Padua University. *Blood* **2016**, *128*, 2527. [CrossRef]
4. Badiee, P.; Hashemizadeh, Z. Opportunistic invasive fungal infections: Diagnosis & clinical management. *Indian J. Med. Res.* **2014**, *139*, 195–204.
5. Loyse, A.; Burry, J.; Cohn, J.; Ford, N.; Chiller, T.; Ribeiro, I.; Koulla-Shiro, S.; Mghamba, J.; Ramadhani, A.; Nyirenda, R.; et al. Leave no one behind: Response to new evidence and guidelines for the management of cryptococcal meningitis in low-income and middle-income countries. *Lancet Infect. Dis.* **2018**. [CrossRef]
6. Baxi, S.N.; Portnoy, J.M.; Larenas-Linnemann, D.; Phipatanakul, W. Exposure and Health Effects of Fungi on Humans. *J. Allergy Clin. Immunol. Pract.* **2016**, *4*, 396–404. [CrossRef]
7. Dogra, S.; Narang, T. Emerging atypical and unusual presentations of dermatophytosis in India. *Clin. Dermatol. Rev.* **2017**, *1*, 12–18. [CrossRef]
8. Singh, A.; Masih, A.; Monroy-Nieto, J.; Singh, P.K.; Bowers, J.; Travis, J.; Khurana, A.; Engelthaler, D.M.; Meis, J.F.; Chowdhary, A. A unique multidrug-resistant clonal Trichophyton population distinct from Trichophyton mentagrophytes/Trichophyton interdigitale complex causing an ongoing alarming dermatophytosis outbreak in India: Genomic insights and resistance profile. *Fungal Genet. Biol.* **2019**, *133*, 103266. [CrossRef]
9. Verma, S.; Madhu, R. The Great Indian Epidemic of Superficial Dermatophytosis: An Appraisal. *Indian J. Dermatol.* **2017**, *62*, 227–236.
10. Agarwal, U.S.; Saran, J.; Agarwal, P. Clinico-mycological study of dermatophytes in a tertiary care centre in Northwest India. *Indian J. Dermatol. Venereol. Leprol.* **2014**, *80*, 194. [CrossRef]
11. Noronha, T.M.; Tophakhane, R.S.; Nadiger, S. Clinico-microbiological study of dermatophytosis in a tertiary-care hospital in North Karnataka. *Indian Dermatol. Online J.* **2016**, *7*, 264–271. [CrossRef] [PubMed]
12. Khanjanasthiti, P. Germination and survival of dermatophyte spores in various environmental conditions. *Chiang Mai Med.* **1984**, *23*, 83–98.
13. Vos, T.; Flaxman, A.D.; Naghavi, M.; Lozano, R.; Michaud, C.; Ezzati, M.; Shibuya, K.; Salomon, J.A.; Abdalla, S.; Aboyans, V.; et al. Years lived with disability (YLDs) for 1160 sequelae of 289 diseases and injuries 1990–2010: A systematic analysis for the Global Burden of Disease Study 2010. *Lancet* **2012**, *380*, 2163–2196. [CrossRef]
14. Denning, D.W. The ambitious '95–95 by 2025' roadmap for the diagnosis and management of fungal diseases. *Thorax* **2015**, *70*, 613–614. [CrossRef] [PubMed]
15. Ethiopian Ministry of Education. *Ethiopia National Education Profile 2014 Update*; Ethiopian Ministry of Education: Addis Ababa, Ethiopia, 2014.
16. Ethiopian Ministry of Education. *Education for All 2015 National Review Report: Ethiopia*; Ethiopian Ministry of Education: Addis Ababa, Ethiopia, 2015.
17. UNAIDS. DATA 2018. Available online: https://wwwunaidsorg/en/resources/documents/2018/unaids-data-2018 (accessed on 10 June 2019).
18. *Global HIV/AIDS Response: Epidemic Update and Health Sector Progress Towards Universal Access WHO, UNICEF, UNAIDS*; Progress Report; WHO: Geneva, Switzerland, 2011.
19. *Estimates of TB and MDR-TB Burden in Ethiopia*; WHO: Geneva, Switzerland, 2017.
20. *Ethiopia Demographic and Health Surve*; WHO: Addis Ababa, Ethiopia, 2011.
21. *Progress Report 2011: Global HIV/AIDS Response*; WHO: Geneva, Switzerland, 2011.
22. Tuberculosis Country Profiles. 2017. Available online: https://wwwwhoint/tb/country/data/profiles/en/ (accessed on 8 June 2019).
23. To, T.; Stanojevic, S.; Moores, G.; Gershon, A.S.; Bateman, E.D.; Cruz, A.A.; Boulet, L.P. Global asthma prevalence in adults: Findings from the cross-sectional world health survey. *BMC Public Health* **2012**, *12*, 204. [CrossRef]

24. Musafiri, S.; van Meerbeeck, J.; Musango, L.; Brusselle, G.; Joos, G.; Seminega, B.; Rutayisire, C. Prevalence of atopy, asthma and COPD in an urban and a rural area of an African country. *Respir. Med.* **2011**, *105*, 1596–1605. [CrossRef]
25. Beyene, T.; Zewde, A.G.; Balcha, A.; Hirpo, B.; Yitbarik, T.; Gebissa, T.; Rajasingham, R.; Boulware, D.R. Inadequacy of High-Dose Fluconazole Monotherapy Among Cerebrospinal Fluid Cryptococcal Antigen (CrAg)-Positive Human Immunodeficiency Virus-Infected Persons in an Ethiopian CrAg Screening Program. *Clin. Infect. Dis.* **2017**, *65*, 2126–2129. [CrossRef]
26. Alemu, A.S.; Kempker, R.R.; Tenna, A.; Smitson, C.; Berhe, N.; Fekade, D.; Blumberg, H.M.; Aseffa, A. High prevalence of Cryptococcal antigenemia among HIV-infected patients receiving antiretroviral therapy in Ethiopia. *PLoS ONE* **2013**, *8*, e58377. [CrossRef]
27. Mamuye, A.T.; Bornstein, E.; Temesgen, O.; Blumberg, H.M.; Kempker, R.R. Point-of-Care Testing for Cryptococcal Disease Among Hospitalized Human Immunodeficiency Virus-Infected Adults in Ethiopia. *Am. J. Trop. Med. Hyg.* **2016**, *95*, 786–792. [CrossRef]
28. Beyene, T.; Woldeamanuel, Y.; Asrat, D.; Ayana, G.; Boulware, D.R. Comparison of cryptococcal antigenemia between antiretroviral naïve and antiretroviral experienced HIV positive patients at two hospitals in Ethiopia. *PLoS ONE* **2013**, *8*, e75585. [CrossRef]
29. Derbie, A.; Ayalew, W.; Mekonnen, D.; Alemu, M.; Mulugeta, Y. Magnitude of Cryptococcal Antigenemia among HIV Infected Patients at a Referral Hospital, Northwest Ethiopia. *Ethiop. J. Health Sci.* **2018**, *28*, 369–374. [PubMed]
30. Aderaye, G.; Bruchfeld, J.; Aseffa, G.; Nigussie, Y.; Melaku, K.; Woldeamanuel, Y.; Asrat, D.; Worku, A.; Gaegziabher, H.; Lebaad, M.; et al. Pneumocystis jiroveci pneumonia and other pulmonary infections in TB smear-negative HIV-positive patients with atypical chest X-ray in Ethiopia. *Scand. J. Infect. Dis.* **2007**, *39*, 1045–1053. [CrossRef] [PubMed]
31. Aderaye, G.; Bruchfeld, J.; Olsson, M.; Lindquist, L. Occurrence of Pneumocystis carinii in HIV-positive patients with suspected pulmonary tuberculosis in Ethiopia. *Aids* **2003**, *17*, 435–440. [CrossRef] [PubMed]
32. Fabian, F.M.; Kahabuka, F.K.; Petersen, P.E.; Shubi, F.M.; Jurgensen, N. Oral manifestations among people living with HIV/AIDS in Tanzania. *Int. Dent. J.* **2009**, *59*, 187–191. [PubMed]
33. Smith, E.; Orholm, M. Trends and patterns of opportunistic diseases in Danish AIDS patients 1980–1990. *Scand. J. Infect. Dis.* **1990**, *22*, 665–672. [CrossRef] [PubMed]
34. Denning, D.W.; Pleuvry, A.; Cole, D.C. Global burden of allergic bronchopulmonary aspergillosis with asthma and its complication chronic pulmonary aspergillosis in adults. *Med. Mycol.* **2013**, *51*, 361–370. [CrossRef] [PubMed]
35. Page, I.D.; Richardson, M.D.; Denning, D.W. Comparison of six Aspergillus-specific IgG assays for the diagnosis of chronic pulmonary aspergillosis (CPA). *J. Infect.* **2016**, *72*, 240–249. [CrossRef]
36. Sobel, J.D. Vulvovaginal candidosis. *Lancet* **2007**, *369*, 1961–1971. [CrossRef]
37. Foxman, B.; Muraglia, R.; Dietz, J.P.; Sobel, J.D.; Wagner, J. Prevalence of recurrent vulvovaginal candidiasis in 5 European countries and the United States: Results from an internet panel survey. *J. Low Genit. Tract. Dis.* **2013**, *17*, 340–345. [CrossRef]
38. Hibstu, D.T.; Kebede, D.L. Epidemiology of Tinea Capitis and Associated Factors among School Age Children in Hawassa Zuria District, Southern Ethiopia, 2016. *J. Bacteriol. Parasitol.* **2017**, *8*, 2. [CrossRef]
39. Figueroa, J.I.; Hawranek, T.; Abraha, A.; Hay, R.J. Tinea capitis in south-western Ethiopia: A study of risk factors for infection and carriage. *Int. J. Dermatol.* **1997**, *36*, 661–666. [CrossRef] [PubMed]
40. Murgia, V.; Bilcha, K.D.; Shibeshi, D. Community dermatology in Debre Markos: An attempt to define children's dermatological needs in a rural area of Ethiopia. *Int. J. Dermatol.* **2010**, *49*, 666–671. [CrossRef] [PubMed]
41. Leiva-Salinas, M.; Marin-Cabanas, I.; Betlloch, I.; Tesfasmariam, A.; Reyes, F.; Belinchon, I.; Ramos, J.M. Tinea capitis in schoolchildren in a rural area in southern Ethiopia. *Int. J. Dermatol.* **2015**, *54*, 800–805. [CrossRef] [PubMed]
42. Kitonsa, J.; Mayanja, Y.; Aling, E.; Kiwanuka, J.; Namutundu, J.; Anywaine, Z.; Ggayi, A.-B.; Kibengo, F.; Kiwanuka, N.; Kaleebu, P. Factors affecting mortality among HIV positive patients two years after completing recommended therapy for Cryptococcal meningitis in Uganda. *PLoS ONE* **2019**, *14*, e0210287. [CrossRef] [PubMed]

43. Rajasingham, R.; Smith, R.M.; Park, B.J.; Jarvis, J.N.; Govender, N.P.; Chiller, T.M.; Denning, D.W.; Loyse, A.; Boulware, D.R. Global burden of disease of HIV-associated cryptococcal meningitis: An updated analysis. *Lancet Infect. Dis.* **2017**, *17*, 873–881. [CrossRef]
44. Denning, D.W. Minimizing fungal disease deaths will allow the UNAIDS target of reducing annual AIDS deaths below 500 000 by 2020 to be realized. *Philos. Trans. R. Soc. Lond. B Biol. Sci.* **2016**, *371*, 20150468. [CrossRef] [PubMed]
45. De Armas Rodríguez, Y.; Wissmann, G.; Müller, A.L.; Pederiva, M.A.; Brum, M.C.; Brackmann, R.L.; Capó de Paz, V.; Calderón, E.J. Pneumocystis jirovecii pneumonia in developing countries. *Parasite* **2011**, *18*, 219–228. [CrossRef]
46. Aderaye, G.; Woldeamanuel, Y.; Asrat, D.; Lebbad, M.; Beser, J.; Worku, A.; Fernandez, V.; Lindquist, L. Evaluation of Toluidine Blue O staining for the diagnosis of Pneumocystis jiroveci in expectorated sputum sample and bronchoalveolar lavage from HIV-infected patients in a tertiary care referral center in Ethiopia. *Infection* **2008**, *36*, 237–243. [CrossRef]
47. Mulu, A.; Kassu, A.; Anagaw, B.; Moges, B.; Gelaw, A.; Alemayehu, M.; Belyhun, Y.; Biadglegne, F.; Hurissa, Z.; Moges, F.; et al. Frequent detection of 'azole' resistant Candida species among late presenting AIDS patients in northwest Ethiopia. *BMC Infect. Dis.* **2013**, *13*, 82. [CrossRef]
48. Xiao, J.; Gao, G.; Li, Y.; Zhang, W.; Tian, Y.; Huang, Y.; Su, W.; Han, N.; Yang, D.; Zhao, H. Correction: Spectrums of Opportunistic Infections and Malignancies in HIV-Infected Patients in Tertiary Care Hospital, China. *PLoS ONE* **2014**, *9*. [CrossRef]
49. Matee, M.I.; Scheutz, F.; Moshy, J. Occurrence of oral lesions in relation to clinical and immunological status among HIV-infected adult Tanzanians. *Oral Dis.* **2000**, *6*, 106–111. [CrossRef] [PubMed]
50. Amin, R.; Dupuis, A.; Aaron, S.D.; Ratjen, F. The effect of chronic infection with Aspergillus fumigatus on lung function and hospitalization in patients with cystic fibrosis. *Chest* **2010**, *137*, 171–176. [CrossRef] [PubMed]
51. Schweer, K.E.; Bangard, C.; Hekmat, K.; Cornely, O.A. Chronic pulmonary aspergillosis. *Mycoses* **2014**, *57*, 257–270. [CrossRef] [PubMed]
52. Singh, M.; Das, S.; Chauhan, A.; Paul, N.; Sodhi, K.S.; Mathew, J.; Chakrabarti, A. The diagnostic criteria for allergic bronchopulmonary aspergillosis in children with poorly controlled asthma need to be re-evaluated. *Acta Paediatr.* **2015**, *104*, e206–e209. [CrossRef]
53. Denning, D. How Common are Fungal Diseases? 2016. Available online: http://wwwfungalinfectiontrustorg/How%20Common%20are%20Fungal%20Diseases5pdf (accessed on 18 March 2019).
54. Pohl, C.; Jugheli, L.; Haraka, F.; Mfinanga, E.; Said, K.; Reither, K. Pulmonary aspergilloma: A treatment challenge in sub-Saharan Africa. *PLoS Negl. Trop. Dis.* **2013**, *7*, e2352. [CrossRef]
55. Lortholary, O.; Gangneux, J.P.; Sitbon, K.; Lebeau, B.; de Monbrison, F.; Le Strat, Y.; Coignard, B.; Dromer, F.; Bretagne, S. Epidemiological trends in invasive aspergillosis in France: The SAIF network (2005–2007). *Clin. Microbiol. Infect.* **2011**, *17*, 1882–1889. [CrossRef]
56. Yan, X.; Li, M.; Jiang, M.; Zou, L.Q.; Luo, F.; Jiang, Y. Clinical characteristics of 45 patients with invasive pulmonary aspergillosis: Retrospective analysis of 1711 lung cancer cases. *Cancer* **2009**, *115*, 5018–5025. [CrossRef]
57. Guinea, J.; Torres-Narbona, M.; Gijon, P.; Munoz, P.; Pozo, F.; Pelaez, T.; de Miguel, J.; Bouza, E. Pulmonary aspergillosis in patients with chronic obstructive pulmonary disease: Incidence, risk factors, and outcome. *Clin. Microbiol. Infect.* **2010**, *16*, 870–877. [CrossRef]
58. Denning, D.W.; Kneale, M.; Sobel, J.D.; Rautemaa-Richardson, R. Global burden of recurrent vulvovaginal candidiasis: A systematic review. *Lancet Infect. Dis.* **2018**, *18*, e339–e347. [CrossRef]
59. Rathod, S.D.; Buffler, P.A. Highly-cited estimates of the cumulative incidence and recurrence of vulvovaginal candidiasis are inadequately documented. *BMC Womens Health* **2014**, *14*, 43. [CrossRef]
60. Amouri, I.; Sellami, H.; Borji, N.; Abbes, S.; Sellami, A.; Cheikhrouhou, F.; Maazoun, L.; Khaled, S.; Khrouf, S.; Boujelben, Y.; et al. Epidemiological survey of vulvovaginal candidosis in Sfax, Tunisia. *Mycoses* **2011**, *54*, e499–e505. [CrossRef] [PubMed]
61. Aderaye, G.; Seifu, D. African histoplasmosis in Ethiopia: A case report. *East Afr. Med. J.* **1987**, *64*, 428–430. [PubMed]
62. Von Eiff, M.; Roos, N.; Schulten, R.; Hesse, M.; Zuhlsdorf, M.; van de Loo, J. Pulmonary aspergillosis: Early diagnosis improves survival. *Respiration* **1995**, *62*, 341–347. [CrossRef] [PubMed]

63. Vandewoude, K.H.; Blot, S.I.; Depuydt, P.; Benoit, D.; Temmerman, W.; Colardyn, F.; Vogelaers, D. Clinical relevance of Aspergillus isolation from respiratory tract samples in critically ill patients. *Crit. Care* **2006**, *10*, R31. [CrossRef] [PubMed]
64. Kreusch, A.; Karstaedt, A.S. Candidemia among adults in Soweto, South Africa, 1990–2007. *Int. J. Infect. Dis.* **2013**, *17*, e621–e623. [CrossRef] [PubMed]
65. Anonymous. Global, regional, and national age-sex specific all-cause and cause-specific mortality for 240 causes of death, 1990–2013: A systematic analysis for the Global Burden of Disease Study 2013. *Lancet* **2015**, *385*, 117–171. [CrossRef]
66. Kwizera, R.; Musaazi, J.; Meya, D.B.; Worodria, W.; Bwanga, F.; Kajumbula, H.; Fowler, S.J.; Kirenga, B.J.; Gore, R.; Denning, D.W. Burden of fungal asthma in Africa: A systematic review and meta-analysis. *PLoS ONE* **2019**, *14*, e0216568. [CrossRef]
67. Faini, D.; Maokola, W.; Furrer, H.; Hatz, C.; Battegay, M.; Tanner, M.; Denning, D.W.; Letang, E. Burden of serious fungal infections in Tanzania. *Mycoses* **2015**, *58*, 70–79. [CrossRef]
68. Guto, J.A.; Bii, C.C.; Denning, D.W. Estimated burden of fungal infections in Kenya. *J. Infect. Dev. Ctries.* **2016**, *10*, 777–784. [CrossRef]
69. Guidelines for Managing Advanced HIV Disease and Rapid Initiation of Antiretroviral Therapy. 2017. Available online: https://wwwwhoint/hiv/pub/guidelines/advanced-HIV-disease/en/ (accessed on 25 October 2019).
70. Boulware, D.R.; Meya, D.B.; Muzoora, C.; Rolfes, M.A.; Huppler Hullsiek, K.; Musubire, A.; Taseera, K.; Nabeta, H.W.; Schutz, C.; Williams, D.A.; et al. Timing of antiretroviral therapy after diagnosis of cryptococcal meningitis. *N. Engl. J. Med.* **2014**, *370*, 2487–2498. [CrossRef]
71. Federal Ministry of Health. *National Guidelines for Comprehensive HIV Prevention, Care and Treatment*; Federal Ministry of Health: Addis Ababa, Ethiopia, 2018.
72. Mekonnen, D.; Derbie, A.; Mekonnen, H.; Zenebe, Y. Profile and treatment outcomes of patients with tuberculosis in Northeastern Ethiopia: A cross sectional study. *Afr. Health Sci.* **2016**, *16*, 663–670. [CrossRef] [PubMed]
73. Denning, D.W.; Page, I.D.; Chakaya, J.; Jabeen, K.; Jude, C.M.; Cornet, M.; Alastruey-Izquierdo, A.; Bongomin, F.; Bowyer, P.; Chakrabarti, A.; et al. Case Definition of Chronic Pulmonary Aspergillosis in Resource-Constrained Settings. *Emerg. Infect. Dis.* **2018**, *24*, e171312. [CrossRef] [PubMed]
74. Stucky Hunter, E.; Richardson, M.D.; Denning, D.W. Evaluation of LDBio Aspergillus ICT Lateral Flow Assay for IgG and IgM Antibody Detection in Chronic Pulmonary Aspergillosis. *J. Clin. Microbiol.* **2019**, *57*, e00538. [CrossRef] [PubMed]
75. Adeloye, D.; Chan, K.Y.; Rudan, I.; Campbell, H. An estimate of asthma prevalence in Africa: A systematic analysis. *Croat. Med. J.* **2013**, *54*, 519–531. [CrossRef] [PubMed]
76. Woldeamanuel, Y.; Leekassa, R.; Chryssanthou, E.; Menghistu, Y.; Petrini, B. Prevalence of tinea capitis in Ethiopian schoolchildren. *Mycoses* **2005**, *48*, 137–141. [CrossRef] [PubMed]
77. Coulibaly, O.; L'Ollivier, C.; Piarroux, R.; Ranque, S. Epidemiology of human dermatophytoses in Africa. *Med. Mycol.* **2018**, *56*, 145–161. [CrossRef] [PubMed]
78. Adesiji, Y.O.; Omolade, F.B.; Aderibigbe, I.A.; Ogungbe, O.; Adefioye, O.A.; Adedokun, S.A.; Adekanle, M.A.; Ojedele, R. Prevalence of Tinea Capitis among Children in Osogbo, Nigeria, and the Associated Risk Factors. *Diseases* **2019**, *7*, 13. [CrossRef]
79. Wisplinghoff, H.; Ebbers, J.; Geurtz, L.; Stefanik, D.; Major, Y.; Edmond, M.B.; Wenzel, R.P.; Seifert, H. Nosocomial bloodstream infections due to Candida spp. in the USA: Species distribution, clinical features and antifungal susceptibilities. *Int. J. Antimicrob. Agents* **2014**, *43*, 78–81. [CrossRef]

2

Detection of *Fusarium* Species in Clinical Specimens by Probe-Based Real-Time PCR

Jan Springer [1,*], Grit Walther [2], Volker Rickerts [3], Axel Hamprecht [4,5], Birgit Willinger [6], Daniel Teschner [7], Hermann Einsele [1], Oliver Kurzai [2,8] and Juergen Loeffler [1]

1 Department for Internal Medicine II, University Hospital of Wuerzburg, 97080 Wuerzburg, Germany; einsele_h@ukw.de (H.E.); loeffler_j@ukw.de (J.L.)
2 National Reference Center for Invasive Fungal Infections (NRZMyk), Leibniz Institute for Natural Product Research and Infection Biology, Hans Knöll Institute, 07745 Jena, Germany; Grit.Walther@hki-jena.de (G.W.); oliver.kurzai@leibniz-hki.de or okurzai@hygiene.uni-wuerzburg.de (O.K.)
3 Robert Koch Institute Berlin, 13353 Berlin, Germany; RickertsV@rki.de
4 Institute for Medical Microbiology, Immunology and Hygiene, University Hospital of Cologne, University of Cologne, 50935 Cologne, Germany; axel.hamprecht@uk-koeln.de
5 Institute for Medical Microbiology and Virology, Carl von Ossietzky University of Oldenburg, 26129 Oldenburg, Germany
6 Division of Clinical Microbiology, Institute of Hygiene and Medical Microbiology of the University, Vienna University Hospital, 1090 Vienna, Austria; birgit.willinger@meduniwien.ac.at
7 Department of Hematology, Medical Oncology, and Pneumology, University Medical Center of the Johannes Gutenberg University, 55122 Mainz, Germany; Daniel.Teschner@unimedizin-mainz.de
8 Institute for Hygiene and Microbiology, University Wuerzburg, 97080 Wuerzburg, Germany
* Correspondence: springer_j@ukw.de

Abstract: The mold *Fusarium* is a ubiquitous fungus causing plant, animal and human infections. In humans, *Fusarium* spp. are the major cause of eye infections in patients wearing contact lenses or after local trauma. Systemic infections by *Fusarium* spp. mainly occur in immunosuppressed patients and can disseminate throughout the human body. Due to high levels of resistance to antifungals a fast identification of the causative agent is an urgent need. By using a probe-based real-time PCR assay specific for the genus *Fusarium* we analysed several different clinical specimens detecting *Fusarium* spp. commonly found in clinical samples in Germany. Also, a large collection of lung fluid samples of haematological patients was analysed ($n = 243$). In these, two samples (0.8%) were reproducibly positive, but only one could be confirmed by sequencing. For this case of probable invasive fungal disease (IFD) culture was positive for *Fusarium* species. Here we describe a rapid, probe-based real-time PCR assay to specifically detect DNA from a broad range of *Fusarium* species and its application to clinically relevant specimens.

Keywords: probe-based real-time PCR; Fusarium; bronchoalveolar lavage fluid; fungal molecular diagnostics

---

1. Introduction

The mold *Fusarium* is a ubiquitous fungus well known as a plant pathogen and mycotoxin producer [1]. There are more than 300 phylogenetically distinct species known [2]. At least 70 are involved in invasive fusariosis. Within these, the *Fusarium solani* species complex (FSSC) is responsible for the most fusariosis cases [3,4], followed by other complexes causing human infections (*Fusarium oxysporum* species complex (FOSC), *Fusarium dimerum* species complex (FDSC), *Fusarium fujikuroi* species complex (FFSC; also known as *Gibberella fujikuroi* species complex GFSC), and *Fusarium incarnatum–Fusarium equiseti* species complex (FIESC)) [3]. Invasive fusariosis is a life-threatening invasive fungal disease (IFD) with poor outcome that mostly occurs in immunocompromised patients [5] with mainly haematological malignancies [6]. Improved fungal diagnostics and treatment has led to a decrease in the number of infections caused by *Candida* and *Aspergillus*, but also to a rise of so-called rare fungal pathogens, including members of the genus *Fusarium* [7–10]. As *Fusarium* may display high levels of resistance to most classes of antifungals [11], a fast identification of the causative agent is mandatory for effective treatment leading to a good patients' outcome. The drug recommended for first-line treatment is voriconazole [12].

To improve *Fusarium* identification, DNA detection via polymerase chain reaction (PCR) is a rapid and sensitive tool. There are different methods to detect *Fusarium* by PCR including conventional and real-time (hybridization or hydrolysis probe based) PCR [6,13–15], which are limited by their high turnaround time, detection of some selected species, or uncommon real-time PCR formats. Here we describe a rapid, probe-based real-time PCR assay to specifically detect DNA from a broad range of *Fusarium* species and its application to clinically relevant specimens.

2. Materials and Methods

2.1. DNA from Clinical Specimens Positive for Fusarium spp. and Isolates

From 1998 to 2017, clinical specimens were sent to German laboratories to detect fungi. Fungal DNA extracts of clinical samples ($n = 10$) or clinical isolates ($n = 12$) containing DNA of *Fusarium* species were kindly provided (National Reference Center for Invasive Fungal Infections, Jena, Robert Koch Institute, Berlin, and University Hospital of Cologne, Institute for Medical Microbiology, Immunology and Hygiene) reflecting the most common causative fungi isolated from disseminated and local infections [16]. Samples comprised several different *Fusarium* spp. (*F. dimerum complex*, $n = 2$; *F. keratoplasticum*, $n = 2$; *F. musae*, $n = 2$; *F. oxysporum* complex, $n = 5$; *F. petroliphilum*, $n = 6$; *F. proliferatum*, $n = 2$; *F. sacchari*, $n = 1$; *F. verticilloides*, $n = 1$). Twelve were related to the eye (contact lens fluid, cornea tissue, eye fluid), 5 were derived from blood cultures, 2 from bronchoalveolar lavage fluid (BALF), and 3 from skin or mucosal tissue (sinus).

2.2. Bronchoalveolar Lavage Fluid (BALF)

From July 2016 to December 2018, BALF samples taken for routine clinical investigation of chest infection (new or progressive lung infiltrates) in adult patients (≥ 18 years old) with haematological malignancies (HM) across ten hospitals, 9 centers from Germany and one from Austria, were retained. DNA eluates of BALF samples were stored at −20 °C for retrospective PCR testing. In addition to standard of care procedures, each sample was tested retrospectively for the presence of fungal DNA by a newly developed *Fusarium*–specific real-time PCR. Patients were categorized according to revised European Organization for the Research and Treatment of Cancer (EORTC)/Mycoses Study Group (MSG) criteria [17] resulting in 7 proven IFD (3.2%; *Aspergillus*, $n = 3$; *Rhizopus*, $n = 1$; not defined, $n = 3$), 72 probable IFD (32.6%), 108 possible IFD (48.9%), 29 undetermined IFD (13.1%), and 5 unknown (2.3%). Bronchoscopy was performed in accordance with institutional protocols. The study was approved by the local ethics committees of the UKW (Ethikommission des Universitätsklinikums Würzburg, 270/15), and elsewhere as appropriate.

2.3. DNA Extraction from BALF

All steps for extracting DNA from BALF were performed in a class II laminar-flow cabinet. Briefly, samples were vortexed, and 0.5 ml of BAL fluid was centrifuged at 5000× *g* for 7 min. The supernatant was transferred to a new tube. The remaining pellet was bead-beaten after adding 50 μL of BALF supernatant for 90 secs using 1.4-mm (diameter) ceramic beads. Using a commercial extraction kit (High Pure template preparation kit, Roche) both fractions were combined and extracted as described before [18]. Elution volume was adjusted to 70 μL.

2.4. 28S-Based Fusarium-Specific Real-Time PCR

The 28S-based assay described by Muraosa et al. [13] was adapted by designing a specific hydrolysis probe including the originally used nucleotides. The original reverse primer was modified in one nucleotide (5-GCTATCGGTCTCTGGCC**R**G-3; R for G or A) and a novel locked nucleic acid (LNA nucleotides in bold and brackets) probe (Sigma Life Science; qFUS-LNA76 5- FAM-CC[G][T]CT[G][G]T[T][G]GA-BHQ-3) was designed. Where possible, DNA eluates were analysed in duplicate (226 BALF, 16 others). Amplifications were performed in a 20 μL mixture using a StepOnePlus thermocycler (Applied Biosystems). Each reaction mixture contained 10 μL 2× Takyon Rox Probe MasterMix UNG (Eurogentec), 450 nM forward and reverse primer, 150 nM probe, and 5 μL of extracted DNA. The assay, described by Muraosa et al., was specific for *Fusarium* confirmed by testing other fungi including *Aspergillus* and *Candida* [13]. Amplification was carried out applying a standard thermocycling protocol: Uracil-DNA glycosylase (UNG) activation was at 50 °C for 2 min, and initial *Taq* polymerase activation was at 95 °C for 3 min, followed by 50 cycles of 95 °C for 10 s, 55 °C for 30 s, and 72 °C for 20 s (standard ramp speed and standard cycling conditions). In each run, negative (molecular grade water) and positive controls (DNA of *Fusarium* sp.) were included. Amplicons of clinical samples were purified, sequenced (the classical dye chain-termination sequencing method ("Sanger sequencing") by a commercial company (LGC, Berlin)), and analyzed by using BLAST analysis (National Center of Biotechnology Information, Washington DC, www.ncbi.nlm.nih.gov/BLAST) as described before [19].

To determine the limit of detection (LoD) of qPCR assay, DNA was measured using a NanoDrop (ND-1000, Peqlab) and serially diluted. Exemplarily, the LoD using DNA of *F. solanii* was determined to be 15 fg, fitting perfectly to the originally described LoD (one copy of standard DNA which corresponds to approximately 30 fg) [13]. PCR efficiency was 91.1% using 5 ten-fold dilutions in triplicates ranging from 1.2 to 12,000 copies.

3. Results

3.1. Clinical Specimens Positive for Fusarium spp.

In total, 22 DNA eluates from clinical isolates ($n = 12$) and clinical samples ($n = 10$) were tested for the presence of fungal DNA. In 20 eluates comprising a variety of *Fusarium* spp., DNA of the genus *Fusarium* could be detected (*F. dimerum* complex, *F. keratoplasticum*, *F. musae*, *F. oxysporum* complex, *F. petroliphilum*, *F. proliferatum*, *F. sacchari*, *F. verticilloides*). All *Fusarium* spp. commonly found in clinical samples in Germany [16] could be detected by using this real-time PCR assay. Two of 10 clinical samples were not detected. For one negatively tested sample, the eluate volume was limited and no further testing was possible, neither for a duplicate using the *Fusarium*-specific PCR assay nor for testing of PCR inhibition. The second negative sample was reproducibly negative and showed no PCR inhibition. Interestingly, both originally contained *F. oxysporum* complex as determined by not-yet-published PCR assays (personal communication, G. Walther), which can be generally detected by our PCR assay as shown by testing other specimens ($n = 3$). Unsuitable storage or transport conditions of tested DNA samples cannot be excluded as a reason for PCR negativity.

3.2. Bronchoalveolar Lavage Fluid (BALF)

In total, 243 BALF samples from 221 patients were collected and retrospectively analyzed for the presence of fungal DNA. Two samples (0.8%) showed positive PCR results for *Fusarium* DNA, one possible (Cq mean 33.8) and one probable IFD case (Cq mean 24.2). Sequencing revealed the genus *Fusarium* for the probable IFD case, but no homology to fungi was found for the possible case using forward or reverse primer for sequencing. Interestingly, the probable case was also positive for GM testing and *Aspergillus*-specific PCR, suggesting a fungal coinfection. This patient was a 53-year-old man suffering from non-Hodgkin lymphoma (diffuse large B-cell). Because of a relapse, he was treated with irutinib (very good partial remission). Two months later, he was admitted for stem cell transplantation (SCT). Three weeks after transplantation, pulmonary aspergillosis was diagnosed because of positive imaging and GM detection (serum). However, *Aspergillus* sp. was never detected in any of the multiple cultures (blood and BALF), but *Fusarium* species was cultured from BALF. The patient was treated successfully with voriconazole, and GM levels decreased under the cut-off (0.5) within two weeks of treatment. A possible double infection of *Aspergillus* and *Fusarium* could have been treated successfully by administering voriconazole, as both pathogens are often susceptible to this antifungal drug.

The possible IFD case was a 66-year-old male patient with mantle cell lymphoma scheduled for a high-dose (HD) chemotherapy with autologous SCT (aSCT). Initially, he presented with a good performance status with no significant clinical findings. After HD chemotherapy with rituximab, bis-*chloroethyl*-nitrosourea (BCNU), etoposide, cytarabine, and melphalan, the patient received aSCT and developed neutropenia. On day 5 after aSCT, fever occurred and empirical antibiotic treatment with piperacillin/tazobactam was initiated. However, the patient still remained febrile and consequently a pulmonary CT scan of the lung was performed showing signs of atypical pneumonia triggering antifungal treatment with voriconazole. A bronchoscopy was performed and BALF was found to be positive for Herpes simplex virus, *Escherichia coli*, and *Pseudomonas aeruginosa*. After adapting the antibiotic treatment to imipenem according to the microbiological susceptibility testing, the patient recovered and became afebrile within two days. A fungal infection seems therefore unlikely, but we cannot exclude it.

4. Discussion

PCR is an established, very sensitive molecular tool, which has shown its potential to detect fast and specific pathogens in many fields, leading to earlier diagnosis and improved patient outcome. Here we describe the application of a *Fusarium*-specific probe-based real-time PCR assay to clinical specimens. This assay was able to detect all *Fusarium* species commonly found in clinical samples derived from Germany [16].

In our high-risk cohort for IFD (HM patients with lung infiltrates), we found two BALF samples (0.8%) containing DNA of *Fusarium* spp. One probable IFD case also showed signs for invasive aspergillosis (positive GM assay in serum). The second case (possible IFD) could not be confirmed on sequence level. Similar frequencies of *Fusarium* in BALF were recently described by two studies, ranging from 0.6 to 2% [20,21]. Because of this low frequency, clinical diagnostic studies regarding pulmonary fusariosis are difficult to perform, as huge patient numbers are necessary. Both studies used a broad-range PCR to detect fungal DNA, meaning that *Fusarium* is only one detectable fungus beside many others. One could speculate that specific PCR assays are more sensitive than broad-range ones [22], but also the type of investigated patient cohort and the region play a role. This concerns the fungal distribution on genus level, but also on the species level. FSSC is described to be responsible for the most cases of invasive fusariosis in Japan (73%; [4]) and the United States (60%, [23]), but not in Turkey with 42% [24], where FFSC is the most reported *Fusarium* complex (52%). Similar results are reported for the epidemiology of *Aspergillus terreus*, as this fungus is usually accusing a small proportion of invasive aspergillosis while in specific regions the detection rate is much higher [25].

As sequencing of the possible IFD patient could not confirm the presence of *Fusarium* DNA and also the clinical course was not typical for an IFD, the major involvement of a fungal pathogen is unlikely in this patient. However, in the probable IFD patient different fungal biomarkers were found (culture, GM, PCR), increasing the probability of IFD. As even biomarkers of two different fungal species wère detected which can be easily performed by specific molecular tools, e.g. real-time PCR assays, a co-infection of *Aspergillus* and *Fusarium* in this patient is likely. In consequence, the number of co-infections may be underestimated in general, as other studies reported up to 33% of fungal co-infections, which is especially described for *Aspergillus* and Mucorales [22,26–28]. GM testing is described to detect *Aspergillus*, but also to cross-react with other fungi including *Penicillium*, *Geotrichum*, yeasts, and *Fusarium* [29]. Therefore, a positive GM test could indicate the presence of *Aspergillus* but also of *Fusarium*.

Using the described qPCR assay enables fast and specific identification of *Fusarium*, but only on genus level; for some authors, identification at species level is necessary [30], whereas others stated that in clinical practice, species identification is not necessary to find suitable treatment options [3]. A positive test result could be used to trigger or re-evaluate an antifungal treatment regimen because all members of the order *Fusarium* show intrinsic resistances. Therefore, remaining treatment options are limited and should be applied as early as possible. In contrast to our assay, previously described assays to detect *Fusarium* DNA have some disadvantages. Conventional PCR assays are highly prone to contamination, are time-consuming, and cannot quantify fungal load, whereas real-time assays are performed in a closed system, minimizing contamination risk (no necessity to handle amplicons to perform a second, nested PCR assay or to visualize PCR results by gel electrophoresis). Furthermore, quantification is possible and monitoring of *Fusarium* DNA, e.g., in serum samples, could guide treatment effectively and improve patients' outcome.

As fusariosis is a rare disease and is caused by many different species, large future studies have to evaluate this issue by screening many clinical samples with a highly sensitive method. Pretest probability can be increased by analyzing high risk patient cohorts or specimens directly taken from the focus of the disease.

5. Conclusions

Here we describe a rapid, probe-based real-time PCR assay to specifically detect DNA from a broad range of *Fusarium* species and a first pilot application to clinical samples. Validation of positive PCR assays should be confirmed by sequencing. The occurrence of fungal co-infections might be underestimated. This assay is most suitable to confirm the diagnosis of fusariosis.

Author Contributions: Conceptualization, J.S., J.L., and V.R.; methodology, J.S. and G.W.; formal analysis, J.S., G.W., O.K.; resources, H.E. and O.K.; writing—original draft preparation, J.S.; writing—review and editing, J.S., G.W., B.W., D.T., V.R., A.H., H.E., O.K., and J.L.; supervision, J.L.; project administration, J.L., V.R; funding acquisition, J.L., V.R.

Acknowledgments: We thank all providers of clinical specimens or DNA, amongst others (in alphabetic order) Oliver A. Cornely, Sandra Fuhrmann, Werner J. Heinz, Johanna Kessel, Michael G. Kiehl, Stefan W. Krause, Tobias Liebregts, Georg Maschmeyer, Stefan Schwartz and Jörg Janne Vehreschild. Work in the German reference center for invasive fungal infections NRZMyk is supported by the Robert Koch Institute from funds provided by the German Ministry of Health (grant 1369-240).

References

1. Nelson, P.E.; Dignani, M.C.; Anaissie, E.J. Taxonomy, biology, and clinical aspects of Fusarium species. *Clin. Microbiol. Rev.* **1994**, *7*, 479–504. [CrossRef] [PubMed]
2. O'Donnell, K.; Ward, T.J.; Robert, V.A.R.G.; Crous, P.W.; Geiser, D.M.; Kang, S. DNA sequence-based identification of Fusarium: Current status and future directions. *Phytoparasitica* **2015**, *43*, 583–595. [CrossRef]
3. Guarro, J. Fusariosis a complex infection caused by a high diversity of fungal species refractory to treatment. *Eur. J. Clin. Microbiol. Infect. Dis. Off. Publ. Eur. Soc. Clin. Microbiol.* **2013**, *32*, 1491–1500. [CrossRef] [PubMed]
4. Muraosa, Y.; Oguchi, M.; Yahiro, M.; Watanabe, A.; Yaguchi, T.; Kamei, K. Epidemiological Study of Fusarium Species Causing Invasive and Superficial Fusariosis in Japan. *Med. Mycol. J.* **2017**, *58*, E5–E13. [CrossRef] [PubMed]

5. Meletiadis, J.; Roilides, E. Rare Invasive Fungal Infections: Epidemiology, Diagnosis and Management. *Curr. Fungal Infect. Rep.* **2013**, *7*, 351–360. [CrossRef]
6. Kapp, M.; Schargus, M.; Deuchert, T.; Springer, J.; Wendel, F.; Loeffler, J.; Grigoleit, G.U.; Kurzai, O.; Heinz, W.; Einsele, H.; et al. Endophthalmitis as primary clinical manifestation of fatal fusariosis in an allogeneic stem cell recipient. *Transpl. Infect. Dis.* **2011**, *13*, 374–379. [CrossRef] [PubMed]
7. Bitar, D.; Van Cauteren, D.; Lanternier, F.; Dannaoui, E.; Che, D.; Dromer, F.; Desenclos, J.-C.; Lortholary, O. Increasing incidence of zygomycosis (mucormycosis), France, 1997–2006. *Emerg. Infect. Dis.* **2009**, *15*, 1395–1401. [CrossRef] [PubMed]
8. Auberger, J.; Lass-Florl, C.; Aigner, M.; Clausen, J.; Gastl, G.; Nachbaur, D. Invasive fungal breakthrough infections, fungal colonization and emergence of resistant strains in high-risk patients receiving antifungal prophylaxis with posaconazole: real-life data from a single-centre institutional retrospective observational study. *J. Antimicrob. Chemother.* **2012**, *67*, 2268–2273. [CrossRef] [PubMed]
9. Walther, G.; Stasch, S.; Kaerger, K.; Hamprecht, A.; Roth, M.; Cornely, O.A.; Geerling, G.; Mackenzie, C.R.; Kurzai, O.; von Lilienfeld-Toal, M. Fusarium Keratitis in Germany. *J. Clin. Microbiol.* **2017**, *55*, 2983–2995. [CrossRef] [PubMed]
10. Roth, M.; Daas, L.; Renner-Wilde, A.; Cvetkova-Fischer, N.; Saeger, M.; Herwig-Carl, M.; Matthaei, M.; Fekete, A.; Kakkassery, V.; Walther, G.; et al. The German keratomycosis registry: Initial results of amulticenter survey. *Ophthalmol. Z. Dtsch. Ophthalmol. Ges.* **2019**, *116*, 957–966.
11. McCarthy, M.W.; Katragkou, A.; Iosifidis, E.; Roilides, E.; Walsh, T.J. Recent Advances in the Treatment of Scedosporiosis and Fusariosis. *J. Fungi* **2018**, *4*, 73. [CrossRef] [PubMed]
12. 12. Tortorano, A.M.; Richardson, M.; Roilides, E.; van Diepeningen, A.; Caira, M.; Munoz, P.; Johnson, E.; Meletiadis, J.; Pana, Z.D.; Lackner, M.; et al. ESCMID and ECMM joint guidelines on diagnosis and management of hyalohyphomycosis: *Fusarium* spp., *Scedosporium* spp. and others. *Clin. Microbiol. Infect.* **2014**, *20* (Suppl. 3), 27–46. [CrossRef] [PubMed]
13. Muraosa, Y.; Schreiber, A.Z.; Trabasso, P.; Matsuzawa, T.; Taguchi, H.; Moretti, M.L.; Mikami, Y.; Kamei, K. Development of cycling probe-based real-time PCR system to detect Fusarium species and Fusarium solani species complex (FSSC). *Int. J. Med. Microbiol. IJMM* **2014**, *304*, 505–511. [CrossRef] [PubMed]
14. Hue, F.X.; Huerre, M.; Rouffault, M.A.; de Bievre, C. Specific detection of fusarium species in blood and tissues by a PCR technique. *J. Clin. Microbiol.* **1999**, *37*, 2434–2438. [PubMed]
15. Grube, S.; Schonling, J.; Prange, A. Evaluation of a triplex real-time PCR system to detect the plant-pathogenic molds *Alternaria* spp., *Fusarium* spp. and *C. purpurea*. *J. Microbiol. Methods* **2015**, *119*, 180–188. [CrossRef] [PubMed]
16. Hamprecht, A.G.; Goettig, S.; Haas, A.; Held, J.; Koeppel, M.B.; Kurzai, O.; Saleh, A.; Seibold, M.; Steinmann, J.; Tintelnot, K.; et al. Epidemiology and in vitro susceptibility of Fusarium species from human infections in Germany-results of a retrospective multicenter study. *Med. Mycol.* **2018**, *56*, S64.
17. De Pauw, B.; Walsh, T.J.; Donnelly, J.P.; Stevens, D.A.; Edwards, J.E.; Calandra, T.; Pappas, P.G.; Maertens, J.; Lortholary, O.; Kauffman, C.A.; et al. Revised definitions of invasive fungal disease from the European Organization for Research and Treatment of Cancer/Invasive Fungal Infections Cooperative Group and the National Institute of Allergy and Infectious Diseases Mycoses Study Group (EORTC/MSG) Consensus Group. *Clin. Infect. Dis.* **2008**, *46*, 1813–1821. [PubMed]
18. Springer, J.; White, P.L.; Kessel, J.; Wieters, I.; Teschner, D.; Korczynski, D.; Liebregts, T.; Cornely, O.A.; Schwartz, S.; Elgeti, T.; et al. A Comparison of Aspergillus and Mucorales PCR Testing of Different Bronchoalveolar Lavage Fluid Fractions from Patients with Suspected Invasive Pulmonary Fungal Disease. *J. Clin. Microbiol.* **2018**, *56*, e01655-17. [PubMed]
19. Springer, J.; Goldenberger, D.; Schmidt, F.; Weisser, M.; Wehrle-Wieland, E.; Einsele, H.; Frei, R.; Löffler, J. Development and application of two independent real-time PCR assays to detect clinically relevant Mucorales species. *J. Med. Microbiol.* **2016**, *65*, 227–234. [CrossRef] [PubMed]
20. Ricna, D.; Lengerova, M.; Bezdicek, M.; Kocmanova, I.; Drgona, L.; Weinbergerova, B.; Mayer, J.; Racil, Z. Detection and identification of fungi in bronchoalveolar lavage fluid from immunocompromised patients using panfungal PCR. *Folia Microbiol.* **2019**, *64*, 421–428. [CrossRef] [PubMed]

21. Wehrle-Wieland, E.; Affolter, K.; Goldenberger, D.; Tschudin Sutter, S.; Halter, J.; Passweg, J.; Tamm, M.; Khanna, N.; Stolz, D. Diagnosis of invasive mold diseases in patients with hematological malignancies using Aspergillus, Mucorales, and panfungal PCR in BAL. *Transpl. Infect. Dis. Off. J. Transplant. Soc.* **2018**, *20*, e12953. [CrossRef] [PubMed]
22. Springer, J.; McCormick Smith, I.; Hartmann, S.; Winkelmann, R.; Wilmes, D.; Cornely, O.; Kessel, J.; Löffler, J.; Rickerts, V. Identification of Aspergillus and Mucorales in formalin-fixed, paraffin-embedded tissue samples, Comparison of specific and broad-range fungal qPCR assays. *Med. Mycol.* **2019**, *57*, 308–313. [CrossRef] [PubMed]
23. O'Donnell, K.; Sutton, D.A.; Rinaldi, M.G.; Gueidan, C.; Crous, P.W.; Geiser, D.M. Novel multilocus sequence typing scheme reveals high genetic diversity of human pathogenic members of the Fusarium incarnatum-F. equiseti and F. chlamydosporum species complexes within the United States. *J. Clin. Microbiol.* **2009**, *47*, 3851–3861. [CrossRef] [PubMed]
24. Dalyan Cilo, B.; Al-Hatmi, A.M.S.; Seyedmousavi, S.; Rijs, A.J.; Verweij, P.E.; Ener, B.; de Hoog, G.S.; van Diepeningen, A.D. Emergence of fusarioses in a university hospital in Turkey during a 20-year period. *Eur. J. Clin. Microbiol. Infect. Dis. Off. Publ. Eur. Soc. Clin. Microbiol.* **2015**, *34*, 1683–1691.
25. Lass-Florl, C.; Griff, K.; Mayr, A.; Gueidan, C.; Crous, P.W.; Geiser, D.M. Epidemiology and outcome of infections due to Aspergillus terreus: 10-year single centre experience. *Br. J. Haematol.* **2005**, *131*, 201–207. [CrossRef] [PubMed]
26. Rickerts, V.; Just-Nubling, G.; Konrad, F.; Kern, J.; Lambrecht, E.; Böhme, A.; Jacobi, V.; Bialek, R. Diagnosis of invasive aspergillosis and mucormycosis in immunocompromised patients by seminested PCR assay of tissue samples. *Eur. J. Clin. Microbiol. Infect. Dis.* **2006**, *25*, 8–13. [CrossRef] [PubMed]
27. Millon, L.; Herbrecht, R.; Grenouillet, F.; Morio, F.; Alanio, A.; Letscher-Bru, V.; Cassaing, S.; Chouaki, T.; Kauffmann-Lacroix, C.; Poirier, P.; et al. Early diagnosis and monitoring of mucormycosis by detection of circulating DNA in serum: retrospective analysis of 44 cases collected through the French Surveillance Network of Invasive Fungal Infections (RESSIF). *Clin. Microbiol. Infect.* **2016**, *22*, 810-e1–810-e8. [CrossRef] [PubMed]
28. Kontoyiannis, D.P.; Wessel, V.C.; Bodey, G.P.; Rolston, K.V. Zygomycosis in the 1990s in a tertiary-care cancer center. *Clin. Infect. Dis.* **2000**, *30*, 851–856. [CrossRef] [PubMed]
29. Tortorano, A.M.; Esposto, M.C.; Prigitano, A.; Grancini, A.; Ossi, C.; Cavanna, C.; Cascio, G.L. Cross-reactivity of *Fusarium* spp. in the Aspergillus Galactomannan enzyme-linked immunosorbent assay. *J. Clin. Microbiol.* **2012**, *50*, 1051–1053. [CrossRef] [PubMed]
30. Perfect, J.R. Treatment of non-Aspergillus moulds in immunocompromised patients, with amphotericin B lipid complex. *Clin. Infect. Dis. Off. Publ. Infect. Dis. Soc. Am.* **2005**, *40*, S401–S408. [CrossRef] [PubMed]

3

Development and Applications of Prognostic Risk Models in the Management of Invasive Mold Disease

Marta Stanzani [1] and Russell E. Lewis [2,*]

[1] Institute of Hematology "Lorenzo e Ariosto Seràgnoli", Department of Hematology and Clinical Oncology, S. Orsola-Malpighi Hospital, University of Bologna, 40138 Bologna, Italy; marta.stanzani2@unibo.it

[2] Clinic of Infectious Diseases, Department of Medical and Surgical Sciences, S. Orsola-Malpighi Hospital, University of Bologna, 40138 Bologna, Italy

* Correspondence: russeledward.lewis@unibo.it

Abstract: Prognostic models or risk scores are frequently used to aid individualize risk assessment for diseases with multiple, complex risk factors and diagnostic challenges. However, relatively little attention has been paid to the development of risk models for invasive mold diseases encountered in patients with hematological malignancies, despite a large body of epidemiological research. Herein we review recent studies that have described the development of prognostic models for mold disease, summarize our experience with the development and clinical use of one such model (BOSCORE), and discuss the potential impact of prognostic risk scores for individualized therapy, diagnostic and antifungal stewardship, as well as clinical and epidemiological research.

Keywords: prognostic risk model; prediction models; risk score; invasive mold disease; hematological malignancy; risk assessment; antifungal stewardship

---

1. Introduction

Many decisions involved in the prevention, diagnosis and treatment of invasive mold disease (IMD) depend on an accurate estimate of the patient's future risk for developing the infection [1]. This prediction can be challenging given the multivariate and dynamic nature of risk factors that predispose patients to these infections [2–4]. Surprisingly little attention has been given to the development of prediction models or risk scores to aid individualized IMD risk assessment, even though such models have been developed for invasive candidiasis in non-neutropenic patients and incorporated in clinical trial design [5–8]. The concept of developing and validating clinical prediction models for IMD seems logical given that such models have proven to be useful for diseases in other areas of medicine characterized by multivariate and complex risk factors, as well as diagnostic challenges [9,10]. Individualized risk assessment is also a key component of diagnostic and antifungal stewardship efforts, because many evidence-based interventions such as antifungal prophylaxis have only been proven to be clinically beneficial in select high-risk subpopulations [11].

In this review, we will review key risk factors that predispose patients to IMD during the treatment of hematological malignancies, describe recent attempts towards the development prognostic risk models, and explore how these risk models can be incorporated to improve future clinical and epidemiological research. This review is primarily applicable to the development of models for predicting invasive aspergillosis rather than less common molds given the much higher prevalence of this disease, clinical availability of biomarkers for diagnostic-driven management, and evidence-based recommendations for prophylaxis in select patient groups.

2. Risk Factors for Invasive Mold Disease

Epidemiological studies performed over the last four decades have identified many risk factors that predispose patients with hematological malignancies to developing an IMD [3]. These include host-specific factors of the (i) type of underlying malignancy and status, whether in remission or active; (ii) Type of immunosuppressive chemotherapy and associated conditions such as neutropenia and damage to integument; (iii) The type of hematopoietic stem cell transplantation (HSCT) (autologous versus allogeneic graft), stem cell source, status of the malignancy at the time of transplant, and genetic risk factors for fungal disease in the donor; (iv) immunosuppressive therapy required to manage graft versus host disease (GVHD); (iv) Patient comorbidities and age; (v) Environmental or occupational risk factors associated with fungal spore exposure; and (vi) A prior history of IMD [3,4].

Although many of these risk factors are discussed in current treatment guidelines [12,13], most diagnostic and treatment algorithms are still generally based on only a few host risk factors used in epidemiological definitions for probable or proven IMD or in drug registration trials [14]. As a result, patients are generally separated into heterogenous pools of high-risk versus low-risk at the time of a newly-diagnosed malignancy or following HSCT [15]. This approach often falls short in the "real-life" management of patients who receive multiple lines of chemotherapy with relapsed malignancy, genetic or occupational predisposition for mold infections, a prior history of mold disease, or receive novel biological agents or immunosuppressive chemotherapy. Therefore, a goal for any prognostic model is to provide a practical approach for improving the precision and accuracy of risk prediction for all patients so clinicians can make better informed decisions. Before discussing specific risk models, however, it is important to briefly review the major risk factors that predispose patients with hematological malignancies to developing an IMD.

2.1. *Underlying Malignancy and Status*

Acute myeloid leukemia (AML) and myelodysplastic syndromes (MDS) have historically been associated with the highest reported rates of IMD, ranging from 5–25% [4,16,17]. The period at greatest risk for IMD is typically during initial induction chemotherapy, which typically results in prolonged (>21 days) and profound (<500 PMN/mm^3) neutropenia [18]. Other factors in AML patients that may be associated with higher rates of IMD include older age, poor prognosis for achieving complete remission (CR) due to unfavorable cytogenetics or relapsed malignancy, and presence of multiple baseline comorbidities or poor performance status [4]. Patients who receive induction chemotherapy in non-HEPA filtered rooms, or an occupational history of heavy spore exposure (e.g., farming, construction) may also be at higher risk. Relapse of IMD is also a concern in any patient undergoing consolidation chemotherapy with a previous history of fungal infection during their induction regimen [19]. Survival rates among patients with AML have improved in recent years despite relatively few changes in frontline chemotherapy protocols due in part to improved supportive care measures and the introduction of more effective prophylaxis options such as posaconazole [20].

Older patients with transformed MDS are at high risk for IMD if they receive AML-like treatment regimens. However, hypomethylating agents such as azacytidine or decitabine are increasingly being used in place of cytosine arabinoside (ARA-C), resulting in lower rates of infection complications, including a probable or proven IMD of 2–5% [21–23].

Adult patients with acute lymphoblastic leukemia (ALL) are generally considered to be at moderate risk for developing IMD, with most case series having reported rates of probable or proven IMD between 2–5% [17]. A recent randomized study comparing prophylaxis with liposomal amphotericin B to placebo in adult patients with ALL reported rates of probable IMD of 7.5% and 9%, respectively [24]. The relatively higher incidence of probable IMD observed in this study may have reflected recent trends in the use of more intensive chemotherapy regimens in adults designed to improve long-term survival, which are associated with higher rates of infection during induction chemotherapy [25]. The risk of IMD may also be increased in patients with relapsed ALL, especially in patients who receive regimens with high doses of dexamethasone [26]. In contrast, patients with

Philadelphia-positive ALL receiving treatment with tyrosine kinase inhibitors (imatinib, dasatinib, nilotinib, and bosutinib) as part of standard or reduced-intensity regimens appear to have a lower risk of developing an IMD (3–5% incidence) [27–29].

Patients with chronic lymphoproliferative disorders such as non-Hodgkin's and Hodgkin's lymphoma, chronic myelogenous leukemia, or multiple myeloma are generally considered to be at low risk for IMD (<2% incidence). However, select subsets of patients with extensively-treated lymphoma who receive intensive chemotherapy regimens of high-dose corticosteroids followed by autologous HSCT often experience prolonged neutropenia and with rates of IMD like patients with AML/MDS undergoing induction chemotherapy [30]. Patients who receive intensive chemotherapy regimens for CNS lymphomas in combination with drugs that target B-lymphocyte pathways, particularly the Bruton's tyrosine kinase inhibitor ibrutinib, may be at especially high risk for cryptococcosis, pneumocystis pneumonia, and aspergillosis involving the central nervous system [31]. In one case series the use of ibrutinib in combination with temozolomide, etoposide, cytarabine and liposomal doxorubicin, rituximab and dexamethasone was associated with rates of invasive aspergillosis of 44% [30–32]. In contrast, the use of ibrutinib monotherapy in patients with chronic lymphocytic leukemia was associated with low rates of invasive fungal disease (0.5–1.6%) that were comparable to treatment with alkylating agents or monoclonal antibodies, which are no longer considered to be the main standard of care [32,33].

Relatively few data are available describing the risk of IMD among patients with myeloproliferative neoplasms including chronic myelogenous leukemia, polycythemia vera, essential thrombocytopenia, and myelofibrosis [4]. Accurate estimates of IMD risk in these populations are confounded by the increasing use of tyrosine kinase inhibitors (imatinib, dasatinib, nilotinib, bosutinib, and ponatinib) for targeting the BCR-ABL oncoprotein in chronic myelogenous leukemia, which leads to disease control in most patients. Similarly, targeted therapy with JAK (Janus Kinase) inhibitors in patients with myelofibrosis appears to be associated with a low risk of IMD [34,35].

Severe aplastic anemia is characterized by a reduction in the production of hematopoietic progenitor cells resulting in severe pancytopenia [36]. Infection is a major cause of death and is directly related to prolonged neutropenia. The risk of fungal infection is further increased by treatments that reduce T-cells (anti-thymocyte globulin) or function (corticosteroids, calcineurin inhibitors), however *Candida* spp. appear to be much more common than invasive molds [37].

2.2. Conditions Associated with Disease Treatment

Autopsy studies performed in the early 1960s identified prolonged neutropenia as a major predisposing risk factor for IMD [38,39]. Gerson and colleagues [40] later demonstrated that neutropenia persisting longer than three weeks was the most important risk factor for development of invasive pulmonary aspergillosis in patients with acute leukemia. During the first two weeks of neutropenia, patients developed signs of invasive risk of invasive pulmonary aspergillosis at a rate of approximately 1% per day that increased to 4.3% per day between the 24th and 36th days of neutropenia. Of the 13 patients who remained neutropenic at 28 days, 7 (54%) had developed signs of invasive pulmonary aspergillosis.

The European Organization for Research and Treatment of Cancer /Invasive Fungal Infections Cooperative Group and the National Institute of Allergy and Infectious Diseases Mycoses Study Group (EORTC/MSG) Consensus Group have defined neutropenia as a host factor for invasive fungal disease when it presents as <500 cells/mm^3 for >10 days [41]. Typically, the median duration of neutropenia prior to the first signs of IPA ranges from 16–25 days, but for some patients with multiple risk factors, disease onset may occur before 10 days [3].

Lymphopenia (<300 cells/mm^3) and monocytopenia (<10 cells/mm^3) are infrequently the sole predisposing risk factors for IMD, but often indicate delayed immune reconstitution after chemotherapy or allogeneic HSCT [4,42]. In an analysis of 1248 allogeneic HSCT recipients, neutropenia (HR 2.2; 1.3–3.6, $p < 0.01$), lymphocytopenia (1.4, 1–2; $p = 0.05$), and monocytopenia

(HR 1.8, 1.7–3.4, $p < 0.01$) were independently associated with increased risk of mold disease within one year of transplantation [43]. Mikulska et al. identified the presence and duration of lymphopenia as independent risk factors for early mortality from invasive aspergillosis in recipients of allogeneic HSCT from alternative donors [42]. Lewis et al. reported that patients with pulmonary mucormycosis who presented with lymphocyte counts <100 cells/mm^3 had a 4-fold higher rate of mortality versus patients without lymphocytopenia [44].

Glucocorticoid therapy at supraphysiologic doses have long been associated with the development of mold infections [45], but the cumulative dose that places a patient at increased risk varies from study to study and often depends on concomitant chemotherapy, type of allogeneic HSCT and severity of GVHD [46]. The EORTC/MSG consensus definitions for invasive fungal disease include corticosteroids as a host factor for mold disease when a patient has received a mean minimum dose of 0.3 mg/kg/day prednisone equivalent for greater than 3 weeks [41]. Notably, the EORTC/MSG criteria do not consider inhaled corticosteroids to be a host factor even though cases of invasive pulmonary aspergillosis have been described in critically-ill patients with chronic-obstructive pulmonary disease [47,48].

In patients who undergo allogeneic HSCT, high cumulative doses of glucocorticoids are the most frequently identified risk factor associated with invasive aspergillosis after engraftment [49–52]. O'Donnell and colleagues reported that use of high-dose prednisone (0.5–1.0 mg/kg per day) for graft-versus-host-disease increased the risk six-fold versus lower dose prednisone regimens (0.25 mg/kg/day) for developing invasive aspergillosis [53]. Similarly, Marr and colleagues reported that glucocorticoid doses of 1.9 mg/kg per day, 1.9–3.0 mg/kg per day, and greater than 3 mg/kg per day were associated with IMD risks of 5%, 10%, and 14%, respectively [49]. Ribaud and co-workers reported that the 60-day risk of death increased from 12% to 80% if allo-HSCT recipients had received a cumulative prednisolone dose of greater than 7 mg/kg in the week preceding diagnosis of IMD [51].

2.3. Hematopoietic Stem Cell Transplantation

Allogeneic HSCT recipients have among the highest reported incidence of IMD in studies ranging between 7 and 15% [4]. The risk period is bimodal, with early risk for disease (first 40 days) associated with prolonged neutropenia prior to stem cell engraftment, and later invasive mold disease (often after day +70 or +100) associated with immunosuppressive therapy for controlling GVHD. Several additional pre- and post-transplant factors have been reported to influence IMD risk. Pre-transplant risk factors include the type of transplant (matched-related donor, umbilical-cord donor, or haploidentical/mismatched donor) [43,54,55] stem cell dose [56], receipt of T-cell depleting agents (e.g., anti-thymocyte globulin or alemtuzumab) or a T-cell depleted graft [43,57], polymorphisms in donor genes important for detection of fungal antigens and antifungal innate immune responses (i.e., Toll-like receptor 4, Dectin-1, and Pentraxin-3) [58–60], and iron overload associated with frequent transfusions [43,61,62].

Post-allogeneic HSCT risk factors for IMD include the rate of immune reconstitution (time to engraftment and recovery from neutropenia, lymphocytopenia, and monocytopenia), recovery of natural-killer cell populations [63], development of acute graft versus host disease and its treatment with immunosuppressive agents (corticosteroids, anti-T cell therapies), and development/reactivation of viral co-infections, particularly cytomegalovirus (CMV) [43].

The incidence of IMD following autologous HSCT is lower, with reported incidence ranging between 3–8% [64–66]. The incidence is influenced by the underlying malignancy, number and types of chemotherapy cycles prior to transplantation, previous history of IMD, as well as antifungal prophylaxis [4].

2.4. Patient Comorbidities

Besides older age, several underlying comorbidities or poor performance status overall are associated with increased susceptibility to IMD. Patients with uncontrolled diabetes mellitus may exhibit impaired neutrophil migration and fungal cell phagocytosis and T-cell dysfunction [67]. In the setting of metabolic acidosis, uncoupling of free iron from carrier proteins in blood enhances fungal growth and is an important risk factor for disseminated mucormycosis [68,69]. Smoking and chronic pulmonary disease were similarly identified as pre-chemotherapy risk factors for the development of IMD during initial remission-induction therapy [16]. Poor nutritional status or cachexia associated with advanced disease, often manifesting as hypoalbuminemia, was associated with 3-fold lower odds of developing IMD following allogeneic HSCT for each gram/deciliter increase in serum albumin [70].

Viral co-infections, particularly cytomegalovirus (CMV) and influenzae are associated with increased risk of invasive pulmonary aspergillosis. CMV viremia and recipient CMV serostatus have been identified as risk factors following allogeneic HSCT for both early and late-onset IMD, which may be enhanced in patients who developed prolonged neutropenia following treatment with ganciclovir [43,71,72]. However, it is still debated whether CMV replication directly impairs antifungal immunity or is a signal of already impaired cellular immunity that allows permissive growth of molds [73,74]. Nevertheless, the clear temporal association of CMV viremia or infection with the development of IMD suggests CMV replication or disease can be a powerful predictive factor for mold disease [71].

The link between severe influenzae and invasive aspergillosis has been increasingly described in both non-immunocompromised and immunocompromised hosts [75–79]. It has been hypothesized that the evolution of more virulent influenza strains, as exemplified by the pandemic H1N1 strain, are associated with more severe lymphopenia and diffuse damage to the respiratory mucosa during infection that predispose hosts to fungal invasion [79,80]. Influenza preceding IMD is associated with high rates of respiratory failure and mortality, highlighting the importance of prompt diagnosis and initiation of antifungal therapy.

2.5. Environmental and Occupational Risk Factors

Repeated exposures to high fungal spore counts associated with farming, construction work, gardening or composting, and perhaps geoclimatic factors increase colonization and persistence of fungal spores in the respiratory tract and place the patient at increased risk for developing IMD during induction chemotherapy [16,81,82]. Outbreaks of invasive mold disease have been repeatedly described following hospital construction and renovation that results in dust contamination and dispersal of fungal spores [83]. Similarly, some studies have documented a relationship between environmental contamination by *Aspergillus* and other fungal species and the incidence of invasive aspergillosis [84]. This risk may be increased if patients are admitted for intensive chemotherapy or transplantation to rooms without positive pressure high efficiency particulate air (HEPA) filtration [85].

3. Risk Models for Invasive Mold Disease

3.1. Neutropenia-Associated Risk Measured by the D-Index

Given the high frequency and importance of neutropenia as a key risk factor for IMD, several investigators have focused on the development of tools that measure both the intensity and duration of neutropenia to predict risk of IMD. Portugal et al. proposed an index (D-index) to improve the assessment of risk for IMD in neutropenic patients. The D-index represents the difference in the area under the curve (AUC) for neutrophil counts over time versus an area resulting from a normal neutrophil count. This difference is geometrically represented as the area over the neutrophil curve (Figure 1) [86]. The investigators also evaluated the prognostic performance of the cumulative D-index score (c-D-Index), which represents the D-index from the start of neutropenia until the date of the first clinical manifestation of IMD. Compared to just measuring the duration of neutropenia, the D-index and c-D-index better discriminated patients (n = 11) who developed IMD with area under the receiver operator curve (aROC) values of 0.86 and 0.81 versus patients who did not develop an IMD (n = 33). At a cut-off of 6200, the sensitivity and specificity of the D-index was 100% and 58%, respectively and for the c-D-index value of 5800 the sensitivity and specificity were 91% and 58%

respectively. Over an incidence range of 5–15%, the positive predictive value (PPV) of the D-index was relatively low (11–30%) but the negative predictive value was high (97–99%) suggesting that the D-index may be useful for "screening-out" lower risk patients with neutropenia who are unlikely to develop a mold infection [86].

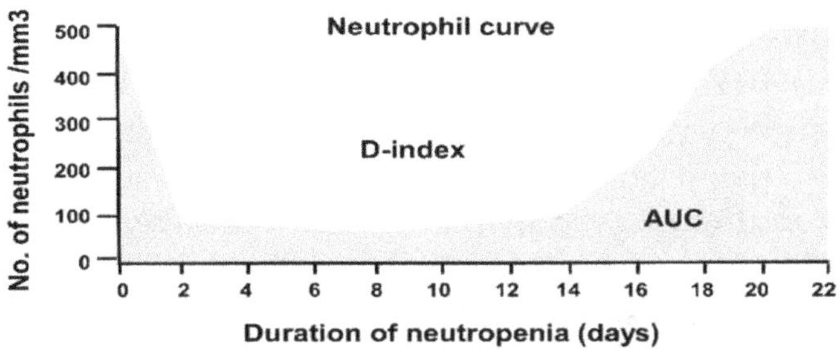

Figure 1. D-index area over the neutrophil curve: AUC areas under the neutrophil curve.

In a follow-up prospective study among 29 patients with acute leukemia undergoing remission-chemotherapy, the investigators utilized the D-index and galactomannan screening to stratify patients as low (<3000), intermediate (3000–5800), and high risk (>5800) for IMD [87]. Although a positive galactomannan result or clinical symptoms triggered a diagnostic workup in similar numbers of patients irrespective of the D-index risk stratification (58–73%), patients in the low risk D-index group were less likely to receive antifungal therapy (17% vs. 54–67%) and no cases of IMD were diagnosed in the low risk group versus 67% and 45% of the patients classified as high and moderate risk, respectively.

3.2. A risk score for Predicting IMD in Lymphoma Patients Receiving Salvage Chemotherapy

Takaoka et al. colleagues retrospectively analyzed 177 consecutive patients who received salvage chemotherapy for active lymphoma (705 courses in total) [88]. The IMD incidence rate was 2.3% (6 probable and 6 possible cases). Multivariate analysis revealed that relapsed refractory disease, receipt of two or more treatment courses, and neutropenia (ANC < 500 cells/mm^3) were independently risk factors associated with the development of IMD. Using these variables, the authors developed a simple weighted risk score: 1 point for refractory therapy, 1 point for two or more treatment lines, 2 points for three or more treatment lines, and 1 point for neutropenia. By applying the score, the authors were able to differentiate a subgroup of lymphoma patients with a higher incidence of IMD by day 80 if the score was above 3 (9% incidence) versus below 2 (0.19% incidence). However, given the retrospective nature of the analysis, it is unclear at what time the score could be applied to predict future IMD. Additionally, the inclusion of EORTC/MSG possible cases of IMD might be questioned as potentially more than half of these cases did not have IMD, especially in the setting of relapsing lymphoma which can produce nodular consolidations in the lung indistinguishable from lymphoma by standard chest CT [89].

3.3. A Risk Score for Predicting IMD Risk Post-Engraftment in Adult Allogeneic HSCT Recipients

Montesinos et al. [90] analyzed risk factors for probable or proven IMD among 404 allogeneic HSCT recipients who engrafted and survived more than 40 days after transplant. The one-year cumulative incidence of IMD in their study cohort was 11%. Five risk factors identified in multivariable analysis (age greater than 40 years, more than one previous HSCT, pre-engraftment neutropenia lasting more than 10 days, extensive and chronic GVHD, and CMV reactivation) were used to construct as risk score for stratifying patients into low risk (0–1 factor, cumulative incidence 0.7%) intermediate risk (2 factors, cumulative incidence 9.9%), and high-risk (3–5 factors, cumulative incidence 24.7%) categories. Although the authors suggest the score could be used to assess risk at patient discharge, two of the five risk factors (extensive chronic GVHD, CMV reactivation) would likely develop later after discharge, therefore patients would need to be reassessed periodically to fully apply the risk score.

3.4. Predicting Invasive Fungal Infection in Pediatric Allogeneic HSCT Recipients

Hol and colleagues retrospectively analyzed pre- and post-transplant predictors of invasive fungal disease among 209 pediatric recipients of allogeneic HSCT with at cumulative incidence of IMD of 12% (mostly molds) [91]. Patients were classified as high or low risk based on pre-transplant risk factors that included: age < 10 years, gender, treatment-related mortality risk predicted by the EBMT risk score, diagnosis type, use of mold-active prophylaxis, prior history of invasive fungal infections, donor type, donor relation and match, conditioning regimen, transplant number, and presence of galactomannan in pre-transplant bronchial alveolar lavage samples. Post-transplant risk factors included duration of neutropenia, aGVHD > grade II, extensive cGVHD, and high-dose corticosteroids (>1 mg/kg/day for at least one week). In multivariate analysis, an EMBT score predicted that treatment related mortality risk >20% was the only factor associated with the occurrence of an IFI, while posttransplant high-dose steroids were the only predictor of invasive fungal infection. After adjustment for pre-transplant treatment related mortality risk and use of corticosteroids, the odds of survival were significantly lower in children who developed IMD versus those who did not (OR 0.30, 95% CI 0.13–0.71, $p = 0.006$).

3.5. Applying Comorbidity Index to Predict IMD after Allogeneic HSCT

Prognostic risk models are frequently used to predict non-relapse mortality among patients undergoing allogeneic HSCT. In 2005, Sorror et al. [92] introduced the hematopoietic stem cell transplantation-comorbidity index (HSCT-CI) assessed prior to transplantation as a means of predicting non-relapse mortality, that was later updated with additional clinical risk factors [93]. Busca et al. recently explored whether the HSCT-CI could have similar utility in predicting the risk for adult patients undergoing allogeneic HSCT for developing fatal IMD [94]. Among 360 retrospectively-analyzed patients who underwent allogeneic HSCT, 8.5% of patients developed EORTC/MSG probable or proven IMD that was significantly higher among patients with and HSCT-CI score of $\geq$3 (12%) compared to patients with HSCT-CI scores of 0–2 (5%). Pulmonary comorbidities were the most common pre-transplant risk factor associated with the development of IMD. Advanced disease at the time of transplant, acute grade II-IV GVHD, and a comorbidity score $\geq$ 3 were independent risk factors for non-relapse mortality.

3.6. Development of a Universal IMD Risk Model for Patients with Hematological Malignancies

Many decisions regarding the management of IMD (e.g., galactomannan screening, antifungal prophylaxis computer tomography in symptomatic febrile patients) are made at the time or soon after admission to the hospital. With this idea in mind, we sought to develop a universal prognostic risk model that could be assessed at the time of each hospital admission to predict an individual patient's risk for developing IMD in the future [15]. Seventeen risk factors assessed at the time of patient admission were first retrospectively analyzed using a data registry of 840 patients with hematological malignancies over 1709 admission episodes lasting more than 5 days from 2005–2008. The data registry was maintained by a dedicated data manager and adjudicated periodically by an attending hematologist with expertise in infectious diseases. Although a total of 11/17 analyzed risk factors correlated with IMD in univariate analysis, only four risk factors were retained in the final multivariable model that were predictive of probable or proven IMD within 90 days of admission: (i) active malignancy (not in remission); (ii) PMN < 500 cells/mm^3 > 10 days or projected prolonged with chemotherapy; (iii) severe lymphocytopenia < 50 cells/mm^3, or lymphocyte-impairing therapies such as calcineurin inhibitors; (iv) and prior history of IMD. These variables were then used to construct a weighted risk score (BOSCORE) with a scale of 0–13. A risk score threshold of < 6 differentiated patients with low (<1%) versus higher (>5%) probability thresholds of IMD. The score was then prospectively validated in our institution in 855 patients over 1746 admissions from 2009–2012

(Figure 2). The discrimination and calibration of the score for predicting IMD were similar in the validation cohort of patients despite introduction of routine posaconazole prophylaxis in AML/MDS patients undergoing induction chemotherapy, with an aROC of 0.84 (95% CI 0.79–0.89) and negative predictive value of 0.99 (95% CI 0.98–0.99) at a 5% predicted probability threshold cut-off.

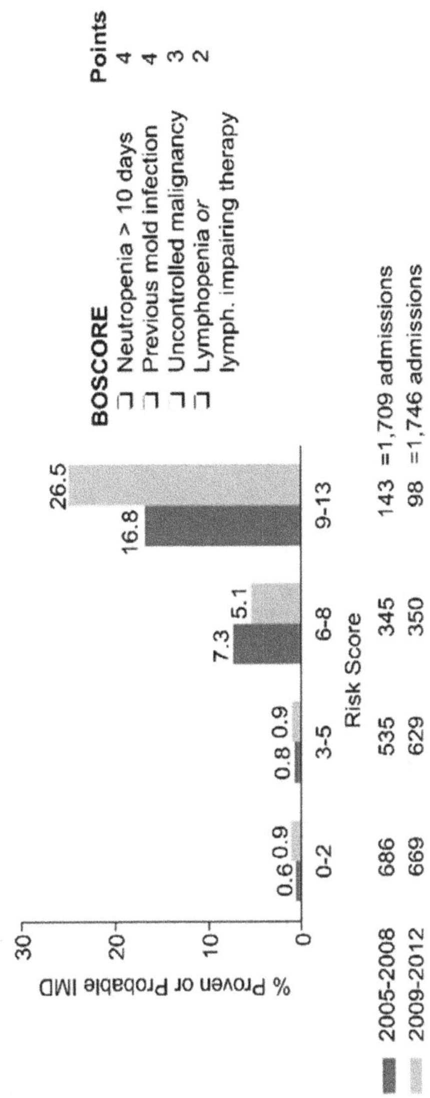

Figure 2. BOSCORE distribution versus observed 90-day cumulative incidence of IMD in the retrospective (2005–2008) development and prospective (2009–2012) validation cohorts.

We recently recalibrated the BOSCORE with additional risk factors to predict the 60-day probability of developing probable or proven IMD using 1944 patients with 4127 admissions from 2007–2016. The overall incidence of probable or proven IMD was 3.3%. Most of the analyzed risk factors were associated with the development of IMD (Figure 3), however only seven risk factors were retained in the final multivariable model: (i) prior history of IMD, (iii) receipt of 0.5 mg/kg prednisone equivalent within 30 days, (iii) uncontrolled malignancy; (iv) receipt of high-risk chemotherapy—e.g., any conditioning for allogeneic HSCT, high-dose ARA-C, fludarabine, and idarubicin (FLAI), or ifosfamide, carboplatin, etoposide (ICE); (v) PMN < 100 cells/mm^3 for >10 days or anticipated prolonged neutropenia; (vi) total lymphocyte count <50 cells/mm^3; and (vii) CMV reactivation (DNA > 1000 IU/mL in serum) or disease.

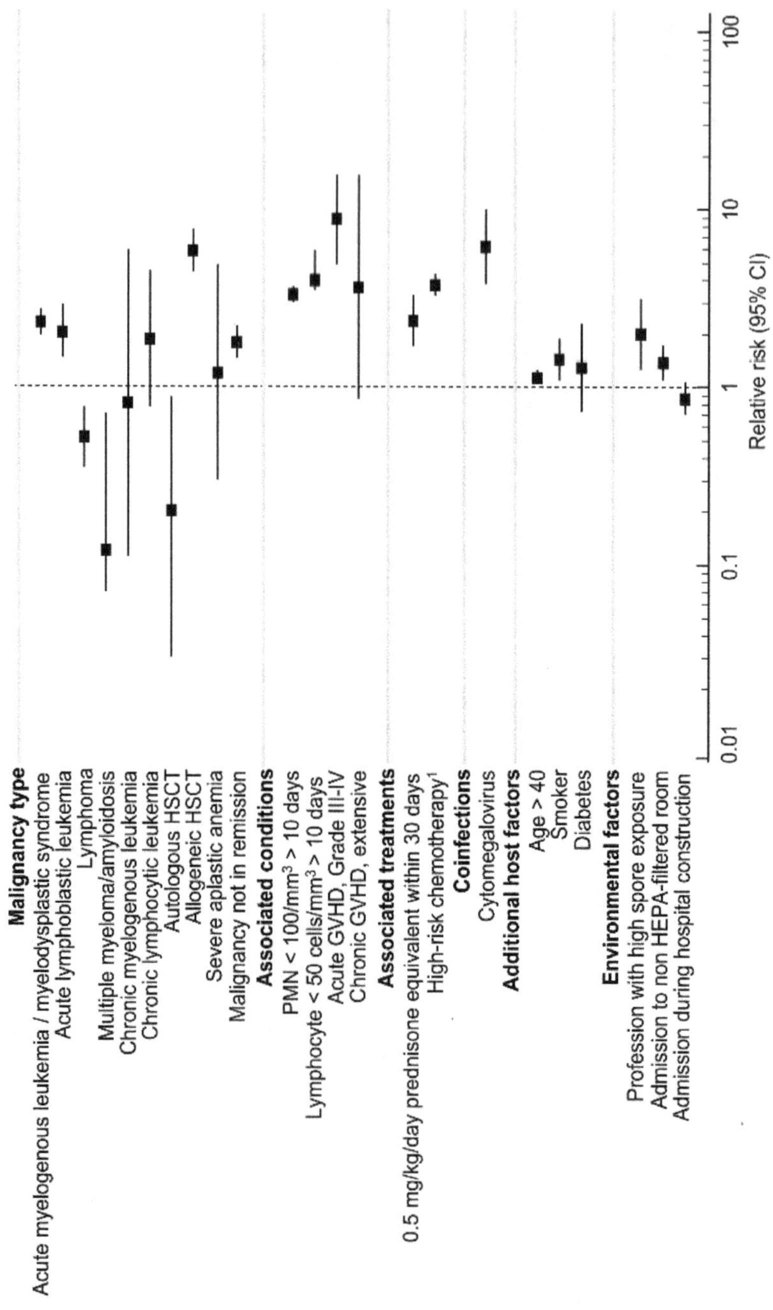

Figure 3. Risk factors in univariate analysis associated with the development of EORTC/MSG defined probable or proven invasive mold disease (n = 133) among 1944 adult inpatients (n = 4127 admissions) undergoing treatment for a hematological malignancy from 2007–2016 at the Seràgnoli Hematology Institute in Bologna, Italy.

The re-calibrated multivariate risk model displayed good calibration and discrimination in both low and higher risk groups and provided consistent predictions during internal validation with bootstrap resampled populations over an IMD incidence range from 2–9% (Figure 4a). When a 5% threshold was applied to differentiate low versus high-risk patients, the risk model correctly identified 60-day IMD outcomes in 85% of patients (Figure 4b). Among patients who developed IMD but were predicted to be low risk at admission, most (74%) fell just below the provisional 5% threshold (i.e., 3.5%–4.9% risk).

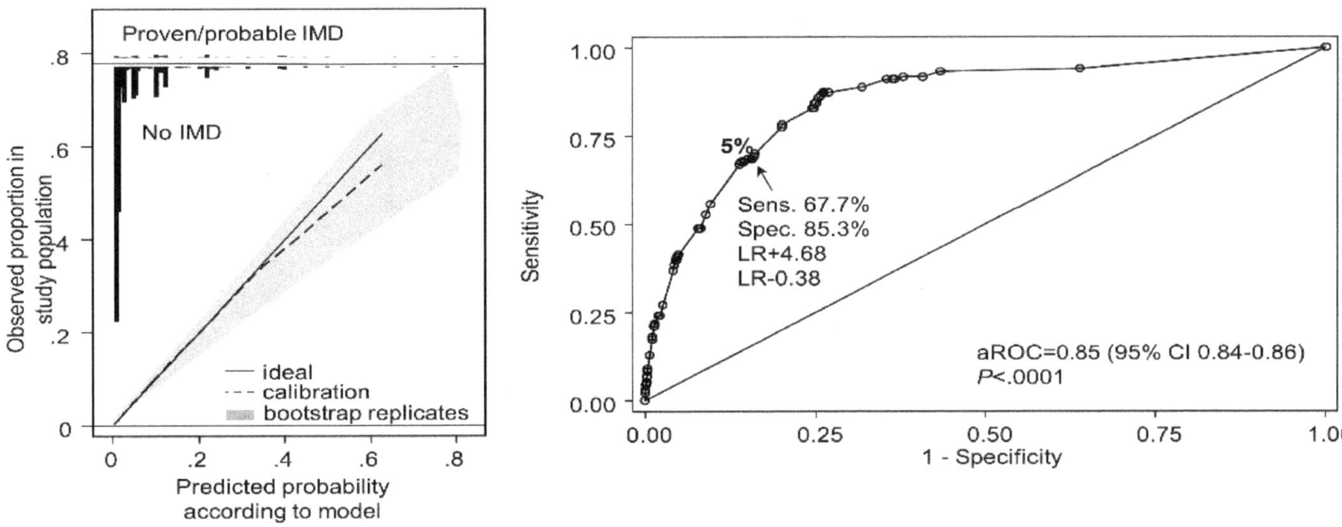

(**a**) (**b**)

Figure 4. Revised BOSCORE model calibration and discrimination. Panel (**a**) shows the relationship between a perfectly calibrated model (solid line) and the observed incidence of EORTC/MSG proven, or probable mold disease fitted using the Loess smoothing algorithm (dashed line). Black bars on the top frame of the graph show the relative risk distribution of admissions without IMD (downward pointing spikes) or patients with proven or probable IMD (upward pointing spikes). The gray shaded area shows observed versus predicted incidence of proven or probable mold disease in 100 bootstrapped resampled datasets with varying IMD incidence of 2–9%. Panel (**b**) shows the area under the receiver operator curve (aROC) and predicted performance for EORTC/MSG probable or proven IMD at a prediction cut-off of 5%. Sens., sensitivity, spec. specificity, LR, likelihood ratio.

The risk model was subsequently developed as a smartphone application (Figure 5) that requires users to only check boxes of each risk factor present on admission and the 60-day risk for IMD is automatically calculated with links to recommendations institutional diagnostic and treatment algorithms based on the patient's estimated risk.

The true test of any prognostic risk model is its acceptance by practitioners and effects on clinical decision making [95]. The high negative-predictive value of the BOSCORE (0.96–1.0) across a wide range of patient groups with varying incidence of IMD (0.4–8%) is used by clinicians in our institute to screen out the majority (> 67%) of patients admitted who are unlikely to benefit from intensive monitoring of serum galactomannan or posaconazole prophylaxis (Figure 6). Indeed, routine serum testing of galactomannan in serum of patients with a low pretest probability of IMD (i.e., <2%) may result in more frequent false-positive rather than true-positive results resulting in potentially unnecessary invasive diagnostic procedures and antifungal therapy [96]. Patients at greater than 5% risk are considered for more intensive management by a diagnostic-driven algorithm. This algorithm consists of twice weekly serum galactomannan screening plus immediate low-dose CT (within 24–48 h of fever or signs of infection) followed by CT pulmonary angiography $\pm$ bronchoscopy with culture or possible biopsy if the patient has evaluable lesions and can tolerate the procedures [97].

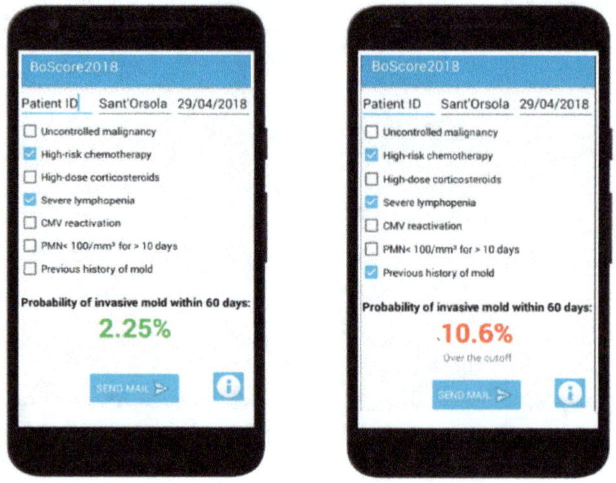

(a) (b)

Figure 5. Smartphone-assisted prognostic model assessments of lower-risk (**a**) and higher-risk (**b**) nonneutropenic patient. The probability of IMD within 60 days is estimated using the formula: Risk = (0.68 × uncontrolled malignancy) + (0.79 × high-risk chemotherapy) + (0.80 × high-dose corticosteroids) + (0.89 × severe lymphopenia) + (1.14 × CMV reactivation) + (1.52 × prolonged neutropenia) + (1.64 × previous mold disease) − 5.45. To calculate the 60-day probability from the formula, the calculated result is first converted from log odds to odds (eRisk); then odds must be converted to probability using the formulae: Risk/(1 + Risk).

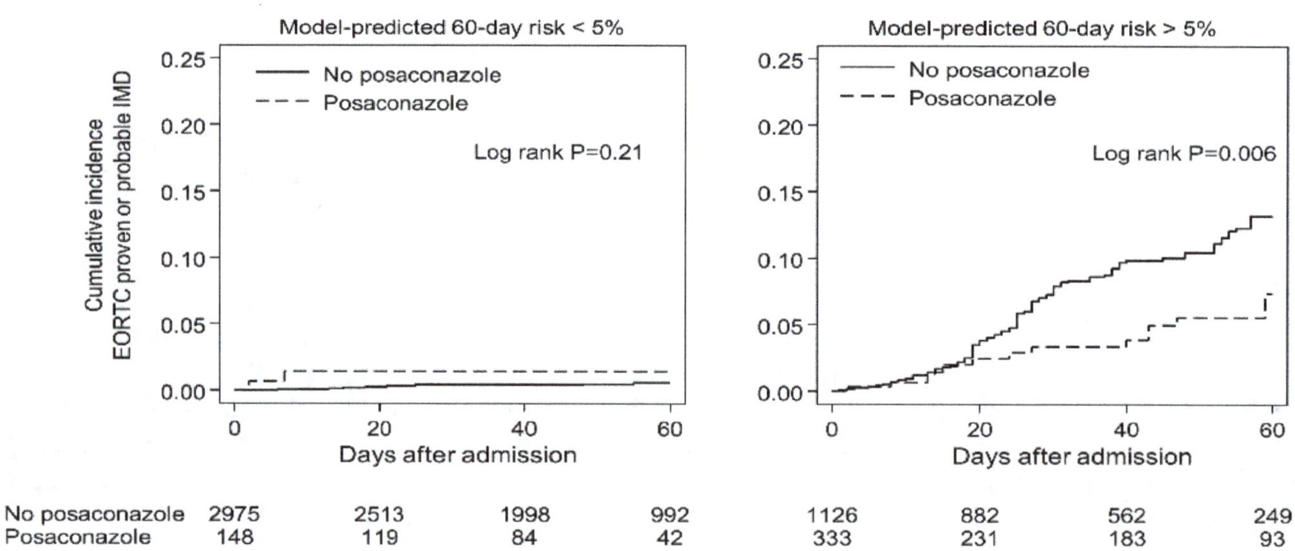

(a) (b)

Figure 6. Impact of posaconazole prophylaxis on the 60-day cumulative incidence of IMD in patients with model predicted risk of IMD <5% (**a**) and >5% (**b**). Note the nonsignificant higher rate of IMD in low risk patients (Panel A) is explained by two patients. One patient had a predicted risk at the risk cut-off (0.5) and prior IMD as the only risk factor (receiving posaconazole secondary prophylaxis). He was diagnosed with breakthrough IMD within 7 days of admission with fever. The second patient receiving posaconazole prophylaxis was admitted for treatment of extensive chronic graft versus host disease (he was not receiving corticosteroids) and only had severe lymphopenia at the time of admission. His predicted risk was 2.5%. During his work-up he had no fever but a serum galactomannan was positive and a CT following admission was consistent with IMD.

Very-high risk patients (>10%) may be considered eligible for posaconazole prophylaxis, even if they do not have AML/MDS or have undergone allogeneic HSCT. For example, we routinely use the risk model to help identify patients with acute leukemia undergoing consolidation chemotherapy who require mold-active antifungal prophylaxis. We have also found that that the risk model identifies small subsets of patients with lymphoma (6%) and myeloma (3.4%) who have equivalent risk for developing IMD as an AML patient undergoing remission/induction chemotherapy. These unique subsets of patients are then targeted for more intensive diagnostic intervention.

4. Future Perspectives

Because accurate risk assessment is fundamental to the effective management of mold infections and stewardship of diagnostic and treatment resources, it is likely that interest in prognostic risk models will increase. However, adherence to several fundamental principles during model development and reporting should be encouraged. First and foremost, there should be a clear explanation of the patient population used to develop the predictive model and the timing of assessment- i.e., when IMD is already present (diagnostic model) or to predict the risk of IMD in the future (prognostic model). Steps involved in the development, analysis and validation of the model should be clearly reported according to standards described in the Transparent Reporting of a Multivariable Prediction Model for Individual Prognosis Or Diagnosis (TRIPOD) Guidelines [98]. Adherence to these guidelines improves the clarity in communication and allows researchers from other institutions to better assess the generalizability and risk of bias of published models [98].

Validation studies are often considered to be the benchmark of whether a developed model is of high quality or clinically useful. The real aim of model validation, however, is to measure the model's predictive performance in either resampled participant data of the development data set (often referred to as internal validation) or in other, independent participant data that were not used for developing the model (often referred to as external validation) [98,99]. In this respect, the key difference is the generalizability of the performance characteristics of the model, which should ideally be confirmed before the model is used in clinical care like any new diagnostic test [95]. Prediction models developed in one institution may not necessarily be equally useful in another setting, as illustrated with recent studies of *Candida* prediction models in non-neutropenic patients [8]. Indeed, it is not uncommon that existing models must be adapted to local circumstances or with new predictors before application in a local setting. This adaption will be impossible if local hospitals do not have surveillance systems in place where these infections are managed. Finally, research on the uptake and effect of prognostic models on clinical decision-making and patients' outcomes (impact studies) are needed to confirm the usefulness of the prognostic model in clinical care.

Outside of daily clinical use, Harrell and colleagues have identified several areas of clinical research where prognostic risk models are applicable [10]. Risk models are useful in the evaluation of new diagnostic technologies, as estimates derived both with and without the new test can be compared to measure the incremental prognostic information provided. White, Parr and Barnes recently used this approach to evaluate how genetic risk factors with early diagnostic markers can improve predictions of which neutropenic patients with hematological malignancies will develop invasive aspergillosis [100]. The investigators found that compared to clinical risk factors alone (allogeneic HSCT, respiratory virus infection), the incorporation of genetic risk factors (DECTIN-1, DC-SIGN mutations) plus a positive PCR result increased the predicted probability of invasive aspergillosis from 7% to 56.7%. This combined prognostic-diagnostic model approach was associated with good discrimination (aROC 0.86) and could substantially reduce the percentage of patients administered preemptive therapy to only 8.4% of the population of patients with febrile neutropenia.

A second means by which a validated prognostic model could benefit clinical research is to enable researchers to better estimate the effect of a single factor (e.g., antifungal prophylaxis) on patients' outcomes in observational data where many uncontrolled confounding factors also affect risk.

Finally, prognostic models can improve the design and enrollment of clinical trials for invasive mold diseases. Both the decision concerning which patients to randomize and the design of the randomization process (for example, stratified randomization using prognostic factors) are improved by more accurate prediction of patient risk before randomization. Accurate prognostic models can be used to test for differential therapeutic benefit or to estimate the clinical benefit for an individual patient in a clinical trial, because low-risk patients are likely to have less absolute benefit. These areas are largely unexplored for prognostic models and clinical studies of IMD.

5. Conclusions

Compared to therapeutic trials and etiological research, prognostic risk models for IMD have received relatively little attention. However, several studies have now shown that development of such models can improve the accuracy of risk prediction, and incorporation of these models into the clinical management of patients has the potential to improve diagnostic and antifungal stewardship, as well as personalized treatment of invasive mold diseases in patients with hematological malignancies.

Author Contributions: M.S. was involved in the writing of the manuscript, study concept and design and collection of data for the BSCORE risk model. R.L. was involved in the writing and editing of the manuscript and statistical analysis of the BOSCORE models.

Acknowledgments: Nicola Vianelli, Giovanni Vianelli and Nicola Semprini helped develop the BOSCORE smartphone application. Riccardo Ragionieri was responsible for the development and maintenance of the data registry used to construct BOSCORE.

References

1. Lamoth, F.; Calandra, T. Early diagnosis of invasive mould infections and disease. *J. Antimicrob. Chemother.* **2017**, *72*, i19–i28. [CrossRef] [PubMed]
2. Pagano, L.; Akova, M.; Dimopoulos, G.; Herbrecht, R.; Drgona, L.; Blijlevens, N. Risk assessment and prognostic factors for mould-related diseases in immunocompromised patients. *J. Antimicrob. Chemother.* **2011**, *66*, i5–i14. [CrossRef] [PubMed]
3. Herbrecht, R.; Bories, P.; Moulin, J.-C.; Ledoux, M.-P.; Letscher-Bru, V. Risk stratification for invasive aspergillosis in immunocompromised patients. *Ann. N. Y. Acad. Sci.* **2012**, *1272*, 23–30. [CrossRef]
4. Pagano, L.; Busca, A.; Candoni, A.; Cattaneo, C.; Cesaro, S.; Fanci, R.; Nadali, G.; Potenza, L.; Russo, D.; Tumbarello, M.; et al. Risk stratification for invasive fungal infections in patients with hematological malignancies: SEIFEM recommendations. *Blood Rev.* **2016**, *31*, 17–29. [CrossRef] [PubMed]
5. Ostrosky-Zeichner, L.; Sable, C.; Sobel, J.; Alexander, B.D.; Donowitz, G.; Kan, V.; Kauffman, C.A.; Kett, D.; Larsen, R.A.; Morrison, V.; et al. Multicenter retrospective development and validation of a clinical prediction rule for nosocomial invasive candidiasis in the intensive care setting. *Eur. J. Clin. Microbiol. Infect. Dis.* **2007**, *26*, 271–276. [CrossRef] [PubMed]
6. Ostrosky-Zeichner, L.; Shoham, S.; Vazquez, J.; Reboli, A.; Betts, R.; Barron, M.A.; Schuster, M.; Judson, M.A.; Revankar, S.G.; Caeiro, J.P.; et al. MSG-01: A randomized, double-blind, placebo-controlled trial of caspofungin prophylaxis followed by preemptive therapy for invasive candidiasis in high-risk adults in the critical care setting. *Clin. Infect. Dis.* **2014**, *58*, 1219–1226. [CrossRef] [PubMed]
7. León, C.; Ruiz-Santana, S.; Saavedra, P.; Almirante, B.; Nolla-Salas, J.; Alvarez-Lerma, F.; Garnacho-Montero, J.; León, M.A.; EPCAN Study Group. A bedside scoring system ("Candida score") for early antifungal treatment in nonneutropenic critically ill patients with Candida colonization. *Crit. Care Med.* **2006**, *34*, 730–737. [CrossRef]
8. Guillamet, C.V.; Vazquez, R.; Micek, S.T.; Ursu, O.; Kollef, M. Development and validation of a clinical prediction rule for candidemia in hospitalized patients with severe sepsis and septic shock. *J. Crit. Care* **2015**, *30*, 715–720. [CrossRef]

9. Moons, K.; Royston, P.; Vergouwe, Y.; Grobbee, D.E. Prognosis and prognostic research: What, why, and how? *BMJ* **2009**, *338*, 1317–1320. [CrossRef]
10. Harrell, F.E.; Lee, K.L.; Mark, D.B. Tutorial in biostatistics multivariable prognostic models: Issues in developing models, evaluating assumptions and adequacy, and measuring and reducing errors. *Stat. Med.* **1996**, *15*, 361–387. [CrossRef]
11. Cornely, O.A.; Koehler, P.; Arenz, D.; C Mellinghoff, S. EQUAL Aspergillosis Score 2018: An ECMM score derived from current guidelines to measure QUALity of the clinical management of invasive pulmonary aspergillosis. *Mycoses* **2018**, *61*, 833–836. [CrossRef] [PubMed]
12. Ullmann, A.J.; Aguado, J.M.; Arikan-Akdagli, S.; Denning, D.W.; Groll, A.H.; Lagrou, K.; Lass-Flörl, C.; Lewis, R.E.; Munoz, P.; Verweij, P.E.; et al. Diagnosis and management of Aspergillus diseases: Executive summary of the 2017 ESCMID-ECMM-ERS guideline. *Clin. Microbiol. Infect.* **2018**, *24* (Suppl. 1), e1–e38. [CrossRef]
13. Patterson, T.F.; Thompson, G.R., 3rd; Denning, D.W.; Fishman, J.A.; Hadley, S.; Herbrecht, R.; Kontoyiannis, D.P.; Marr, K.A.; Morrison, V.A.; Nguyen, M.H.; Segal, B.H.; et al. Practice Guidelines for the Diagnosis and Management of Aspergillosis: 2016 Update by the Infectious Diseases Society of America. *Clin. Infect. Dis.* **2016**, *63*, e1–e60. [CrossRef] [PubMed]
14. Ascioglu, S.; Rex, J.H.; de Pauw, B.; Bennett, J.E.; Bille, J.; Crokaert, F.; Denning, D.W.; Donnelly, J.P.; Edwards, J.E.; Erjavec, Z.; et al. Defining opportunistic invasive fungal infections in immunocompromised patients with cancer and hematopoietic stem cell transplants: An international consensus. *Clin. Infect. Dis.* **2002**, *34*, 7–14. [CrossRef] [PubMed]
15. Stanzani, M.; Lewis, R.E.; Fiacchini, M.; Ricci, P.; Tumietto, F.; Viale, P.; Ambretti, S.; Baccarani, M.; Cavo, M.; Vianelli, N. A risk prediction score for invasive mold disease in patients with hematological malignancies. *PLoS ONE* **2013**, *8*, e75531. [CrossRef] [PubMed]
16. Caira, M.; Candoni, A.; Verga, L.; Busca, A.; Delia, M.; Nosari, A.; Caramatti, C.; Castagnola, C.; Cattaneo, C.; Fanci, R.; et al. Pre-chemotherapy risk factors for invasive fungal diseases: Prospective analysis of 1192 patients with newly diagnosed acute myeloid leukemia (SEIFEM 2010-a multicenter study). *Haematologica* **2015**, *100*, 284–292. [CrossRef] [PubMed]
17. Pagano, L.; Caira, M.; Candoni, A.; Offidani, M.; Fianchi, L.; Martino, B.; Pastore, D.; Picardi, M.; Bonini, A.; Chierichini, A.; et al. The epidemiology of fungal infections in patients with hematologic malignancies: The SEIFEM-2004 study. *Haematologica* **2006**, *91*, 1068–1075.
18. Pagano, L.; Girmenia, C.; Mele, L.; Ricci, P.; Tosti, M.E.; Nosari, A.; Buelli, M.; Picardi, M.; Allione, B.; Corvatta, L.; et al. Infections caused by filamentous fungi in patients with hematologic malignancies. A report of 391 cases by GIMEMA Infection Program. *Haematologica* **2001**, *86*, 862–870.
19. Lionakis, M.S.; Lewis, R.E.; Kontoyiannis, D.P. Breakthrough Invasive Mold Infections in the Hematology Patient: Current Concepts and Future Directions. *Clin. Infect. Dis.* **2018**, *67*, 1621–1630. [CrossRef]
20. Estey, E.H. Acute myeloid leukemia: 2019 update on risk-stratification and management. *Am. J. Hematol.* **2018**, *93*, 1267–1291. [CrossRef]
21. Falantes, J.F.; Calderón, C.; Márquez-Malaver, F.J.; Aguilar-Guisado, M.; Martín-Peña, A.; Martino, M.L.; Montero, I.; González, J.; Parody, R.; Pérez-Simón, J.A.; Espigado, I. Patterns of infection in patients with myelodysplastic syndromes and acute myeloid leukemia receiving azacitidine as salvage therapy. Implications for primary antifungal prophylaxis. *Clin. Lymphoma Myeloma Leuk.* **2014**, *14*, 80–86. [CrossRef] [PubMed]
22. Trubiano, J.A.; Dickinson, M.; Thursky, K.A.; Spelman, T.; Seymour, J.F.; Slavin, M.A.; Worth, L.J. Incidence, etiology and timing of infections following azacitidine therapy for myelodysplastic syndromes. *Leuk. Lymphoma* **2017**, *58*, 2379–2386. [CrossRef] [PubMed]
23. Pomares, H.; Arnan, M.; Sánchez-Ortega, I.; Sureda, A.; Duarte, R.F. Invasive fungal infections in AML/MDS patients treated with azacitidine: A risk worth considering antifungal prophylaxis? *Mycoses* **2016**, *59*, 516–519. [CrossRef] [PubMed]
24. Cornely, O.A.; Leguay, T.; Maertens, J.; Vehreschild, M.J.G.T.; Anagnostopoulos, A.; Castagnola, C.; Verga, L.; Rieger, C.; Kondakci, M.; Härter, G.; et al. Randomized comparison of liposomal amphotericin B versus placebo to prevent invasive mycoses in acute lymphoblastic leukaemia. *J. Antimicrob. Chemother.* **2017**, *72*, 2359–2367. [CrossRef] [PubMed]

25. Storring, J.M.; Minden, M.D.; Kao, S.; Gupta, V.; Schuh, A.C.; Schimmer, A.D.; Yee, K.W.L.; Kamel-Reid, S.; Chang, H.; Lipton, J.H.; et al. Treatment of adults with BCR-ABL negative acute lymphoblastic leukaemia with a modified paediatric regimen. *Br. J. Haematol.* **2009**, *146*, 76–85. [CrossRef] [PubMed]
26. Kadia, T.M.; Cortes, J.; Ravandi, F.; Jabbour, E.; Konopleva, M.; Benton, C.B.; Burger, J.; Sasaki, K.; Borthakur, G.; DiNardo, C.D.; et al. Cladribine and low-dose cytarabine alternating with decitabine as front-line therapy for elderly patients with acute myeloid leukaemia: A phase 2 single-arm trial. *Lancet Haematol* **2018**, *5*, e411–e421. [CrossRef]
27. Bassan, R.; Rossi, G.; Pogliani, E.M.; Di Bona, E.; Angelucci, E.; Cavattoni, I.; Lambertenghi-Deliliers, G.; Mannelli, F.; Levis, A.; Ciceri, F.; et al. Chemotherapy-phased imatinib pulses improve long-term outcome of adult patients with Philadelphia chromosome-positive acute lymphoblastic leukemia: Northern Italy Leukemia Group protocol 09/00. *J. Clin. Oncol.* **2010**, *28*, 3644–3652. [CrossRef]
28. Foà, R.; Vitale, A.; Vignetti, M.; Meloni, G.; Guarini, A.; De Propris, M.S.; Elia, L.; Paoloni, F.; Fazi, P.; Cimino, G.; et al. Dasatinib as first-line treatment for adult patients with Philadelphia chromosome-positive acute lymphoblastic leukemia. *Blood* **2011**, *118*, 6521–6528. [CrossRef]
29. Ottmann, O.G.; Druker, B.J.; Sawyers, C.L.; Goldman, J.M.; Reiffers, J.; Silver, R.T.; Tura, S.; Fischer, T.; Deininger, M.W.; Schiffer, C.A.; et al. A phase 2 study of imatinib in patients with relapsed or refractory Philadelphia chromosome–positive acute lymphoid leukemias. *Blood* **2002**, *100*, 1965–1971. [CrossRef]
30. Teng, J.C.; Slavin, M.A.; Teh, B.W.; Lingaratnam, S.M.; Ananda-Rajah, M.R.; Worth, L.J.; Seymour, J.F.; Thursky, K.A. Epidemiology of invasive fungal disease in lymphoproliferative disorders. *Haematologica* **2015**, *100*, e462–e466. [CrossRef]
31. Chamilos, G.; Lionakis, M.S.; Kontoyiannis, D.P. Call for Action: Invasive Fungal Infections Associated with Ibrutinib and Other Small Molecule Kinase Inhibitors Targeting Immune Signaling Pathways. *Clin. Infect. Dis.* **2018**, *66*, 140–148. [CrossRef] [PubMed]
32. Teh, B.W.; Tam, C.S.; Handunnetti, S.; Worth, L.J.; Slavin, M.A. Infections in patients with chronic lymphocytic leukaemia: Mitigating risk in the era of targeted therapies. *Blood Rev.* **2018**. [CrossRef] [PubMed]
33. Byrd, J.C.; Brown, J.R.; O'Brien, S.; Barrientos, J.C.; Kay, N.E.; Reddy, N.M.; Coutre, S.; Tam, C.S.; Mulligan, S.P.; Jaeger, U.; et al. Ibrutinib versus ofatumumab in previously treated chronic lymphoid leukemia. *N. Engl. J. Med.* **2014**, *371*, 213–223. [CrossRef] [PubMed]
34. Jabbour, E.; Kantarjian, H.M.; Saglio, G.; Steegmann, J.L.; Shah, N.P.; Boqué, C.; Chuah, C.; Pavlovsky, C.; Mayer, J.; Cortes, J.; et al. Early response with dasatinib or imatinib in chronic myeloid leukemia: 3-year follow-up from a randomized phase 3 trial (DASISION). *Blood* **2014**, *123*, 494–500. [CrossRef] [PubMed]
35. Polverelli, N.; Breccia, M.; Benevolo, G.; Martino, B.; Tieghi, A.; Latagliata, R.; Sabattini, E.; Riminucci, M.; Godio, L.; Catani, L.; et al. Risk factors for infections in myelofibrosis: Role of disease status and treatment. A multicenter study of 507 patients. *Am. J. Hematol.* **2017**, *92*, 37–41. [CrossRef]
36. Valdez, J.M.; Scheinberg, P.; Young, N.S.; Walsh, T.J. Infections in patients with aplastic anemia. *Semin. Hematol.* **2009**, *46*, 269–276. [CrossRef]
37. Valdez, J.M.; Scheinberg, P.; Nunez, O.; Wu, C.O.; Young, N.S.; Walsh, T.J. Decreased infection-related mortality and improved survival in severe aplastic anemia in the past two decades. *Clin. Infect. Dis.* **2011**, *52*, 726–735. [CrossRef]
38. Bodey, G.P. The changing face of febrile neutropenia-from monotherapy to moulds to mucositis. Fever and neutropenia: The early years. *J. Antimicrob. Chemother.* **2009**, *63* (Suppl. 1), i3–i13. [CrossRef]
39. Bodey, G.P. Fungal infections complicating acute leukemia. *J. Chronic Dis.* **1966**, *19*, 667–687. [CrossRef]
40. Gerson, S.L.; Talbot, G.H.; Hurwitz, S.; Strom, B.L.; Lusk, E.J.; Cassileth, P.A. Prolonged granulocytopenia: The major risk factor for invasive pulmonary aspergillosis in patients with acute leukemia. *Ann. Intern. Med.* **1984**, *100*, 345–351. [CrossRef]
41. De Pauw, B.; Walsh, T.J.; Donnelly, J.P.; Stevens, D.A.; Edwards, J.E.; Calandra, T.; Pappas, P.G.; Maertens, J.; Lortholary, O.; Kauffman, C.A.; et al. Revised definitions of invasive fungal disease from the European Organization for Research and Treatment of Cancer/Invasive Fungal Infections Cooperative Group and the National Institute of Allergy and Infectious Diseases Mycoses Study Group (EORTC/MSG) Consensus Group. *Clin. Infect. Dis.* **2008**, *46*, 1813–1821. [PubMed]
42. Mikulska, M.; Raiola, A.M.; Bruno, B.; Furfaro, E.; Van Lint, M.T.; Bregante, S.; Ibatici, A.; Del Bono, V.; Bacigalupo, A.; Viscoli, C. Risk factors for invasive aspergillosis and related mortality in recipients of

allogeneic SCT from alternative donors: An analysis of 306 patients. *Bone Marrow Transplant.* **2009**, *44*, 361–370. [CrossRef]

43. Garcia-Vidal, C.; Upton, A.; Kirby, K.A.; Marr, K.A. Epidemiology of invasive mold infections in allogeneic stem cell transplant recipients: Biological risk factors for infection according to time after transplantation. *Clin. Infect. Dis.* **2008**, *47*, 1041–1050. [CrossRef] [PubMed]
44. Lewis, R.E.; Georgiadou, S.P.; Sampsonas, F.; Chamilos, G.; Kontoyiannis, D.P. Risk factors for early mortality in haematological malignancy patients with pulmonary mucormycosis. *Mycoses* **2014**, *57*, 49–55. [CrossRef] [PubMed]
45. Graham, B.S.; Tucker, W.S., Jr. Opportunistic infections in endogenous Cushing's syndrome. *Ann. Intern. Med.* **1984**, *101*, 334–338. [CrossRef]
46. Lionakis, M.S.; Kontoyiannis, D.P. Glucocorticoids and invasive fungal infections. *Lancet* **2003**, *362*, 1828–1838. [CrossRef]
47. Taccone, F.S.; Van den Abeele, A.-M.; Bulpa, P.; Misset, B.; Meersseman, W.; Cardoso, T.; Paiva, J.-A.; Blasco-Navalpotro, M.; De Laere, E.; Dimopoulos, G.; et al. Epidemiology of invasive aspergillosis in critically ill patients: Clinical presentation, underlying conditions, and outcomes. *Crit. Care* **2015**, *19*, 7. [CrossRef]
48. Bassetti, M.; Garnacho-Montero, J.; Calandra, T.; Kullberg, B.; Dimopoulos, G.; Azoulay, E.; Chakrabarti, A.; Kett, D.; Leon, C.; Ostrosky-Zeichner, L.; et al. Intensive care medicine research agenda on invasive fungal infection in critically ill patients. *Intensive Care Med.* **2017**, 1–14. [CrossRef] [PubMed]
49. Marr, K.A.; Carter, R.A.; Boeckh, M.; Martin, P.; Corey, L. Invasive aspergillosis in allogeneic stem cell transplant recipients: Changes in epidemiology and risk factors. *Blood* **2002**, *100*, 4358–4366. [CrossRef]
50. Wald, A.; Leisenring, W.; van Burik, J.A.; Bowden, R.A. Epidemiology of *Aspergillus* infections in a large cohort of patients undergoing bone marrow transplantation. *J. Infect. Dis.* **1997**, *175*, 1459–1466. [CrossRef]
51. Ribaud, P.; Chastang, C.; Latgé, J.P.; Baffroy-Lafitte, L.; Parquet, N.; Devergie, A.; Espérou, H.; Sélimi, F.; Rocha, V.; Espérou, H.; et al. Survival and prognostic factors of invasive aspergillosis after allogeneic bone marrow transplantation. *Clin. Infect. Dis.* **1999**, *28*, 322–330. [CrossRef] [PubMed]
52. Hovi, L.; Saarinen-Pihkala, U.M.; Vettenranta, K.; Saxen, H. Invasive fungal infections in pediatric bone marrow transplant recipients: Single center experience of 10 years. *Bone Marrow Transplant.* **2000**, *26*, 999–1004. [CrossRef] [PubMed]
53. O'Donnell, M.R.; Schmidt, G.M.; Tegtmeier, B.R.; Faucett, C.; Fahey, J.L.; Ito, J.; Nademanee, A.; Niland, J.; Parker, P.; Smith, E.P. Prediction of systemic fungal infection in allogeneic marrow recipients: Impact of amphotericin prophylaxis in high-risk patients. *J. Clin. Oncol.* **1994**, *12*, 827–834. [CrossRef] [PubMed]
54. Girmenia, C.; Raiola, A.M.; Piciocchi, A.; Algarotti, A.; Stanzani, M.; Cudillo, L.; Pecoraro, C.; Guidi, S.; Iori, A.P.; Montante, B.; et al. Incidence and outcome of invasive fungal diseases after allogeneic stem cell transplantation: A prospective study of the Gruppo Italiano Trapianto Midollo Osseo (GITMO). *Biol. Blood Marrow Transplant.* **2014**, *20*, 872–880. [CrossRef] [PubMed]
55. Atalla, A.; Garnica, M.; Maiolino, A.; Nucci, M. Risk factors for invasive mold diseases in allogeneic hematopoietic cell transplant recipients. *Transpl. Infect. Dis.* **2015**, *17*, 7–13. [CrossRef] [PubMed]
56. Bittencourt, H.; Rocha, V.; Chevret, S.; Socié, G.; Espérou, H.; Devergie, A.; Dal Cortivo, L.; Marolleau, J.-P.; Garnier, F.; Ribaud, P.; Gluckman, E. Association of CD34 cell dose with hematopoietic recovery, infections, and other outcomes after HLA-identical sibling bone marrow transplantation. *Blood* **2002**, *99*, 2726–2733. [CrossRef] [PubMed]
57. Kuster, S.; Stampf, S.; Gerber, B.; Baettig, V.; Weisser, M.; Gerull, S.; Medinger, M.; Passweg, J.; Schanz, U.; Garzoni, C.; et al. Incidence and outcome of invasive fungal diseases after allogeneic hematopoietic stem cell transplantation: A Swiss transplant cohort study. *Transpl. Infect. Dis.* **2018**, e12981. [CrossRef] [PubMed]
58. Bochud, P.-Y.; Chien, J.W.; Marr, K.A.; Leisenring, W.M.; Upton, A.; Janer, M.; Rodrigues, S.D.; Li, S.; Hansen, J.A.; Zhao, L.P.; et al. Toll-like receptor 4 polymorphisms and aspergillosis in stem-cell transplantation. *N. Engl. J. Med.* **2008**, *359*, 1766–1777. [CrossRef] [PubMed]
59. Cunha, C.; Di Ianni, M.; Bozza, S.; Giovannini, G.; Zagarella, S.; Zelante, T.; D'Angelo, C.; Pierini, A.; Pitzurra, L.; Falzetti, F.; et al. Dectin-1 Y238X polymorphism associates with susceptibility to invasive aspergillosis in hematopoietic transplantation through impairment of both recipient- and donor-dependent mechanisms of antifungal immunity. *Blood* **2010**, *116*, 5394–5402. [CrossRef]

60. Cunha, C.; Aversa, F.; Lacerda, J.F.; Busca, A.; Kurzai, O.; Grube, M.; Löffler, J.; Maertens, J.A.; Bell, A.S.; Inforzato, A.; et al. Genetic PTX3 deficiency and aspergillosis in stem-cell transplantation. *N. Engl. J. Med.* **2014**, *370*, 421–432. [CrossRef]
61. Sucak, G.T.; Yegin, Z.A.; Ozkurt, Z.N.; Aki, S.Z.; Karakan, T.; Akyol, G. The role of liver biopsy in the workup of liver dysfunction late after SCT: Is the role of iron overload underestimated? *Bone Marrow Transplant.* **2008**, *42*, 461–467. [CrossRef] [PubMed]
62. Kontoyiannis, D.P.; Chamilos, G.; Lewis, R.E.; Giralt, S.; Cortes, J.; Raad, I.I.; Manning, J.T.; Han, X. Increased bone marrow iron stores is an independent risk factor for invasive aspergillosis in patients with high-risk hematologic malignancies and recipients of allogeneic hematopoietic stem cell transplantation. *Cancer* **2007**, *110*, 1303–1306. [CrossRef] [PubMed]
63. Stuehler, C.; Kuenzli, E.; Jaeger, V.K.; Baettig, V.; Ferracin, F.; Rajacic, Z.; Kaiser, D.; Bernardini, C.; Forrer, P.; Weisser, M.; et al. Immune reconstitution after allogeneic hematopoietic stem cell transplantation and association with occurrence and outcome of invasive aspergillosis. *J. Infect. Dis.* **2015**, *212*, 959–967. [CrossRef] [PubMed]
64. Kontoyiannis, D.P.; Marr, K.A.; Park, B.J. Prospective surveillance for invasive fungal infections in hematopoietic stem cell transplant recipients, 2001–2006: Overview of the Transplant-Associated Infection Surveillance Network (TRANSET). *Clin. Infect. Dis.* **2010**, *50*, 1091–1100. [CrossRef] [PubMed]
65. Gil, L.; Kozlowska-Skrzypczak, M.; Mol, A.; Poplawski, D.; Styczynski, J.; Komarnicki, M. Increased risk for invasive aspergillosis in patients with lymphoproliferative diseases after autologous hematopoietic SCT. *Bone Marrow Transplant.* **2009**, *43*, 121–126. [CrossRef] [PubMed]
66. Teh, B.W.; Teng, J.C.; Urbancic, K.; Grigg, A.; Harrison, S.J.; Worth, L.J.; Slavin, M.A.; Thursky, K.A. Invasive fungal infections in patients with multiple myeloma: A multi-center study in the era of novel myeloma therapies. *Haematologica* **2015**, *100*, e28–e31. [CrossRef] [PubMed]
67. Peleg, A.Y.; Weerarathna, T.; McCarthy, J.S.; Davis, T.M.E. Common infections in diabetes: Pathogenesis, management and relationship to glycaemic control. *Diabetes. Metab. Res. Rev.* **2007**, *23*, 3–13. [CrossRef]
68. Ibrahim, A.S. Host cell invasion in mucormycosis: Role of iron. *Curr. Opin. Microbiol.* **2011**, *14*, 406–411. [CrossRef] [PubMed]
69. Artis, W.M.; Fountain, J.A.; Delcher, H.K.; Jones, H.E. A mechanism of susceptibility to mucormycosis in diabetic ketoacidosis: Transferrin and iron availability. *Diabetes* **1982**, *31*, 1109–1114. [CrossRef] [PubMed]
70. Corzo-León, D.E.; Satlin, M.J.; Soave, R.; Shore, T.B.; Schuetz, A.N.; Jacobs, S.E.; Walsh, T.J. Epidemiology and outcomes of invasive fungal infections in allogeneic haematopoietic stem cell transplant recipients in the era of antifungal prophylaxis: A single-centre study with focus on emerging pathogens. *Mycoses* **2015**, *58*, 325–336. [CrossRef] [PubMed]
71. Yong, M.K.; Slavin, M.A.; Kontoyiannis, D.P. Invasive fungal disease and cytomegalovirus infection: Is there an association? *Curr. Opin. Infect. Dis.* **2018**, *31*, 481. [CrossRef] [PubMed]
72. Martino, R.; Piñana, J.L.; Parody, R.; Valcarcel, D.; Sureda, A.; Brunet, S.; Briones, J.; Delgado, J.; Sánchez, F.; Rabella, N.; Sierra, J. Lower respiratory tract respiratory virus infections increase the risk of invasive aspergillosis after a reduced-intensity allogeneic hematopoietic SCT. *Bone Marrow Transplant.* **2009**, *44*, 749–756. [CrossRef] [PubMed]
73. Giménez, E.; Solano, C.; Nieto, J.; Remigia, M.J.; Clari, M.Á.; Costa, E.; Muñoz-Cobo, B.; Amat, P.; Bravo, D.; Benet, I.; Navarro, D. An investigation on the relationship between the occurrence of CMV DNAemia and the development of invasive aspergillosis in the allogeneic stem cell transplantation setting. *J. Med. Virol.* **2014**, *86*, 568–575. [CrossRef] [PubMed]
74. Yong, M.K.; Lewin, S.R.; Manuel, O. Immune Monitoring for CMV in Transplantation. *Curr. Infect. Dis. Rep.* **2018**, *20*, 4. [CrossRef] [PubMed]
75. Lamoth, F.; Calandra, T. Let's add invasive aspergillosis to the list of influenza complications. *Lancet Respir. Med.* **2018**, *6*, 733–735. [CrossRef]
76. Schauwvlieghe, A.F.A.D.; Rijnders, B.J.A.; Philips, N.; Verwijs, R.; Vanderbeke, L.; Van Tienen, C.; Lagrou, K.; Verweij, P.E.; Van de Veerdonk, F.L.; Gommers, D.; et al. Invasive aspergillosis in patients admitted to the intensive care unit with severe influenza: A retrospective cohort study. *Lancet Respir. Med.* **2018**, *6*, 782–792. [CrossRef]
77. Garnacho-Montero, J.; León-Moya, C.; Gutiérrez-Pizarraya, A.; Arenzana-Seisdedos, A.; Vidaur, L.; Guerrero, J.E.; Gordón, M.; Martín-Loeches, I.; Rodriguez, A. Clinical characteristics, evolution,

and treatment-related risk factors for mortality among immunosuppressed patients with influenza A (H1N1) virus admitted to the intensive care unit. *J. Crit. Care* **2018**, *48*, 172–177. [CrossRef]
78. Garcia-Vidal, C.; Barba, P.; Arnan, M.; Moreno, A.; Ruiz-Camps, I.; Gudiol, C.; Ayats, J.; Ortí, G.; Carratalà, J. Invasive aspergillosis complicating pandemic influenza A (H1N1) infection in severely immunocompromised patients. *Clin. Infect. Dis.* **2011**, *53*, e16–e19. [CrossRef]
79. Crum-Cianflone, N.F. Invasive Aspergillosis associated with severe influenza infections. *Open Forum Infect. Dis.* **2016**, *3*, ofw171. [CrossRef]
80. Guarner, J.; Falcón-Escobedo, R. Comparison of the pathology caused by H1N1, H5N1, and H3N2 influenza viruses. *Arch. Med. Res.* **2009**, *40*, 655–661. [CrossRef]
81. Panackal, A.A.; Li, H.; Kontoyiannis, D.P.; Mori, M.; Perego, C.A.; Boeckh, M.; Marr, K.A. Geoclimatic influences on invasive aspergillosis after hematopoietic stem cell transplantation. *Clin. Infect. Dis.* **2010**, *50*, 1588–1597. [CrossRef] [PubMed]
82. Tanaka, R.J.; Boon, N.J.; Vrcelj, K.; Nguyen, A.; Vinci, C.; Armstrong-James, D.; Bignell, E. In silico modeling of spore inhalation reveals fungal persistence following low dose exposure. *Sci. Rep.* **2015**, *5*, 13958. [CrossRef]
83. Kanamori, H.; Rutala, W.A.; Sickbert-Bennett, E.E.; Weber, D.J. Review of Fungal Outbreaks and Infection Prevention in Healthcare Settings during Construction and Renovation. *Clin. Infect. Dis.* **2015**, *61*, 433–444. [CrossRef]
84. Alberti, C.; Bouakline, A.; Ribaud, P.; Lacroix, C.; Rousselot, P.; Leblanc, T.; Derouin, F.; Aspergillus Study Group. Relationship between environmental fungal contamination and the incidence of invasive aspergillosis in haematology patients. *J. Hosp. Infect.* **2001**, *48*, 198–206. [CrossRef] [PubMed]
85. Cornet, M.; Levy, V.; Fleury, L.; Lortholary, J.; Barquins, S.; Coureul, M.H.; Deliere, E.; Zittoun, R.; Brücker, G.; Bouvet, A. Efficacy of prevention by high-efficiency particulate air filtration or laminar airflow against Aspergillus airborne contamination during hospital renovation. *Infect. Control Hosp. Epidemiol.* **1999**, *20*, 508–513. [CrossRef]
86. Portugal, R.D.; Garnica, M.; Nucci, M. Index to predict invasive mold infection in high-risk neutropenic patients based on the area over the neutrophil curve. *J. Clin. Oncol.* **2009**, *27*, 3849–3854. [CrossRef] [PubMed]
87. Garnica, M.; Sinhorelo, A.; Madeira, L.; Portugal, R.; Nucci, M. Diagnostic-driven antifungal therapy in neutropenic patients using the D-index and serial serum galactomannan testing. *Braz. J. Infect. Dis.* **2016**, *20*, 354–359. [CrossRef]
88. Takaoka, K.; Nannya, Y.; Shinohara, A.; Arai, S.; Nakamura, F.; Kurokawa, M. A novel scoring system to predict the incidence of invasive fungal disease in salvage chemotherapies for malignant lymphoma. *Ann. Hematol.* **2014**, *93*, 1637–1644. [CrossRef]
89. Sassi, C.; Stanzani, M.; Lewis, R.E. Computerized tomographic pulmonary angiography discriminates invasive mould disease of the lung from lymphoma. *Br. J. Haematol.* **2015**, *169*, 462. [CrossRef]
90. Montesinos, P.; Rodríguez-Veiga, R.; Boluda, B.; Martínez-Cuadrón, D.; Cano, I.; Lancharro, A.; Sanz, J.; Arilla, M.J.; López-Chuliá, F.; Navarro, I.; et al. Incidence and risk factors of post-engraftment invasive fungal disease in adult allogeneic hematopoietic stem cell transplant recipients receiving oral azoles prophylaxis. *Bone Marrow Transpl.* **2015**, *50*, 1465–1472. [CrossRef]
91. Hol, J.A.; Wolfs, T.F.W.; Bierings, M.B.; Lindemans, C.A.; Versluys, A.B.J.; Wildt de, A.; Gerhardt, C.E.; Boelens, J.J. Predictors of invasive fungal infection in pediatric allogeneic hematopoietic SCT recipients. *Bone Marrow Transpl.* **2014**, *49*, 95–101. [CrossRef] [PubMed]
92. Sorror, M.L.; Maris, M.B.; Storb, R.; Baron, F.; Sandmaier, B.M.; Maloney, D.G.; Storer, B. Hematopoietic cell transplantation (HCT)-specific comorbidity index: A new tool for risk assessment before allogeneic HCT. *Blood* **2005**, *106*, 2912–2919. [CrossRef] [PubMed]
93. Sorror, M.L.; Storb, R.F.; Sandmaier, B.M.; Maziarz, R.T.; Pulsipher, M.A.; Maris, M.B.; Bhatia, S.; Ostronoff, F.; Deeg, H.J.; Syrjala, K.L.; et al. Comorbidity-age index: A clinical measure of biologic age before allogeneic hematopoietic cell transplantation. *J. Clin. Oncol.* **2014**, *32*, 3249–3256. [CrossRef]
94. Busca, A.; Passera, R.; Maffini, E.; Festuccia, M.; Brunello, L.; Dellacasa, C.M.; Aydin, S.; Frairia, C.; Manetta, S.; Butera, S.; et al. Hematopoietic cell transplantation comorbidity index and risk of developing invasive fungal infections after allografting. *Bone Marrow Transpl.* **2018**, *53*, 1304–1310. [CrossRef] [PubMed]
95. Moons, K.G.M.; Altman, D.G.; Vergouwe, Y.; Royston, P. Prognosis and prognostic research: Application and impact of prognostic models in clinical practice. *BMJ* **2009**, *338*, 1487–1490. [CrossRef] [PubMed]

96. Duarte, R.F.; Sánchez-Ortega, I.; Cuesta, I.; Arnan, M.; Patiño, B.; Fernández de Sevilla, A.; Gudiol, C.; Ayats, J.; Cuenca-Estrella, M. Serum galactomannan-based early detection of invasive aspergillosis in hematology patients receiving effective anti-mold prophylaxis. *Clin. Infect. Dis.* **2014**, *59*, 1696–1702. [CrossRef]
97. Stanzani, M.; Sassi, C.; Lewis, R.E.; Tolomelli, G.; Bazzocchi, A.; Cavo, M.; Vianelli, N.; Battista, G. High resolution computed tomography angiography improves the radiographic diagnosis of invasive mold disease in patients with hematological malignancies. *Clin. Infect. Dis.* **2015**, *60*, 1603–1610. [CrossRef] [PubMed]
98. Moons, K.G.M.; Altman, D.G.; Reitsma, J.B.; Ioannidis, J.P.A.; Macaskill, P.; Steyerberg, E.W.; Vickers, A.J.; Ransohoff, D.F.; Collins, G.S. Transparent Reporting of a multivariable prediction model for Individual Prognosis or Diagnosis (TRIPOD): Explanation and elaboration. *Ann. Intern. Med.* **2015**, *162*, W1–W73. [CrossRef]
99. Altman, D.G.; Vergouwe, Y.; Royston, P.; Moons, K.G.M. Prognosis and prognostic research: Validating a prognostic model. *BMJ* **2009**, *338*, b605. [CrossRef]
100. White, P.L.; Parr, C.; Barnes, R.A. Predicting Invasive Aspergillosis in Hematology Patients by Combining Clinical and Genetic Risk Factors with Early Diagnostic Biomarkers. *J. Clin. Microbiol.* **2018**, *56*, e01122-17. [CrossRef]

4

Understanding Pathogenesis and Care Challenges of Immune Reconstitution Inflammatory Syndrome in Fungal Infections

Sarah Dellière [1], Romain Guery [1], Sophie Candon [2], Blandine Rammaert [3], Claire Aguilar [1], Fanny Lanternier [1,4], Lucienne Chatenoud [2] and Olivier Lortholary [1,4,*]

1 Medical School, Paris-Descartes University, APHP, Necker-Enfants Malades Hospital, Infectious Disease Center Necker-Pasteur, IHU Imagine, 75015 Paris, France; sarah.delliere@gmail.com (S.D.); romain.guery@aphp.fr (R.G.); ag_claire@yahoo.fr (C.A.); fanny.lanternier@aphp.fr (F.L.)

2 Medical School, Paris-Descartes University, INSERM U1151-CNRS UMR 8253APHP, Necker-Enfants Malades Hospital, APHP, Clinical Immunology, 75015 Paris, France; sophie.candon@inserm.fr (S.C.); lucienne.chatenoud@inserm.fr (L.C.)

3 Medical School, Poitiers University, Poitiers, France; Poitiers University Hospital, Infectious Disease Unit, Poitiers, France; INSERM U1070, 86022 Poitiers, France; blandine.rammaert.paltrie@univ-poitiers.fr

4 Pasteur Institute, Molecular Mycology Unit, National Reference Center for Invasive Fungal Disease and Antifungals, CNRS UMR 2000, 75015 Paris, France

* Correspondence: olivier.lortholary@aphp.fr

Received: 19 November 2018; Accepted: 15 December 2018; Published: 17 December 2018

Abstract: Immune deficiency of diverse etiology, including human immunodeficiency virus (HIV), antineoplastic agents, immunosuppressive agents used in solid organ recipients, immunomodulatory therapy, and other biologics, all promote invasive fungal infections. Subsequent voluntary or unintended immune recovery may induce an exaggerated inflammatory response defining immune reconstitution inflammatory syndrome (IRIS), which causes significant mortality and morbidity. Fungal-associated IRIS raises several diagnostic and management issues. Mostly studied with *Cryptococcus*, it has also been described with other major fungi implicated in human invasive fungal infections, such as *Pneumocystis*, *Aspergillus*, *Candida*, and *Histoplasma*. Furthermore, the understanding of IRIS pathogenesis remains in its infancy. This review summarizes current knowledge regarding the clinical characteristics of IRIS depending on fungal species and existing strategies to predict, prevent, and treat IRIS in this patient population, and tries to propose a common immunological background to fungal IRIS.

Keywords: invasive fungal infections; mycoses; immune reconstitution inflammatory syndrome; fungal immunity

---

1. Introduction

The increasing prevalence of acquired immunodeficiency, subsequent to the human immunodeficiency virus (HIV) pandemic and medical advances, such as organ transplant, stem cell transplant, intensive anti-neoplastic chemotherapy, or immunomodulatory biological agents, has tremendously raised the prevalence of opportunistic infectious diseases, including fungal ones [1]. Further progress, such as anti-retroviral therapy (ART) in HIV patients, has managed to restore immunity, therefore shedding light on a new syndrome: immune reconstitution inflammatory syndrome (IRIS). IRIS is now known to occur during the course of various invasive fungal diseases (IFD). It can be defined as a clinical worsening, or the new presentation, of infectious disease after reversal of immune deficiency. This reversal can be driven by the introduction of ART in HIV patients, neutrophil recovery after chemotherapy and/or stem cell transplant, inadequate balancing of immunosuppressive therapy after solid organ transplantation (SOT) [2,3], and even by post-partum immunological changes after pregnancy [4]. IRIS is triggered by the recovery of immune cells, resulting in a "cytokine storm" and an exaggerated host inflammatory response. IRIS has been best described in HIV-infected patients as a syndrome occurring in the first 6 months of ART and associated with a wide range of opportunistic pathogens, such as JC virus, cytomegalovirus, non-tuberculous mycobacteria, *Mycobacterium tuberculosis*, cryptococci, and *Histoplasma* species [5]. IRIS is commonly divided into two clinical pictures. "Paradoxical" IRIS refers to a primarily diagnosed and treated infectious disease with a secondary inflammatory increase occurring during antimicrobial treatment and immunodeficiency reversal [6]. "Unmasking" IRIS refers to disease symptoms that first appear after immune recovery [6]. When occurring during fungal infections, these entities have been extensively studied in the context of cryptococcosis. Cryptococcal IRIS develops in 8-49% of patients with known cryptococcal disease before ART [6]. The panel and clinical presentation of IFD responsible for IRIS after immune recovery varies with the underlying primary or acquired immunodeficiency. It depends on multifactorial conditions, including the nature of the immune defect, host genetics, and fungal pathogenesis and exposure. Our understanding of IRIS's pathogenesis remains poor. It is a true diagnosis challenge to distinguish IRIS from sole fungal infection or treatment failure due to a similar clinical presentation. Misdiagnosis and the resulting ineffective treatment with antifungals instead of anti-inflammatory drugs may result in the disease having a fatal course [7]. Furthermore, the therapeutics attempted for IRIS include many anti-inflammatory agents and biologic immunomodulators; however, these remain poorly codified in guidelines. In this review, we will summarize current knowledge on the risk factors and the clinical and biological manifestations of IRIS associated with various fungal infections. Current knowledge and cues to understanding the immunopathogenesis of IRIS will be detailed. Finally, IRIS management, including therapeutics and prevention strategies, will be discussed and research priorities highlighted.

2. Fungal-Pathogen-Associated IRIS Characteristics

2.1. *Cryptococcus*

The yeast *Cryptococcus* is the most frequently described genus in IRIS [6]. The difference between paradoxical and unmasking IRIS is also best described and defined for this pathogen [6]. In cases where cryptococcal disease was not recognized at ART initiation, it may be difficult to differentiate between IRIS (caused by the restoration of immune functions then called unmasking IRIS) and the progression of a disease in the context of persisting immunodeficiency. Therefore, Haddow et al. proposed a panel of criteria to support this controversial entity [6]. These criteria mainly include unusual, exaggerated, and heightened inflammatory features. The epidemiology of cryptococcal IRIS may describe various incidence rates. In a review, including 12 studies and 598 patients with diagnosed cryptococcal disease before ART initiation, paradoxical IRIS developed in 8–49% of patients [6]. Interestingly, it appears that the incidence is lower in high-income countries (i.e., 8% in France, 13% in Thailand) while the highest incidence is found in low-income countries (i.e., 49% in Uganda). Furthermore, it seems that cryptococcal IRIS is seen less frequently in the most recent studies [6,8]. The increase in access to improved antifungal therapies may explain such figures. The incidence of unmasking IRIS is much lower, ranging from 0 to 7%; however, a case definition has not been uniformly addressed. Cryptococcal paradoxical IRIS has been described in HIV, SOT (mostly in kidney and liver transplant recipients) [3,9,10], and in early post-partum after pregnancy [4]. IRIS may occur a few days or several months after ART initiation in HIV-infected patients. In SOT recipients, a mean occurrence of 6 weeks after the introduction of antifungal treatment has been described and is triggered by a reduction in immunosuppressive treatment [11]. In those cases, patients may experience allograft loss temporally related to the onset of IRIS through Th1 upregulation. IRIS seems to occur more frequently in patients receiving a combination of tacrolimus, mycophenolate mofetil, and prednisone than in patients receiving another immunosuppressive regimen [2,12]. Clinical manifestations are described in

Table 1. IRIS non-specific symptoms may occur in organs that were not apparently initially infected by the fungus, resulting from exuberant tissue inflammation [13]. Diagnosis remains clinical and requires exclusion of other diagnoses, including worsening or relapse of infection, other opportunistic infections, tumors, and drug-related adverse effects. Cerebrospinal fluid (CSF) culture is typically sterile in IRIS; however, if IRIS arises shortly after antifungal treatment, culture may remain positive. In this case, comparing the fungal burden to CSF at the initial diagnosis of cryptococcosis can help to differentiate IRIS from relapse; however, this technique is not part of routine management. Moreover, it has been suggested that monitoring (1-3)-β-D-glucan (BDG) in CSF could be helpful [14]. Indeed, it has been shown in a recent Ugandan and South African cohort of HIV-infected patients with cryptococcal meningitis that BDG measured in CSF could contribute to the differentiation of fungal progression (i.e., positive BDG) from cryptococcal paradoxical IRIS (i.e., negative BDG) [14]. Furthermore, a PCR-based assay might also be useful: the FilmArray system was evaluated in 39 HIV-infected patients from Uganda with suspected cryptococcal meningitis and was able to detect *Cryptococcus* with 100% sensitivity and to distinguish relapse from IRIS in a limited number of patients [15]. IRIS-like syndrome has been described in immunocompetent patients. Cases have been described with both *Cryptococcus neoformans* and *Cryptococcus gattii* [16–18]. They report an extended overwhelming inflammatory immune response despite CSF culture sterilization with a poor prognosis and subsequent neurological sequelae. In one case, thalidomide was successfully used to decrease inflammation when corticosteroids were inefficient [17]. It is possible that antifungal therapy reduces the burden of *Cryptococcus*, thereby facilitating the reversion of a Th2 response to a Th1 response. However, all of these cases failed to study if the strains may belong to a hypervirulent clade and if a host immune polymorphism could have led to this specific clinical presentation.

2.2. *Candida*

Chronic disseminated candidiasis (CDC), also called hepato-splenic candidiasis, has been suspected to be a form of candidiasis-related IRIS [19]. This clinical entity develops in patients who recently experienced profound and prolonged neutropenia, especially at neutrophil recovery after chemotherapy for acute leukemia. Before the introduction of posaconazole as the primary antifungal prophylaxis, its incidence ranged from 3 to 29% in this population [19], and a diagnosis is usually obtained within 2 weeks following immune recovery but can sometimes be diagnosed as late as 165 days thereafter [19]. Symptoms, which are described in Table 1, usually persist despite antifungal therapy. MRI has a much better sensitivity than ultrasonography and computed tomography (CT) to detect micro-abscesses, which are most frequently localized in the liver and the spleen and result from an exuberant inflammatory response [20]. Positron emission tomography (PET) has been increasingly used and shows promising results in CDC diagnosis [21,22]. At a histopathological level, epithelioid granulomas and micro-abscesses are encountered in most cases [19]. Blood cultures are negative in more than 80% of cases, and microscopy shows the presence of the yeast in less than 50% of cases [19,23]. Biomarkers could be useful in diagnosing CDC. BDG are usually highly increased (>500 ng/L); however, serum detection of mannan antigens and antibodies (Platelia®Candida) appears to be more sensitive to detect the disease and monitor treatment efficacy [24]. Ongoing pathophysiological and imaging studies from our group aim to better decipher the CDC entity. To our knowledge, no form of paradoxical candida-related IRIS after ART initiation in HIV-infected patient has ever been reported.

2.3. *Aspergillus*

Aspergillus-related IRIS also occurs during neutrophil recovery, especially after a course of chemotherapy to treat acute leukemia, or after stem cell recipients [25]. The mean time to clinical and radiological findings of IRIS from an absolute neutrophil count >100/µL and >500/µL was 3.5 days and 2 days, respectively, in a cohort of 19 patients [26]. A few cases of *Aspergillus*-related IRIS have also been described in lung transplant recipients [27]. The clinical manifestations, which are summarized in Table 1, include non-specific worsening, or new onset, of hypoxia, chest pain, cough, dyspnea, and hemoptysis [26]. A CT scan can show a size increase in pulmonary infiltrates, a pleural effusion, nodular lesions, and/or cavitation of a pre-existing lesion [26]. As with all fungi-related IRIS, it remains a diagnosis of exclusion. However, a decrease in serum galactomannan together with a perceived clinical and radiological worsening is good supporting evidence [28]. Overall, *Aspergillus*-related IRIS in neutropenic patients appears to have a good prognosis [28].

2.4. *Histoplasma*

The dimorphic yeast *Histoplasma capsulatum* is represented by two species found in endemic regions: *Histoplasma capsulatum* variety *capsulatum* is mostly encountered in North and South America as well as a few regions in Africa and Asia, while *capsulatum* var. *duboisii* is found in Africa only. Immunocompetent patients infected with *Histoplasma capsulatum* are mostly asymptomatic (>90%), while in immunocompromised patients, a reactivation of infection is common and may lead to a disseminated disease associated with a poor prognosis. *Histoplasma*-related IRIS may present as "unmasking" or "paradoxical". Most cases have been described with *H. capsulatum* var. *capsulatum* in HIV patients [29–31], solid organ transplant recipients [32], and patients receiving TNFα inhibitors [33]. To our knowledge, only one case was described with *H. capsulatum* var. *duboisii* in a HIV patient [34]. The HIV patient population has been the most studied. The incidence of histoplasmosis appears to be higher in patients treated with anti-TNF monoclonal antibodies (e.g., infliximab) than in patients receiving soluble TNF-α receptors (e.g., etanercept) [33]. Overall, IRIS occurs in 9.2% of this patient population [33]. The median time of onset of IRIS symptoms from TNF-α inhibitors discontinuation was 6 weeks (1–45) in 9 patients [33]. Clinical presentations are described in Table 1.

2.5. *Pneumocystis jiroveci*

Pneumocystis jiroveci is a unique fungal organism and was only recently reclassified from a protozoan to an ascomycetous fungus after an analysis of the ribosomal DNA (rDNA) subunit [35]. It is a common opportunistic fungal pathogen and causes pneumonitis in immunocompromised patients. While *P. jirovecii* transmission occurs via person-to-person contact during the first years of life and is controlled by the immune system, it may rapidly multiply in the lungs of immunocompromised patients and lead to severe hypoxia and death [36]. Cases of *Pneumocystis*-associated IRIS have been described mostly in HIV-infected patients and patients receiving high-dose corticosteroids secondarily tapered [37–39]. In an analysis of 15 reports, time to IRIS symptom onset following ART initiation was 15 days (3–301 days) [40]. *P. jiroveci* pneumonia (PJP)-IRIS presents as a recurrence of fever, dyspnea, cough, and night sweat in patients treated for PJP. When performed, a CT scan often shows a recurrence of ground glass opacities; however, many cases also report atypical radiologic manifestations, including nodules, consolidations, and organizing pneumonia [37,41,42]. No adequate diagnostic criteria have been described for this entity. Similarly to other fungi-associated IRIS, microbiological tests (a direct examination of the broncho-alveolar lavage, PCR) are more likely to be negative. Nowadays, a PJP diagnosis often relies on quantitative PCR performed on the bronchoalveolar lavage or induced-sputum [43]. However, the lack of consensus on molecular threshold values for fungal load makes the PCR results difficult to interpret, even more so in the case of IRIS. Furthermore, the lack of a culture technique for *P. jiroveci* creates an additional challenge to distinguish relapse from IRIS. When performed, especially in organizing pneumonia forms, biopsies also showed granulomatous inflammation [37,41,42,44]. These histopathological results have also been described in liver and renal transplant recipients; however, whether a decrease in immunosuppression was responsible or not for IRIS was unclear [45,46].

2.6. *Other Fungi*

Fungi-related IRIS has also been described during infections with *Talaromyces marneffei* (ex-*Penicillium marneffei*) [47–51], *Coccidioides* spp. [52], *Paracoccidioides* spp. [53], *Sporothrix schenckii* [54], *Fusarium* spp. [55], or the newly described *Emergomyces africanus* [56]. To the best of our knowledge, no case of IRIS has been described with any of the Mucorales and phaeohyphomycetes. All IRIS cases related to these more unusual fungi occurred in HIV-infected patients after introduction of ART except for the case involving *Fusarium*, which occurred after neutrophil recovery in a patient treated for acute myeloid leukemia.

3. Is There a Common Background for Fungal IRIS?

Finding a common pathophysiological explanation for all fungi-associated IRIS may appear to be impossible in the light of the diversity of organisms, clinical presentation, and immunological mechanisms underlying a sudden increase in immune response. Although all data come from an isolated clinical picture and a limited series, the histopathological hallmarks when a biopsy is performed seem to consistently involve numerous non-growing fungi, necrosis, macrophages, and, more specifically, granuloma (Table 1). However, objective histopathological data are lacking concerning *Aspergillus*-associated IRIS [26,28]. This granulomatous reaction is described as clusters of epithelioid macrophages, which are sometimes vacuolated and always CD68-positive [57,58]. A lymphocytic infiltrate can also be observed, predominantly at the periphery of granulomatous lesions. Hence, a common immunological explanation might link the underlying mechanisms of fungal IRIS in these very different clinical pictures.

An inadequate balance between pro-inflammatory Th1 response and anti-inflammatory Th2 response was commonly admitted to be the origin of IRIS. With the recent discovery of Th17 and regulatory T cell (Treg) responses, this model evolved to an inbalance between pro-inflammatory Th1/Th17 and anti-inflammatory Th2/Treg axes [3,59–61]. Cytokines driving the differentiation of naïve Th0 cells into Th1, Th2, Th17, and Treg stimulated by cytokines are summarized in Figure 1. Specific transcription factor pathways are detailed for each subset (Figure 1) [3]. IRIS is now believed to arise from an unregulated Th1/Th17 leading to increased production of interferon-γ (IFNγ) [3].

Table 1. Clinical presentation and characteristics of fungi-associated immune reconstitution inflammatory syndrome (IRIS) by fungal species.

Pathogen	Patient Background	Symptoms	Diagnostic Test	Histopathology	Reference
Cryptococcus species	HIV SOT Pregnancy	Headaches, seizures, neurological deficits Lymphadenopathy, pneumonitis, chorioretinitis, skin and soft tissues lesions	**Diagnosis of exclusion** * **No consensual diagnostic test** Sterile CSF culture BDG- CSF PCR-	Granulomatous lesions	[7,14,15]
Candida species	Neutropenia (acute leukemia, lymphoma, stem cell transplant)	Fever, abdominal pain, liver and spleen enlargement MRI: mm-sized abscesses in liver, spleen, kidney, and/or lungs	**Diagnosis of exclusion** * ↑ liver enzymes ↑ BDG Mannan/anti-mannan antibody detection	Epithelioid granuloma, necrosis with minimal inflammatory reaction, micro-abscesses with major inflammatory reaction	[19,22,24]
Aspergillus species	Neutropenia (Stem cell transplant and acute leukemia)	Hypoxia, chest pain, dyspnea, hemoptysis CT scan: ↑ pulmonary infiltrates	**Diagnosis of exclusion** * ↓ galactomannan	Insufficiently studied	[25,26,28]
Histoplasma capsulatum	HIV SOT TNF-α receptor inhibitors	Hemoptysis, dyspnea, lymphadenopathy, skin nodules CT scan: pulmonary bilateral nodules and ground-glass opacities	**Diagnosis of exclusion** * ↓ *Histoplasma* serum antigen Sterile culture	Well-formed granulomatous inflammation	[29–33]
Pneumocystis jiroveci	HIV Corticosteroid-treated patients	Fever, cough, dyspnea, night sweat	**Diagnosis of exclusion** *	Organizing pneumonia: organizing granulation tissue	[39–42,44]

* Exclusion of other diagnosis: microbial progression, other opportunistic infection, tumors, a drug-related adverse effect. SOT, Solid Organ Transplant; BDG, (1-3)-β-D-glucan; CSF, cerebral spinal fluid; HIV, human immunodeficiency virus.

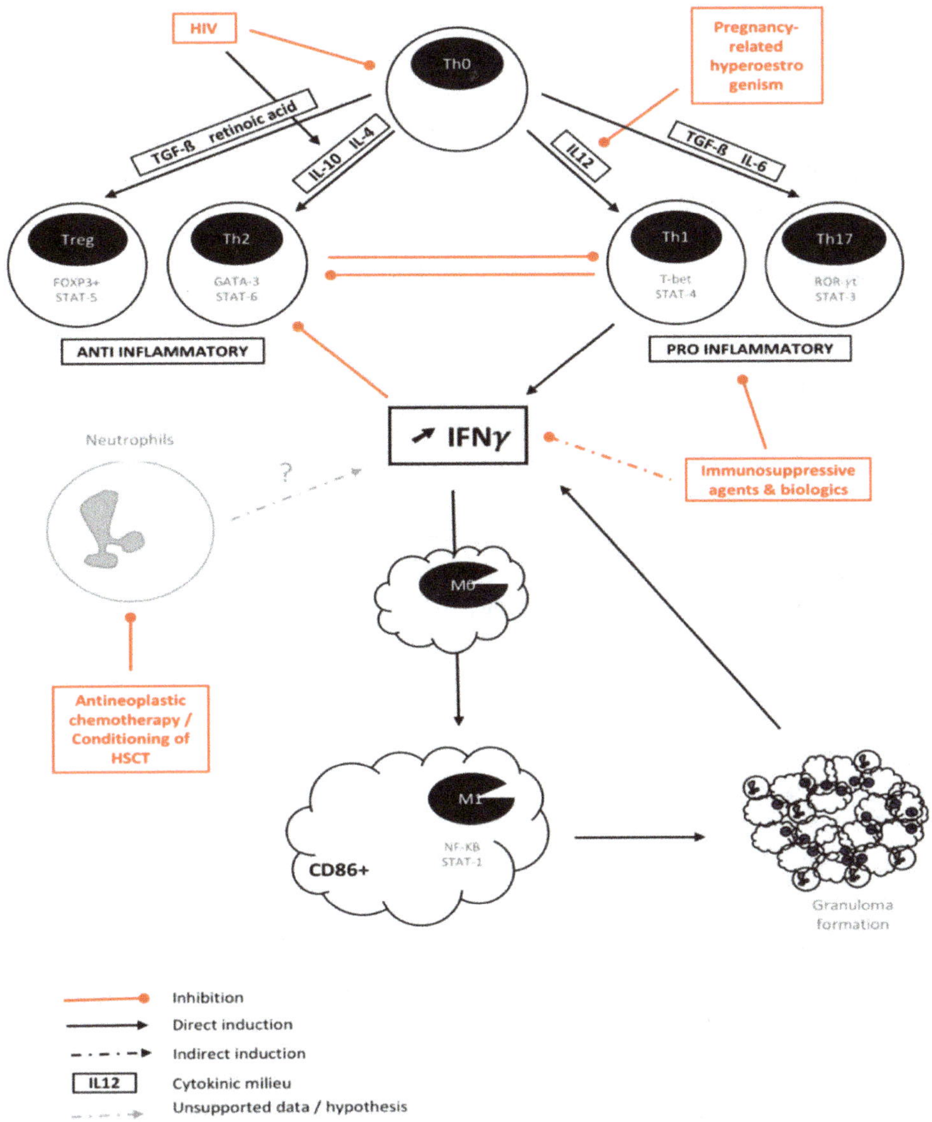

Figure 1. Proposed immune pathophysiology of IRIS. Precursor T helper cells (Th0) differentiate into Th1, Th17, or Th2 cells or Tregs according to cytokines produced in the surrounding milieu through induction of specific transcription factor expression: FOXP3/STAT-5, GATA-3/STAT-6, T-bet/STAT-4, and ROR-γt/STAT-3 for Treg, Th2, Th1, and Th17, respectively [60,61]. Th1 and Th17 cells are pro-inflammatory cells and produce IFN-γ driving macrophage differentiation into M1 macrophages and their activation. M1 macrophages promote granuloma formation and subsequently produce more IFNγ, thus creating an amplification loop leading to an inflammation burst [62]. HIV drives depletion of all Th cell subsets and favors an anti-inflammatory response in remaining cells through a change in cytokine balance [63,64]. Pregnancy hormones inhibit differentiation of naive Th0 cells into Th1 cells, thus promoting a Th2 environment [65]. Biologic agents, such as infliximab, inhibit the pro-inflammatory cytokine TNFα [66]. Immunosuppressive therapeutics inhibit Th1/Th17 response and allow graft acceptance in solid organ transplant [3]. Neutropenia resulting from chemotherapy or conditioning for hematopoeitic stem cell therapy leads to a decrease in IFNγ production through cytokinic interaction with T-cell production; however, data are lacking [67]. Many feedback loops exist between these different players depending on cytokine production. Sudden dysregulation at any level may create an exaggerated inflammatory response with an IFN-γ-unregulated increase leading to IRIS. FOXP3, fox head box P3; IFN, interferon; IL, interleukin; PMN, polymorphonuclear; TGF, transforming growth factor; ROR, retinoid orphan receptor; STAT, signal transducer and activation of transcription; HSCT, Hematopoietic Stem Cell Therapy.

Overall, this exaggerated inflammatory response translates in radiological findings as edema and abnormal contrast medium uptake into pulmonary and brain lesions [58]. Cells of the innate immune system, such as monocytes, macrophages, and neutrophils, are of increasing interest in IRIS pathophysiology, since granuloma appears to be frequently found in IRIS lesions [19,41,47]. Indeed, granuloma is the histopathology hallmark in chronic disseminated candidiasis [19] and is commonly found in other fungi-related IRIS [37,41,48,49,56]. An extended description of granuloma in fungi-related IRIS is unavailable, and should be better studied in particular through immune staining to understand which cell types are implicated and their degree of differentiation/activation. Granulomas may display very distinct features, may be activated or latent, and their cell-type composition may vary according to the situation and pathogen [68]. In a simplistic approach, excess IFNγ produced by Th1 cells, neutrophils, or activated macrophages will elicit the differentiation of monocytes towards macrophages and activate their phagocytic activity as well as stimulate granuloma formation. IFNγ favors the classical activation of macrophages into M1-phenotype macrophages [62]. These macrophages secrete large amounts of pro-inflammatory cytokines, such as IL-1β, TNFα, IL-12, IL-18, and IL-23, driving in return a Th1/Th17 cell inflammatory response. Phenotypically, M1 macrophages express high levels of histocompatibility complex class II and the CD86 marker. M1 macrophages are implicated in initiating and sustaining inflammation, and can, therefore, be detrimental. Furthermore, M1 polarization appears to be predominant in granuloma formation [69]. Conversely, M2-polarized or alternately activated macrophages produce IL-4, IL-13, and IL-10 and are prone to immune regulation and tissue remodeling [70]. A further analysis would provide significant data to help us understand fungi-associated IRIS.

The immune pathophysiology appears to vary according to the underlying type of immunosuppression before immune recovery. HIV, in addition to depleting the total pool of CD4+ T-cells by apoptosis, including Th0 cells, induces preferential death of Th1 cells and differentiation of the remaining Th0 into Th2 cells through a critical change in cytokine balance [63,64]. Introduction of ART leads to an initial redistribution of CD4+ T-cells to the blood rather than proliferation. After 4–6 weeks, the production of naive CD4+ T-cells and memory T-cells coincides with the mean onset of paradoxical IRIS [71]. A concomitant infection responsible for increased circulating pro-inflammatory cytokines may also contribute to dominant Th1 differentiation and IRIS. In addition, HIV induces Tregs to migrate and accumulate in peripheral and mucosal lymphoid tissues [72]. Montes et al. have described an initial redistribution of Tregs to the blood at ART initiation [73]. This tissular depletion in Tregs may also participate in a locally uncontrolled inflammatory response. Moreover, the functional capacities of Tregs appear to be reduced [74].

After solid organ transplantation, graft survival relies on the inhibition of alloreactive Th1/Th17 responses by immunosuppressive drugs (i.e., mycophenolate mofetil, calcineurin inhibitors, corticosteroids ...) through different mechanisms [3]. Calcineurin inhibitors, especially tacrolimus, strongly suppress the Th1 response while rapamycin promotes Treg survival and function and suppresses the differentiation of Th17 cells [3]. Corticosteroids decrease Th1 responses but also expand Th2 cells and Tregs [3]. Post-transplant IRIS is subsequent to a decrease in immunosuppression due to drug–drug interactions or an intentional modification in drug dosage in the context of an ongoing infection, therefore increasing Th1/Th17 responses. However, a recent study showed that only a discontinuation of calcineurin inhibitors influenced the development of IRIS in cryptococcosis by a 5-fold higher risk [11]. The excessive Th1 response observed in IRIS may also lead to collateral damage to the graft. Indeed, in a prospective study involving 54 renal allograft recipients with cryptococcosis, 5.5% of patients presented with IRIS and the renal graft was lost due to chronic rejection in 66% of patients with IRIS as compared to 5.9% of IRIS-free patients [12].

Immunomodulatory biologic agents are increasingly being used to treat chronic autoimmune and inflammatory conditions, such as rheumatoid arthritis and inflammatory colitis. Tumor necrosis factor (TNF)-α, a cytokine mainly produced by activated macrophages, is involved in systemic inflammation and plays a key role in the recruitment of immune cells and granuloma formation. Histoplasmosis is the most prevalent IFD in patients undergoing TNFα inhibitors therapy, followed by candidiasis and aspergillosis [66]. Most mycoses described in those patients were associated with the use of the monoclonal antibodies infliximab/adalimumab rather than the soluble TNFα receptor etanercept, reflecting the difference in the mechanism of action between those drugs [66]. Discontinuation of TNFα inhibitors results in IRIS in 9.2% of patients with histoplasmosis [33]. Alemtuzumab, a humanized CD52 monoclonal antibody that depletes T and B cell populations, has also been involved in fungi-related IRIS with *C. neoformans* and *P. jiroveci* upon its withdrawal [75,76].

A prompt recovery of neutrophils after a stem-cell transplant or a chemotherapy cycle has been linked to a severe pulmonary complication subsequent to inflammation during invasive pulmonary aspergillosis [25]. Likewise, chronic disseminated candidiasis manifests during neutrophil recovery [19]. Despite the lack of studies and data concerning this IRIS-like syndrome following the fast expansion of neutrophils after a stem-cell transplantation, it could be expected that a direct or indirect increase in IFNγ plays a role in pathogenesis. Indeed, a subset of neutrophils, Gr-1+/CD11b+ cells, has been shown in mice to produce IFNγ and mediate early graft loss or take part in severe renal ischemia reperfusion injury [67,77]. However, production of IFNγ by human neutrophils is controversial [78]. They may, nonetheless, participate through indirect mechanisms, especially through a crosstalk with Th17 cells, in cytokine production to increase IFNγ levels [79]. More data are needed to understand IRIS following neutrophil recovery, and its pathogenesis is currently being studied in the CANPHARI study (NCT01916057) headed by our group.

During pregnancy, mechanisms of fetal tolerance lead to downregulation of the Th1/Th17 axis. Interestingly, regulation of M2 macrophage polarization is required for successful pregnancy, and is sustained by pregnancy hormones, such as estrogen and HCG [65]. A shift in cytokine pattern is observed during the post-partum period that may be associated with pathological inflammatory syndrome and has been documented 3–6 weeks after delivery [4,80].

In addition to this immune dysregulation, commonly used antifungals are known to bear some immunomodulatory properties that could contribute to IRIS. These data only supported by in vitro studies, and the few in vivo studies in mice are to be taken with caution. Amphotericin B deoxycholate upregulates Th1 response through toll-like receptor 2 (TLR-2)-mediated transcription and inflammatory cytokine transcription [81,82]. Conversely, the lipid formulation of polyene has no effect on, or even downregulates, the inflammatory response directly due to the intrinsic properties of the liposomes [82]. However, it may confer an increase in the phagocytic properties of macrophages and neutrophils against numerous fungi [82–85]. Echinocandins unmask β-glucan from the fungal cell wall, eliciting pro-inflammatory cytokine release upon its recognition through pattern recognition receptors (PRR). Azoles seem to be the least active with respect to modulation of the host's immune system [82]. However, fluconazole and voriconazole have been shown to enhance phagocytic pro-inflammatory activity through a TLR2 interaction [82]. Overall, the initial choice of antifungal could influence the subsequent inflammatory response; however, their immunomodulatory effects have not been studied in the context of IRIS.

Lastly, three more elements, often omitted and far less studied, may be discussed to explain IRIS's pathophysiology: fungal strain immunomodulatory characteristics, host immune system features, and autoimmunity disorders. Firstly, *Cryptococcus* itself inhibits the Th1 response while inducing a Th2 response that compromises the host's resistance in mice [86]. Furthermore, the cryptococcal genotype has been shown to influence the immune response and human clinical outcome after meningitis [87]. In addition, Desnos-Ollivier et al. showed that mixed strain infections are seen in 20% of patients and could drive overstimulation of the immune system [88]. Similarly, infection by *P. jiroveci* often results from mixed strain genotypes [89]. However, the impact of strain genotype in IRIS has not been studied. Secondly, on the host side, human immune system genetics is a growing field of interest and may be involved in IRIS development. Polymorphisms in cytokine genes may play a role in host susceptibility to IRIS [90]. For instance, a non-synonymous polymorphism in IL-23R is associated with a reduced risk of schistosomiasis-associated IRIS in a Kenyan population [91]. Similarly, a common haplotype of the IL-4 promoter was over-represented in patients with CDC [92]. Also, a single nucleotide polymorphism in the promoter of leukotriene A4 hydroxylase (LTA4H) regulating the balance between anti-inflammatory lipoxins and the pro-inflammatory LTB4 is responsible for a higher incidence of severe tuberculosis-associated IRIS [93]. One could easily hypothesize that polymorphisms of the human IFNγ receptor may lead to different susceptibility patterns to IRIS. Third, opportunistic infection results in tissue damage and the epitope spreading that is known to predispose to autoimmunity [71]. Furthermore, various autoimmune disorders have been discovered in HIV-infected patients after ART initiation that may play a role in the excessive inflammatory response [71]. Nevertheless, these hypotheses require further investigations, which are currently ongoing through a collaborative work about chronic disseminated candidiasis between the group of Lausanne and ours.

Overall, any rapid immune recovery can lead to IRIS, driven by multifactorial factors, such as patient response to drugs (ART, antifungals, ...), host immune genetics, and the microbial strain. Fungal pathogen immunogenicity may trigger an overshoot of IFNγ production either through an enhancement of the Th1/Th17 axis and/or rapid neutrophil reconstitution leading to overproduction/activation of CD68+ macrophages and promoting granuloma formation and inflammatory disease.

4. A Limited Therapeutic Arsenal Against IRIS

The ideal management of fungi-associated IRIS in general remains unknown. No recognized clinical guidelines have been dedicated to this challenging subject matter except those from IDSA for the management of IRIS in cryptococcal disease [7]. They do not recommend a specific treatment for minor IRIS manifestations that usually resolve within a few days or weeks. However, for complications involving central nervous system (CNS) inflammation associated with increased intracranial pressure, they advise corticosteroids (0.5–1 mg/kg/day of prednisone equivalent) and dexamethasone at higher doses for more severe CNS signs and symptoms. No data support recommendations for the length of treatment; however, a 2–6-week course with close monitoring and concomitant antifungal treatment is widely accepted [7].

Corticosteroids are the only drug class that has been recognized for the treatment of IRIS so far [94]. They show an anti-inflammatory effect on most immune cells by altering the transcription of inflammatory mediators, interfering with the nuclear factor-KB, and directly enhancing the effect of the anti-inflammatory proteins [95]. An evaluation of the efficacy of corticosteroids compared to a placebo in a randomized controlled trial has only been done in TB-associated IRIS, and showed a reduced length of hospitalization and surgical procedure [96,97]. Regarding fungal infections, only case reports and small series account for the benefit of corticosteroids in fungi-associated IRIS, especially in patients with impending respiratory failure after neutrophil recovery and aspergillosis [26,98], chronic disseminated candidiasis [57], and cryptococcosis [13,58,99]. Also, despite the lack of formal diagnostic criteria for IRIS, old studies support the adjunction of corticosteroids to prevent early deterioration in patients with moderately severe *P. jiroveci* pneumonia and HIV [100]. In cryptococcal meningitis, adjunction of dexamethasone at baseline did not reduce mortality among patients with HIV, nor was it associated with a reduced incidence of IRIS in a large cohort of 451 patients [8]. On the contrary, it was correlated with more adverse effects and disability than a placebo [8]. Indeed, complications associated with the use of corticosteroids must be considered. Their non-specific immunosuppressive effect can lead to subsequent infectious complications, such as herpes virus reactivation, strongyloides hyperinfection, worsening of chronic hepatitis B, and Kaposi sarcoma progression [94,101,102]. In addition, corticosteroids can cause metabolic complications, such as dysglycemia, hypertension, and cushingoïd features, or be responsible for other adverse effects, such as worsening psychiatric disorders and drug interactions [94].

TNF-α is a pro-inflammatory cytokine required for macrophage activation and granuloma formation. The anti-TNF-α antibodies infliximab and adalimumab have been used in several case reports to reduce inflammation in IRIS. Etanercept is a soluble TNFα receptor; however, it has never been reported to be effective in IRIS treatment. Infliximab has primarily been used [103,104]; however, adalimumab has shown the ability to treat corticosteroid- and/or infliximab-resistant IRIS associated with TB and Cryptococcus [105–107]. Although the optimal length of treatment with such therapy has not been determined yet, the successful management of IRIS has been reported to require several months of treatment. Overall, adalimumab should probably be preferred when considering anti-TNF-α for treating IRIS, since more fungal complications have been reported with infliximab [66].

Thalidomide also acts as an immunomodulatory drug inhibiting TNFα synthesis among other cytokines (i.e. IFNγ, IL-10, and IL-12 and cyclooxygenase 2 (COX-2)) [17]. In several cases, it has been shown to be an interesting molecule for corticosteroid-dependent IRIS in cryptococcal meningitis that allows for steroid tapering [17,58,108]. The treatment duration in these studies ranged from 4 weeks to 14 months with no relapse [19].

Non-steroidal anti-inflammatory drugs (NSAIDs) inhibit cyclooxygenase, an enzyme required for prostaglandin synthesis and inflammation mediation. Many cases report the use of NSAIDs in TB-IRIS [94], and some clinical guidelines recommend their use for mild IRIS related to mycobacterial infection [109]. Nonetheless, no clinical trial supports these recommendations and data are lacking regarding fungi-associated IRIS. Moreover, nephrotoxicity is a concern with long-term use and concomitant administration of other nephrotoxic drugs, such as amphotericin B or calcineurin inhibitors.

Statins inhibit 3-hydroxy-3-methyl-glutary-CoA (HMG-CoA) reductase. It has been hypothesized that, considering the close homology between fungal and human HMG-CoA reductase, statins may have a potential antifungal effect. However, a meta-analysis of five retrospective studies showed no positive effects during fungal infections [110]. Nevertheless, statins display immunomodulatory activity promoting the Th2/Treg axis through various mechanisms [111]. Subsequently, many authors speculate that they could play a role in the management of IRIS; however, data is still lacking [111,112].

Finally, intravenous immunoglobulins have been successfully used in virus-related IRIS [113,114]; however, they have never been tried in the fungal context.

To conclude, the best-studied and most-used therapy for IRIS is corticosteroids despite their several drawbacks. Anti-TNFα, especially adalimumab, as well as thalidomide, appear to be promising in treating fungi-associated IRIS or corticosteroid-dependent IRIS. However, more studies are required. Symptomatic treatment alone, including analgesia and anti-epileptic treatment, is often sufficient to manage symptoms and should not be underestimated.

5. Predict and Prevent: The Cornerstone of IRIS Management Today

Since treating IRIS remains uncertain and challenging with no guidelines to rely on, patient care has been focusing on identifying risk factors and developing preventive strategies.

5.1. Prediction with Diagnostic Markers

The identification of risk factors mostly depends on biological markers assessed in diagnostic labs and a few clinical risk factors, especially information concerning patient treatment. Once again, cryptococcal-related paradoxical IRIS in HIV-infected patients has been the most studied situation. Therefore, our current knowledge on predictive markers is limited to these circumstances in predictive markers as well. Risk factors for cryptococcal-associated IRIS can be divided into three categories: (i) host-related factors, (ii) pathogen-related factors, and (iii) treatment-related factors. Host-related factors include various measurable immunological blood and cerebrospinal fluid (CSF) parameters. A lower pre-ART CD4 count has been demonstrated many times in bacterial- or viral-associated IRIS as well [115–118]. However, no cut-off has been established. Other blood parameters reflecting a lack of an immune response toward cryptococcosis at diagnosis appear to be relevant to predict the occurrence of IRIS. A lower plasma total IgM, a specific anti-fungal IgM (glucuronoxylomannan-IgM and β-glucan-binding IgM), and a specific IgG prior to initiation of ART were observed in patients who developed IRIS [119]. A lack of pro-inflammatory cytokines in a serum, such as TNFα, IFNγ, granulocyte-colony stimulating factor (G-CSF), and granulocyte-macrophage CSF (GM-CSF), predicted future IRIS [120]. An increase in Th2 response reflected by the IL-4 level was also associated with IRIS [120]. The use of a modified IFNγ release assay of whole blood stimulated with a cryptococcal mannoprotein has confirmed that lower IFNγ responses before ART initiation are associated with a higher risk to develop IRIS [117]. Similarly, a lack of an immune response in CSF with a decrease in the leucocytes count to ≤25 cells/μL and a reduced level of IFNγ, IL-6, IL-8, and TNF-α were associated with the development of IRIS [118,121]. In these circumstances, a global CSF protein level ≤50 mg/dL was also an independent risk factor [121]. A higher CSF ratio of CCL2/CXCL10 and CCL3/CXCL10 were also found in patients who subsequently developed IRIS [122]. CCL2 and CCL3 are chemokines known to attract monocytes, macrophages, neutrophils, and T-cells, whereas CXCL10 is only chemotactic to CXCR3+ lymphocytes (Th1 cells) [122]. Thus, an increase in the former chemokines may promote the infiltration of macrophages and neutrophils into the CSF and be responsible for IRIS.

Pathogen-related risk factors correspond to the fungal burden, which can be assessed by a serum cryptococcal antigen (CrAg) titer, the colony forming unit (CFU)/mL of CSF, and the presence of fungemia [58,118,123]. Patients with IRIS had a 4-fold higher median CrAg level pre-ART [120]. In addition, patients with a negative cryptococcal culture from a CSF sample pre-ART initiation experienced fewer CNS deterioration symptoms and a lower IRIS rate than patients with a positive culture [118].

Treatment-related risk factors include a shorter duration of antifungal treatment prior to starting ART and/or a rapid suppression of HIV viral load. Indeed, a decrease in HIV viral RNA to >2.5 log at the time of IRIS compared with RNA levels before the initiation of ART was associated with subsequent IRIS [116]. In addition, a rapid immunologic response to ART reflected by a more important rise in CD4 cells over a 6-month period was associated with IRIS [124,125]. Furthermore, some ART regimens, especially those using a boosted protease inhibitor, were a risk factor for developing IRIS [116]. Boosted protease inhibitors appear to have direct immunomodulatory effects, including anti-apoptotic effects and an increase in pro-inflammatory cytokines [116]. Recent European studies found that the use of integrase inhibitors, especially dolutegravir, increases the risk of IRIS by an odds ratio of 1.96–3.25 [126–128].

Regarding *Aspergillus*-related IRIS, the use of a colony-stimulating factor appears to be associated with the occurrence of IRIS in patients with invasive pulmonary aspergillosis with neutropenia [28]. Similarly, a personal case describes a severe exacerbation of CDC after G-CSF administration [129]. Concerning other fungal pathogens, no factors have been studied to predict IRIS to our knowledge. Yet, in *Aspergillus*-related IRIS, one can expect higher galactomannan titers by analogy to CrAg titers. Similarly, β-D-glucans may be higher during fungemia before chronic disseminated candidiasis. However, these statements remain hypotheses and require proof.

To conclude, no markers are yet consensual among the community, and more studies are needed to include one or several of them with proper cut-offs in standard patient care guidelines. A selection of a few of these markers, based on ease of use in the laboratory, reproducibility, price, and effectiveness to predict IRIS, should provide a strong algorithm and robust tool for stratifying patients with high, moderate, and low risk to develop IRIS.

5.2. Prevention by Delaying and/or Tapering Immune Restoration

IRIS depends on the critical time point when the immune system is restored. It seems that the shorter this period is, the more likely the occurrence of IRIS [25,116]. In many situations, this period cannot be controlled and only monitored to identify patients at risk to develop IRIS secondarily (i.e., neutrophil recovery, unbalanced immunosuppressive treatment in SOT). However, in HIV-infected patients, immune recovery is elicited by ART and can be adjusted. Two pioneer studies on IRIS in cryptococcal meningitis showed that initiation of ART closer to the diagnosis of the fungal disease was associated with subsequent development of IRIS [58,125]. This suggests that the inflammatory response is likely higher when the fungal burden or its remnants (i.e., antigen titers) is still substantial. Interestingly, the timing of ART appears to be more essential in *Cryptococcus*-IRIS than in TB-IRIS, in which early ART increased survival [130]. Nonetheless, this was not the case when TB meningitis was present, highlighting that CNS involvement in IRIS is the most deleterious form, and requires extra caution and specific guidelines [131].

The timing of ART initiation has been studied in four trials involving HIV-infected patients [132–135]. In the oldest one, all opportunistic infections combined, ART initiation after 2 weeks was associated with a reduced likelihood of progression or death compared to ART initiation after 6–7 weeks [132]. Opportunistic infections were mostly fungal, including 63% of *Pneumocystis* pneumonia, 12% of cryptococcal meningitis, and 4% histoplasmosis. No subanalysis was made in those groups. Surprisingly, IRIS was uncommon (7%) and was not more prevalent in the early or delayed therapy group [132]. This may be related to the smaller incidence of IRIS in *Pneumocystis* pneumonia, where corticosteroids are frequently used in severe cases. The second study focused on cryptococcal meningitis in a cohort of 54 patients in Zimbabwe, in which ART was initiated at 72-h after diagnosis versus 10 weeks later [133]. The 3-year mortality rate was significantly higher in the early ART group (88% versus 54%; p <0.006), and could be attributed to IRIS according to the authors [133]. Similarly, the third study concerned a small cohort of patients from Botswana ($n = 27$) with cryptococcal meningitis [134]. Initiation of ART within 7 days following diagnosis of fungal disease, as compared to 28 days after, was associated with a significantly increased risk of IRIS; however, there was no difference in mortality [134]. Lastly, Boulware et al. conducted an open-label randomized trial in Uganda and South Africa that enrolled HIV patients diagnosed with cryptococcal meningitis [135]. Early ART was given between 1 and 2 weeks after diagnosis, while deferred ART was given after 5 weeks. The 6-month mortality rate was significantly higher in the early ART arm (45% versus 30%; $p = 0.03$), which prematurely ended the study. The rate of IRIS was increased in the early ART arm, but not significantly different from the delayed one (20% versus 13%; $p = 0.32$). No other cause (i.e., antifungal toxicity) could explain the difference [135]. Scriven et al. attempted to explain the difference in mortality by exploring CSF macrophage activation, and found an increase of activation markers (CD206+, CD163+) on monocytes and macrophages in the early ART arm versus the delayed ART arm [136]. More data are required to determine the implications of recent ART initiation for the immune system; however, these results point to the possible involvement of innate immune response mechanisms [136].

While the IDSA guidelines had previously recommended the introduction of ART 2–10 weeks after diagnosis [7], this gap has narrowed to 4–6 weeks in newer recommendations taking into account these studies [137,138]. Though delaying ART is recommended, predictive factors should not be underestimated. Achieving a negative CSF culture prior to starting ART might be a better target to aim for to reduce IRIS risk than considering a consensual time limit, since the immune response may differ among patients. Regarding other forms of IRIS, no studies have been done concerning preventive strategies. Close monitoring of inflammation and clinical worsening is recommended to enable early care in those specific cases.

6. Conclusions/Perspective

IRIS is certainly underdiagnosed and many times considered as a failure of antifungal treatment. No consensual diagnostic test is used and the diagnosis remains clinical. As far as we know, the three following criteria need to be satisfied: (1) the new appearance, or worsening, of clinical or radiographic manifestations consistent with an inflammatory process, (2) symptoms that cannot be explained by a newly acquired infection, and (3) negative culture results and/or a decrease in the fungal antigen level (BDG, galactomannan, histoplasma antigen, cryptococcal antigen ...). Granuloma appear to be the histopathology hallmark, and hypercalcemia subsequent to endogenous production of 1,25 dihydroxyvitamin D by macrophages in granulomas should perhaps be sought more frequently [139]. Existing research bioassays need to be translated into clinical practice to support diagnosis. Until thorough diagnostic markers and a clear definition for fungal-associated IRIS are consensually acknowledged by the medical and scientific community, all studies included in this review ought to be considered with caution.

Regarding treatment, given the drawbacks of corticosteroid treatment, the benefit from such therapy might still be argued in cases where IRIS symptoms do not usually result in lethal complications. Furthermore, the optimal dose and length of treatment for a reasonable risk/benefit ratio need to be discussed. More studies, including randomized trials, are needed to evaluate the relevance of other anti-inflammatory drugs and to propose guidelines for the management of IRIS in fungal diseases.

The prevention of IRIS in HIV relies mostly on the timing of introduction of ART, which appears to be critical in IRIS involving the CNS compartment, such as cryptococcal IRIS resulting in significant morbidity and mortality. Other forms of IRIS, especially involving the lungs or skin, appear to be less life-threatening and have been set aside in research protocols. However, these forms of IRIS bear morbidity, a longer length of stay in the hospital, a high cost investigation, and unnecessary medications, thus requiring attention by the research community to improve the standard of care.

Our understanding of the pathogenesis of IRIS remains in its infancy. More data are available on TB-IRIS; however, additional research is needed to know if these results are applicable to fungi-associated IRIS. The heterogeneity of fungal infections and immunosuppression types contributes to the complexity of understanding IRIS occurring during fungal infections. Multifactorial approaches must be taken to understand its pathogenesis, including host genetics, fungal strain specificities, immunology, and histopathology, which could subsequently lead us to uncover new treatment options.

Author Contributions: O.L., R.G., and S.D. contributed to the conception and design of the review. O.L. and S.D. drafted the manuscript. All authors critically revised the entire manuscript, agreed to be fully accountable for ensuring the integrity and accuracy of the work, and read and approved the final submission.

References

1. Enoch, D.A.; Yang, H.; Aliyu, S.H.; Micallef, C. The changing epidemiology of invasive fungal infections. *Meth. Mol. Biol.* **2017**, *1508*, 17–65.
2. Singh, N.; Lortholary, O.; Alexander, B.D.; Gupta, K.L.; John, G.T.; Pursell, K.; Muñoz, P.; Klintmalm, G.B.; Stosor, V.; del Busto, R.; et al. An immune reconstitution syndrome-like illness associated with *Cryptococcus neoformans* infection in organ transplant recipients. *Clin. Infect. Dis.* **2005**, *40*, 1756–1761. [CrossRef] [PubMed]
3. Sun, H.Y.; Singh, N. Immune reconstitution inflammatory syndrome in non-HIV immunocompromised patients. *Curr. Opin. Infect. Dis.* **2009**, *22*, 394–402. [CrossRef]
4. Singh, N.; Perfect, J.R. Immune reconstitution syndrome and exacerbation of infections after pregnancy. *Clin. Infect. Dis.* **2007**, *45*, 1192–1199. [CrossRef] [PubMed]
5. French, M.A. Immune reconstitution inflammatory syndrome: A reappraisal. *Clin. Infect. Dis.* **2009**, *48*, 101–107. [CrossRef]
6. Haddow, L.J.; Colebunders, R.; Meintjes, G.; Lawn, S.D.; Elliott, J.H.; Manabe, Y.C.; Bohjanen, P.R.; Sungkanuparph, S.; Easterbrook, P.J.; French, M.A.; et al. Cryptococcal immune reconstitution inflammatory syndrome in HIV-1-infected individuals: Proposed clinical case definitions. *Lancet Infect. Dis.* **2010**, *10*, 791–802. [CrossRef]
7. Perfect, J.R.; Dismukes, W.E.; Dromer, F.; Goldman, D.L.; Graybill, J.R.; Hamill, R.J.; Harrison, T.S.; Larsen, R.A.; Lortholary, O.; Nguyen, M.H.; et al. Clinical practice guidelines for the management of cryptococcal disease: 2010 update by the Infectious Diseases Society of America. *Clin. Infect. Dis.* **2010**, *50*, 291–322. [CrossRef] [PubMed]
8. Beardsley, J.; Wolbers, M.; Kibengo, F.M.; Ggayi, A.-B.M.; Kamali, A.; Cuc, N.T.K.; Binh, T.Q.; Chau, N.V.V.; Farrar, J.; Merson, L.; et al. Adjunctive Dexamethasone in HIV-Associated Cryptococcal Meningitis. *N. Engl. J. Med.* **2016**, *374*, 542–554. [CrossRef] [PubMed]

9. Legris, T.; Massad, M.; Purgus, R.; Vacher-Coponat, H.; Ranque, S.; Girard, N.; Berland, Y.; Moal, V. Immune reconstitution inflammatory syndrome mimicking relapsing cryptococcal meningitis in a renal transplant recipient. *Transplant Infect. Dis.* **2010**, *13*, 303–308. [CrossRef] [PubMed]
10. Singh, N.; Sifri, C.D.; Silveira, F.P.; Miller, R.; Gregg, K.S.; Huprikar, S.; Lease, E.D.; Zimmer, A.; Dummer, J.S.; Spak, C.W.; et al. Cryptococcosis in patients with cirrhosis of the liver and posttransplant outcomes. *Transplantation* **2015**, *99*, 2132–2141. [CrossRef] [PubMed]
11. Sun, H.Y.; Alexander, B.D.; Huprikar, S.; Forrest, G.N.; Bruno, D.; Lyon, G.M.; Wray, D.; Johnson, L.B.; Sifri, C.D.; Razonable, R.R.; et al. Predictors of immune reconstitution syndrome in organ transplant recipients with cryptococcosis: Implications for the management of immunosuppression. *Clin. Infect. Dis.* **2014**, *60*, 36–44. [CrossRef] [PubMed]
12. Singh, N.; Lortholary, O.; Alexander, B.D.; Gupta, K.L.; John, G.T.; Pursell, K.; Muñoz, P.; Klintmalm, G.B.; Stosor, V.; Limaye, A.P.; et al. Allograft loss in renal transplant recipients with *Cryptococcus neoformans* associated immune reconstitution syndrome. *Transplantation* **2005**, *80*, 1131–1133. [CrossRef] [PubMed]
13. Lanternier, F.; Chandesris, M.O.; Poiree, S.; Bougnoux, M.E.; Mechai, F.; Mamzer-Bruneel, M.F.; Viard, J.P.; Galmiche-Rolland, L.; Lecuit, M.; Lortholary, O. Cellulitis revealing a Cryptococcosis-related immune reconstitution inflammatory syndrome in a renal allograft recipient. *Am. J. Transplant.* **2007**, *7*, 2826–2828. [CrossRef]
14. Rhein, J.; Bahr, N.C.; Morawski, B.M.; Schutz, C.; Zhang, Y.; Finkelman, M.; Meya, D.B.; Meintjes, G.; Boulware, D.R. Detection of high cerebrospinal fluid levels of (1→3)-β-d-Glucan in cryptococcal meningitis. *Open Forum Infect. Dis.* **2014**, *1*, 267. [CrossRef]
15. Rhein, J.; Bahr, N.C.; Hemmert, A.C.; Cloud, J.L.; Bellamkonda, S.; Oswald, C.; Lo, E.; Nabeta, H.; Kiggundu, R.; Akampurira, A.; et al. Diagnostic performance of a multiplex PCR assay for meningitis in an HIV-infected population in Uganda. *Diagn. Microbiol. Infect. Dis.* **2015**, *84*, 1–6. [CrossRef] [PubMed]
16. Ecevit, I.Z.; Clancy, C.J.; Schmalfuss, I.M.; Nguyen, M.H. The poor prognosis of central nervous system cryptococcosis among nonimmunosuppressed patients: A call for better disease recognition and evaluation of adjuncts to antifungal therapy. *Clin. Infect. Dis.* **2006**, *42*, 1443–1447. [CrossRef] [PubMed]
17. Somerville, L.K.; Henderson, A.P.; Chen, S.C.A.; Kok, J. Successful treatment of *Cryptococcus neoformans* immune reconstitution inflammatory syndrome in an immunocompetent host using thalidomide. *Med. Mycol. Case Rep.* **2015**, *7*, 12–14. [CrossRef]
18. Chen, S.C.A.; Meyer, W.; Sorrell, T.C. *Cryptococcus gattii* infections. *Clin. Microbiol. Rev.* **2014**, *27*, 980–1024. [CrossRef]
19. Rammaert, B.; Desjardins, A.; Lortholary, O. New insights into hepatosplenic candidosis, a manifestation of chronic disseminated candidosis. *Mycoses* **2012**, *55*, e74–e84. [CrossRef]
20. Anttila, V.J.; Lamminen, A.E.; Bondestam, S.; Korhola, O.; Färkkilä, M.; Sivonen, A.; Ruutu, T.; Ruutu, P. Magnetic resonance imaging is superior to computed tomography and ultrasonography in imaging infectious liver foci in acute leukaemia. *Eur. J. Haematol.* **1996**, *56*, 82–87. [CrossRef]
21. Hot, A.; Maunoury, C.; Poiree, S.; Lanternier, F.; Viard, J.P.; Loulergue, P.; Coignard, H.; Bougnoux, M.E.; Suarez, F.; Rubio, M.T.; et al. Diagnostic contribution of positron emission tomography with [^{18}F]fluorodeoxyglucose for invasive fungal infections. *Clin. Microbiol. Infect.* **2011**, *17*, 409–417. [CrossRef] [PubMed]
22. Rammaert, B.; Candon, S.; Maunoury, C.; Bougnoux, M.-E.; Jouvion, G.; Braun, T.; Correas, J.-M.; Lortholary, O. Thalidomide for steroid-dependent chronic disseminated candidiasis after stem cell transplantation: A case report. *Transplant Infect. Dis.* **2016**, *19*, e12637. [CrossRef]
23. De Castro, N.; Mazoyer, E.; Porcher, R.; Raffoux, E.; Suarez, F.; Ribaud, P.; Lortholary, O.; Molina, J.M. Hepatosplenic candidiasis in the era of new antifungal drugs: A study in Paris 2000-2007. *Clin. Microbiol. Infect.* **2012**, *18*, E185–E187. [CrossRef]
24. Ellis, M.; Al-Ramadi, B.; Bernsen, R.; Kristensen, J.; Alizadeh, H.; Hedstrom, U. Prospective evaluation of mannan and anti-mannan antibodies for diagnosis of invasive *Candida* infections in patients with neutropenic fever. *J. Med. Microbiol.* **2009**, *58*, 606–615. [CrossRef] [PubMed]
25. Todeschini, G.; Murari, C.; Bonesi, R.; Pizzolo, G.; Verlato, G.; Tecchio, C.; Meneghini, V.; Franchini, M.; Giuffrida, C.; Perona, G.; Bellavite, P. Invasive aspergillosis in neutropenic patients: Rapid neutrophil recovery is a risk factor for severe pulmonary complications. *Eur. J. Clin. Investig.* **1999**, *29*, 453–457. [CrossRef]

26. Miceli, M.H.; Maertens, J.; Buvé, K.; Grazziutti, M.; Woods, G.; Rahman, M.; Barlogie, B.; Anaissie, E.J. Immune reconstitution inflammatory syndrome in cancer patients with pulmonary aspergillosis recovering from neutropenia: Proof of principle, description, and clinical and research implications. *Cancer* **2007**, *110*, 112–120. [CrossRef] [PubMed]
27. Singh, N.; Suarez, J.F.; Avery, R.; Lass-Flörl, C.; Geltner, C.; Pasqualotto, A.C.; Lyon, G.M.; Barron, M.; Husain, S.; Wagener, M.M.; Montoya, J.G. Immune reconstitution syndrome-like entity in lung transplant recipients with invasive aspergillosis. *Transplant Immunol.* **2013**, *29*, 109–113. [CrossRef] [PubMed]
28. Jung, J.; Hong, H.-L.; Lee, S.-O.; Choi, S.-H.; Kim, Y.S.; Woo, J.H.; Kim, S.-H. Immune reconstitution inflammatory syndrome in neutropenic patients with invasive pulmonary aspergillosis. *J. Infect.* **2015**, *70*, 1–9. [CrossRef] [PubMed]
29. Kiprono, S.K.; Masenga, J.E. Immune reconstitution inflammatory syndrome: Cutaneous and bone histoplasmosis mimicking leprosy after treatment. *J. Clin. Exp. Dermatol.* **2012**, *03*, 1–3. [CrossRef]
30. Kiggundu, R.; Nabeta, H.W.; Okia, R.; Rhein, J.; Lukande, R. Unmasking histoplasmosis immune reconstitution inflammatory syndrome in a patient recently started on antiretroviral therapy. *ACR* **2016**, *6*, 27–33. [CrossRef]
31. Passos, L.; Talhari, C.; Santos, M.; Ribeiro-Rodrigues, R.; Ferreira, L.C.D.L.; Talhari, S. Histoplasmosis-associated immune reconstitution inflammatory syndrome. *An Bras. Dermatol.* **2011**, *86*, S168–S172. [CrossRef]
32. Jazwinski, A.; Naggie, S.; Perfect, J. Immune reconstitution syndrome in a patient with disseminated histoplasmosis and steroid taper: Maintaining the perfect balance. *Mycoses* **2011**, *54*, 270–272. [CrossRef] [PubMed]
33. Vergidis, P.; Avery, R.K.; Wheat, L.J.; Dotson, J.L.; Assi, M.A.; Antoun, S.A.; Hamoud, K.A.; Burdette, S.D.; Freifeld, A.G.; McKinsey, D.S.; et al. Histoplasmosis complicating tumor necrosis factor–α blocker therapy: A retrospective analysis of 98 cases. *Clin. Infect. Dis.* **2015**, *61*, 409–417. [CrossRef]
34. Breton, G.; Adle-Biassette, H.; Therby, A.; Ramanoelina, J.; Choudat, L.; Bissuel, F.; Huerre, M.; Dromer, F.; Dupont, B.; Lortholary, O. Immune reconstitution inflammatory syndrome in HIV-infected patients with disseminated histoplasmosis. *AIDS* **2006**, *20*, 119–121. [CrossRef] [PubMed]
35. Edman, J.C.; Kovacs, J.A.; Masur, H.; Santi, D.V.; Elwood, H.J.; Sogin, M.L. Ribosomal RNA sequence shows *Pneumocystis carinii* to be a member of the fungi. *Nature* **1988**, *334*, 519–522. [CrossRef] [PubMed]
36. Thomas, C.F.; Limper, A.H. Current insights into the biology and pathogenesis of Pneumocystis pneumonia. *Nat. Rev. Micro.* **2007**, *5*, 298–308. [CrossRef]
37. Kim, H.-W.; Heo, J.Y.; Lee, Y.-M.; Kim, S.J.; Jeong, H.W. Unmasking granulomatous *Pneumocystis jirovecii* pneumonia with nodular opacity in an HIV-infected patient after initiation of antiretroviral therapy. *Yonsei Med. J.* **2016**, *57*, 1042–1045. [CrossRef]
38. Barry, S.M.; Lipman, M.C.I.; Deery, A.R.; Johnson, M.A.; Janossy, G. Immune reconstitution pneumonitis following *Pneumocystis carinii* pneumonia in HIV-infected subjects. *HIV Med.* **2002**, *3*, 207–211. [CrossRef]
39. Wu, A.K.; Cheng, V.C.; Tang, B.S.; Hung, I.F.; Lee, R.A.; Hui, D.S.; Yuen, K.Y. The unmasking of *Pneumocystis jiroveci* pneumonia during reversal of immunosuppression: Case reports and literature review. *BMC Infect. Dis.* **2004**, *4*, 543–548. [CrossRef]
40. Mok, H.P.; Hart, E.; Venkatesan, P. Early development of immune reconstitution inflammatory syndrome related to *Pneumocystis* pneumonia after antiretroviral therapy. *Int J STD AIDS* **2014**, *25*, 373–377. [CrossRef]
41. Godoy, M.C.B.; Silva, C.I.S.; Ellis, J.; Phillips, P.; Müller, N.L. Organizing pneumonia as a manifestation of *Pneumocystis jiroveci* immune reconstitution syndrome in HIV-positive patients: Report of 2 cases. *J. Thorac. Imaging* **2008**, *23*, 39–43. [CrossRef] [PubMed]
42. Wislez, M.; Bergot, E.; Antoine, M.; Parrot, A.; Carette, M.; Mayaud, C.; Cadranel, J. Acute Respiratory Failure Following HAART Introduction in Patients Treated for *Pneumocystis carinii* Pneumonia. *Am. J. Respir. Crit. Care Med.* **2001**, *164*, 847–851. [CrossRef] [PubMed]
43. Alanio, A.; Hauser, P.M.; Lagrou, K.; Melchers, W.J.G.; Helweg-Larsen, J.; Matos, O.; Cesaro, S.; Maschmeyer, G.; Einsele, H.; Donnelly, J.P.; et al. ECIL guidelines for the diagnosis of Pneumocystis jirovecii pneumonia in patients with haematological malignancies and stem cell transplant recipients. *J. Antimicrob. Chemother.* **2016**, *71*, 2386–2396. [CrossRef] [PubMed]

44. Mori, S.; Polatino, S.; Estrada-Y-Martin, R.M. *Pneumocystis*-associated organizing pneumonia as a manifestation of immune reconstitution inflammatory syndrome in an HIV-infected individual with a normal CD4+ T-cell count following antiretroviral therapy. *Int. J. STD AIDS* **2009**, *20*, 662–665. [CrossRef] [PubMed]
45. Kleindienst, R.; Fend, F.; Prior, C.; Margreiter, R.; Vogel, W. Bronchiolitis obliterans organizing pneumonia associated with Pneumocystis carinii infection in a liver transplant patient receiving tacrolimus. *Clin. Transplant.* **1999**, *13*, 65–67. [CrossRef] [PubMed]
46. Verma, N.; Soans, B. Cryptogenic organizing pneumonia associated with Pneumocystis carinii infection and sirolimus therapy in a renal transplant patient. *Australas. Radiol.* **2006**, *50*, 68–70. [CrossRef] [PubMed]
47. Hall, C.; Hajjawi, R.; Barlow, G.; Thaker, H.; Adams, K.; Moss, P. *Penicillium marneffei* presenting as an immune reconstitution inflammatory syndrome (IRIS) in a patient with advanced HIV. *BMJ Case Rep.* **2013**, *2013*, bcr2012007555. [CrossRef] [PubMed]
48. Sudjaritruk, T.; Sirisanthana, T.; Sirisanthana, V. Immune reconstitution inflammatory syndrome from *Penicillium marneffei* in an HIV-infected child: A case report and review of literature. *BMC Infect. Dis.* **2012**, *12*, 28–31. [CrossRef]
49. Saikia, L.; Nath, R.; Hazarika, D.; Mahanta, J. Atypical cutaneous lesions of *Penicillium marneffei* infection as a manifestation of the immune reconstitution inflammatory syndrome after highly active antiretroviral therapy. *Indian J. Dermatol. Venereol. Leprol.* **2010**, *76*, 45–48. [CrossRef]
50. Ho, A.; Shankland, G.S.; Seaton, R.A. *Penicillium marneffei* infection presenting as an immune reconstitution inflammatory syndrome in an HIV patient. *Int. J. STD AIDS* **2010**, *21*, 780–782. [CrossRef]
51. Thanh, N.T.; Vinh, L.D.; Liem, N.T.; Shikuma, C.; Day, J.N.; Thwaites, G.; Le, T. Clinical features of three patients with paradoxical immune reconstitution inflammatory syndrome associated with *Talaromyces marneffei* infection. *Med. Mycol. Case Rep.* **2018**, *19*, 33–37. [CrossRef] [PubMed]
52. Mortimer, R.B.; Libke, R.; Eghbalieh, B.; Bilello, J.F. Immune reconstitution inflammatory syndrome presenting as superior vena cava syndrome secondary to Coccidioides lymphadenopathy in an HIV-infected patient. *J. Int. Assoc. Physicians AIDS Care* **2008**, *7*, 283–285. [CrossRef] [PubMed]
53. Almeida, S.M.; Roza, T.H. HIV Immune Recovery Inflammatory Syndrome and Central Nervous System Paracoccidioidomycosis. *Mycopathologia* **2016**, *182*, 1–4. [CrossRef] [PubMed]
54. Galhardo, M.C.G.; Silva, M.T.T.; Lima, M.A.; Nunes, E.P.; Schettini, L.E.C.; de Freitas, R.F.; de Almeida Paes, R.; de Sousa Neves, E.; do Valle, A.C.F. *Sporothrix schenckii* meningitis in AIDS during immune reconstitution syndrome. *J. Neurol. Neurosurg. Psychiatry* **2010**, *81*, 696–699. [CrossRef]
55. Dony, A.; Perpoint, T.; Ducastelle, S.; Ferry, T. Disseminated fusariosis with immune reconstitution syndrome and cracking mycotic aortic aneurysm in a 55-year-old patient with acute myeloid leukaemia. *BMJ Case Rep.* **2013**. [CrossRef] [PubMed]
56. Crombie, K.; Spengane, Z.; Locketz, M.; Dlamini, S.; Lehloenya, R.; Wasserman, S.; Maphanga, T.G.; Govender, N.P.; Kenyon, C.; Schwartz, I.S. Paradoxical worsening of *Emergomyces africanus* infection in an HIV-infected male on itraconazole and antiretroviral therapy. *PLoS Negl. Trop. Dis.* **2018**, *12*, e0006173. [CrossRef] [PubMed]
57. Legrand, F.; Lecuit, M.; Dupont, B.; Bellaton, E.; Huerre, M.; Rohrlich, P.S.; Lortholary, O. Adjuvant corticosteroid therapy for chronic disseminated candidiasis. *Clin. Infect. Dis.* **2008**, *46*, 696–702. [CrossRef]
58. Lortholary, O.; Fontanet, A.; Mémain, N.; Martin, A.; Sitbon, K.; Dromer, F.; French Cryptococcosis Study Group. Incidence and risk factors of immune reconstitution inflammatory syndrome complicating HIV-associated cryptococcosis in France. *AIDS* **2005**, *19*, 1043–1049. [CrossRef]
59. Bettelli, E.; Korn, T.; Oukka, M.; Kuchroo, V.K. Induction and effector functions of TH17 cells. *Nature* **2008**, *453*, 1051–1057. [CrossRef]
60. Weaver, C.T.; Hatton, R.D. Interplay between the TH17 and TReg cell lineages: A (co-)evolutionary perspective. *Nat. Rev. Immunol.* **2009**, *9*, 883–889. [CrossRef]
61. Weaver, C.T.; Hatton, R.D.; Mangan, P.R.; Harrington, L.E. IL-17 Family Cytokines and the Expanding Diversity of Effector T Cell Lineages. *Ann. Rev. Immunol.* **2007**, *25*, 821–852. [CrossRef] [PubMed]
62. Martinez, F.O.; Gordon, S. The M1 and M2 paradigm of macrophage activation: Time for reassessment. *F1000Prime Rep* **2014**, *6*, 13–19. [CrossRef] [PubMed]
63. Shearer, G.M. HIV-Induced immunopathogenesis. *Immunity* **1998**, *9*, 587–593. [CrossRef]

64. Becker, Y. The changes in the T helper 1 (Th1) and T helper 2 (Th2) cytokine balance during HIV-1 infection are indicative of an allergic response to viral proteins that may be reversed by Th2 cytokine inhibitors and immune response modifiers-a review and hypothesis. *Virus Genes* **2004**, *28*, 5–18. [CrossRef]
65. Zhang, Y.-H.; He, M.; Wang, Y.; Liao, A.-H. Modulators of the Balance between M1 and M2 Macrophages during Pregnancy. *Front. Immunol.* **2017**, *8*, 120. [CrossRef] [PubMed]
66. Tsiodras, S.; Samonis, G.; Boumpas, D.T.; Kontoyiannis, D.P. Fungal Infections Complicating Tumor Necrosis Factor α Blockade Therapy. *Mayo Clin. Proc.* **2008**, *83*, 181–194. [CrossRef]
67. Yasunami, Y.; Kojo, S.; Kitamura, H.; Toyofuku, A.; Satoh, M.; Nakano, M.; Nabeyama, K.; Nakamura, Y.; Matsuoka, N.; Ikeda, S.; et al. Vα14 NK T cell–triggered IFN-γ production by Gr-1 +CD11b +cells mediates early graft loss of syngeneic transplanted islets. *J. Exp. Med.* **2005**, *202*, 913–918. [CrossRef] [PubMed]
68. Flynn, J.L.; Chan, J.; Lin, P.L. Macrophages and control of granulomatous inflammation in tuberculosis. *Mucosal Immunol.* **2011**, *4*, 271–278. [CrossRef] [PubMed]
69. Das, P.; Rampal, R.; Udinia, S.; Kumar, T.; Pilli, S.; Wari, N.; Ahmed, I.K.; Kedia, S.; Gupta, S.D.; Kumar, D.; et al. Selective M1 macrophage polarization in granuloma-positive and granuloma-negative Crohn's disease, in comparison to intestinal tuberculosis. *Intest. Res.* **2018**, *16*, 426–435. [CrossRef] [PubMed]
70. Gordon, S. Alternative activation of macrophages. *Nat. Rev. Immunol.* **2003**, *3*, 23–35. [CrossRef] [PubMed]
71. Martin-Blondel, G.; Mars, L.T.; Liblau, R.S. Pathogenesis of the immune reconstitution inflammatory syndrome in HIV-infected patients. *Curr. Opin. Infect. Dis.* **2012**, *25*, 312–320. [CrossRef]
72. Nilsson, J.; Boasso, A.; Velilla, P.A.; Zhang, R.; Vaccari, M.; Franchini, G.; Shearer, G.M.; Andersson, J.; Chougnet, C. HIV-1-driven regulatory T-cell accumulation in lymphoid tissues is associated with disease progression in HIV/AIDS. *Blood* **2006**, *108*, 3808–3817. [CrossRef] [PubMed]
73. Montes, M.; Sanchez, C.; Lewis, D.E.; Graviss, E.A.; Seas, C.; Gotuzzo, E.; White, A.C. Jr. Normalization of FoxP3+ Regulatory T Cells in Response to Effective Antiretroviral Therapy. *J. Infect. Dis.* **2010**, *203*, 496–499. [CrossRef] [PubMed]
74. Seddiki, N.; Sasson, S.C.; Santner-Nanan, B.; Munier, M.; van Bockel, D.; Ip, S.; Marriott, D.; Pett, S.; Nanan, R.; Cooper, D.A.; et al. Proliferation of weakly suppressive regulatory CD4+ T cells is associated with over-active CD4+ T-cell responses in HIV-positive patients with mycobacterial immune restoration disease. *Eur. J. Immunol.* **2009**, *39*, 391–403. [CrossRef] [PubMed]
75. Ingram, P.R.; Howman, R.; Leahy, M.F.; Dyer, J.R. Cryptococcal Immune Reconstitution Inflammatory Syndrome following Alemtuzumab Therapy. *Clin. Infect. Dis.* **2007**, *44*, e115–e117. [CrossRef] [PubMed]
76. Otahbachi, M.; Nugent, K. Granulomatous *Pneumocystis jiroveci* pneumonia in a patient with chronic lymphocytic leukemia: A literature review and hypothesis on pathogenesis. *Phytochemistry.* **2007**, *333*, 131–135. [CrossRef]
77. Li, L.; Huang, L.; Sung, S.-S.J.; Lobo, P.I.; Brown, M.G.; Gregg, R.K.; Engelhard, V.H.; Okusa, M.D. NKT cell activation mediates neutrophil IFN-gamma production and renal ischemia-reperfusion injury. *J. Immunol.* **2007**, *178*, 5899–5911. [CrossRef]
78. Mantovani, A.; Cassatella, M.A.; Costantini, C.; Jaillon, S. Neutrophils in the activation and regulation of innate and adaptive immunity. *Nat. Rev. Immunol.* **2011**, *11*, 519–531. [CrossRef]
79. Pelletier, M.; Maggi, L.; Micheletti, A.; Lazzeri, E.; Tamassia, N.; Costantini, C.; Cosmi, L.; Lunardi, C.; Annunziato, F.; Romagnani, S.; et al. Evidence for a cross-talk between human neutrophils and Th17 cells. *Blood* **2010**, *115*, 335–343. [CrossRef]
80. Elenkov, I.J.; Wilder, R.L.; Bakalov, V.K.; Link, A.A.; Dimitrov, M.A.; Fisher, S.; Crane, M.; Kanik, K.S.; Chrousos, G.P. IL-12, TNF-alpha, and hormonal changes during late pregnancy and early postpartum: Implications for autoimmune disease activity during these times. *J. Clin. Endocrinol. Metab.* **2001**, *86*, 4933–4938.
81. Bellocchio, S.; Gaziano, R.; Bozza, S.; Rossi, G.; Montagnoli, C.; Perruccio, K.; Calvitti, M.; Pitzurra, L.; Romani, L. Liposomal amphotericin B activates antifungal resistance with reduced toxicity by diverting Toll-like receptor signalling from TLR-2 to TLR-4. *J. Antimicrob. Chemother.* **2005**, *55*, 214–222. [CrossRef] [PubMed]
82. Ben-Ami, R.; Lewis, R.E.; Kontoyiannis, D.P. Immunocompromised Hosts: Immunopharmacology of Modern Antifungals. *Clin. Infect. Dis.* **2008**, *47*, 226–235. [CrossRef]

83. Gil-Lamaignere, C.; Roilides, E.; Maloukou, A.; Georgopoulou, I.; Petrikkos, G.; Walsh, T.J. Amphotericin B lipid complex exerts additive antifungal activity in combination with polymorphonuclear leucocytes against *Scedosporium prolificans* and *Scedosporium apiospermum*. *J. Antimicrob. Chemother.* **2002**, *50*, 1027–1030. [CrossRef]
84. Roilides, E.; Lyman, C.A.; Filioti, J.; Akpogheneta, O.; Sein, T.; Lamaignere, C.G.; Petraitiene, R.; Walsh, T.J. Amphotericin B Formulations Exert Additive Antifungal Activity in Combination with Pulmonary Alveolar Macrophages and Polymorphonuclear Leukocytes against Aspergillus fumigatus. *Antimicrob. Agents Chemother.* **2002**, *46*, 1974–1976. [CrossRef]
85. Simitsopoulou, M.; Roilides, E.; Maloukou, A.; Gil-Lamaignere, C.; Walsh, T.J. Interaction of amphotericin B lipid formulations and triazoles with human polymorphonuclear leucocytes for antifungal activity against Zygomycetes. *Mycoses* **2008**, *51*, 147–154. [CrossRef] [PubMed]
86. Voelz, K.; May, R.C. Cryptococcal Interactions with the Host Immune System. *Eukaryotic Cell* **2010**, *9*, 835–846. [CrossRef] [PubMed]
87. Wiesner, D.L.; Moskalenko, O.; Corcoran, J.M.; McDonald, T.; Rolfes, M.A.; Meya, D.B.; Kajumbula, H.; Kambugu, A.; Bohjanen, P.R.; Knight, J.F.; et al. Cryptococcal genotype influences immunologic response and human clinical outcome after meningitis. *mBio* **2012**, *3*, e00196-12. [CrossRef] [PubMed]
88. Desnos-Ollivier, M.; Patel, S.; Spaulding, A.R.; Charlier, C.; Garcia-Hermoso, D.; Nielsen, K.; Dromer, F. Mixed infections and *in vivo* evolution in the human fungal pathogen *Cryptococcus neoformans*. *mBio* **2010**, *1*, 1–9. [CrossRef] [PubMed]
89. Alanio, A.; Gits-Muselli, M.; Mercier-Delarue, S.; Dromer, F.; Bretagne, S. Diversity of *Pneumocystis jirovecii* during infection revealed by ultra-deep pyrosequencing. *Front. Microbiol.* **2016**, *7*, 733. [CrossRef] [PubMed]
90. Price, P.; Morahan, G.; Huang, D.; Stone, E.; Cheong, K.Y.M.; Castley, A.; Rodgers, M.; McIntyre, M.Q.; Abraham, L.J.; French, M.A. Polymorphisms in cytokine genes define subpopulations of HIV-1 patients who experienced immune restoration diseases. *AIDS* **2002**, *16*, 2043–2047. [CrossRef]
91. Ogola, G.O.; Ouma, C.; Jura, W.G.; Muok, E.O.; Colebunders, R.; Mwinzi, P.N. A non-synonymous polymorphism in IL-23R Gene (rs1884444) is associated with reduced risk to schistosomiasis-associated Immune Reconstitution Inflammatory Syndrome in a Kenyan population. *BMC Infect. Dis.* **2014**, *14*, 1–7. [CrossRef] [PubMed]
92. Choi, E.H.; Foster, C.B.; Taylor, J.G.; Erichsen, H.C.; Chen, R.A.; Walsh, T.J.; Anttila, V.-J.; Ruutu, T.; Palotie, A.; Chanock, S.J. Association between chronic disseminated candidiasis in adult acute leukemia and common IL4 promoter haplotypes. *J. Infect. Dis.* **2003**, *187*, 1153–1156. [CrossRef] [PubMed]
93. Narendran, G.; Kavitha, D.; Karunaianantham, R.; Gil-Santana, L.; Almeida-Junior, J.L.; Reddy, S.D.; Kumar, M.M.; Hemalatha, H.; Jayanthi, N.N.; Ravichandran, N.; et al. Role of LTA4H Polymorphism in Tuberculosis-Associated Immune Reconstitution Inflammatory Syndrome Occurrence and Clinical Severity in Patients Infected with HIV. *PLoS ONE* **2016**, *11*, e0163298. [CrossRef] [PubMed]
94. Meintjes, G.; Scriven, J.; Marais, S. Management of the Immune Reconstitution Inflammatory Syndrome. *Curr HIV/AIDS Rep* **2012**, *9*, 238–250. [CrossRef] [PubMed]
95. Rhen, T.; Cidlowski, J.A. Anti-inflammatory action of glucocorticoids—New mechanisms for old drugs. *N. Engl. J. Med.* **2005**, *353*, 1711–1723. [CrossRef] [PubMed]
96. Nahid, P.; Dorman, S.E.; Alipanah, N.; Barry, P.M.; Brozek, J.L.; Cattamanchi, A.; Chaisson, L.H.; Chaisson, R.E.; Daley, C.L.; Grzemska, M.; et al. Official American Thoracic Society/Centers for Disease Control and Prevention/Infectious Diseases Society of America Clinical Practice Guidelines: Treatment of Drug-Susceptible Tuberculosis. *Clin. Infect. Dis.* **2016**, *63*, e147–e195. [CrossRef] [PubMed]
97. Meintjes, G.; Wilkinson, R.J.; Morroni, C.; Pepper, D.J.; Rebe, K.; Rangaka, M.X.; Oni, T.; Maartens, G. Randomized placebo-controlled trial of prednisone for paradoxical tuberculosis-associated immune reconstitution inflammatory syndrome. *AIDS* **2010**, *24*, 1–19. [CrossRef] [PubMed]
98. Caillot, D.; Couaillier, J.F.; Bernard, A.; Casasnovas, O.; Denning, D.W.; Mannone, L.; Lopez, J.; Couillault, G.; Piard, F.; Vagner, O.; et al. Increasing volume and changing characteristics of invasive pulmonary aspergillosis on sequential thoracic computed tomography scans in patients with neutropenia. *J. Clin. Oncol.* **2001**, *19*, 253–259. [CrossRef] [PubMed]
99. Crespo, G.; Cervera, C.; Michelena, J.; Marco, F.; Moreno, A.; Navasa, M. Immune reconstitution syndrome after voriconazole treatment for cryptococcal meningitis in a liver transplant recipient. *Liver Transplant.* **2008**, *14*, 1671–1674. [CrossRef] [PubMed]

100. Montaner, J.S.G. Corticosteroids Prevent Early Deterioration in Patients with Moderately Severe *Pneumocystis carinii* Pneumonia and the Acquired Immunodeficiency Syndrome (AIDS). *Ann. Intern. Med.* **1990**, *113*, 14–20. [CrossRef] [PubMed]
101. Chabria, S.; Barakat, L.; Ogbuagu, O. Steroid-exacerbated HIV-associated cutaneous Kaposi's sarcoma immune reconstitution inflammatory syndrome: "Where a good intention turns bad." *Int. J. STD AIDS* **2016**, *27*, 1026–1029. [CrossRef] [PubMed]
102. Fernández-Sánchez, M.; Iglesias, M.C.; Ablanedo-Terrazas, Y.; Ormsby, C.E.; Alvarado-De La Barrera, C.; Reyes-Terán, G. Steroids are a risk factor for Kaposi's sarcoma-immune reconstitution inflammatory syndrome and mortality in HIV infection. *AIDS* **2016**, *30*, 909–914. [CrossRef]
103. Blackmore, T.K.; Manning, L.; Taylor, W.J.; Wallis, R.S. Therapeutic Use of Infliximab in Tuberculosis to Control Severe Paradoxical Reaction of the Brain and Lymph Nodes. *Clin. Infect. Dis.* **2008**, *47*, e83–e85. [CrossRef] [PubMed]
104. Hsu, D.C.; Faldetta, K.F.; Pei, L.; Sheikh, V.; Utay, N.S.; Roby, G.; Rupert, A.; Fauci, A.S.; Sereti, I. A paradoxical treatment for a paradoxical condition: Infliximab use in three cases of mycobacterial IRIS. *Clin. Infect. Dis.* **2015**, *62*, 258–261. [CrossRef] [PubMed]
105. Lwin, N.; Boyle, M.; Davis, J.S. Adalimumab for Corticosteroid and Infliximab-Resistant Immune Reconstitution Inflammatory Syndrome in the Setting of TB/HIV Coinfection. *Open Forum Infect. Dis.* **2018**, *5*, ofy027. [CrossRef] [PubMed]
106. Gaube, G.; De Castro, N.; Gueguen, A.; Lascoux, C.; Zagdanski, A.M.; Alanio, A.; Molina, J.M. Treatment with adalimumab for severe immune reconstitution inflammatory syndrome in an HIV-infected patient presenting with cryptococcal meningitis. *Medecine et Maladies Infectieuses* **2016**, *46*, 154–156. [CrossRef] [PubMed]
107. Sitapati, A.M.; Kao, C.L.; Cachay, E.R.; Masoumi, H.; Wallis, R.S.; Mathews, W.C. Treatment of HIV-Related Inflammatory Cerebral Cryptococcoma with Adalimumab. *Clin. Infect. Dis.* **2010**, *50*, e7–e10. [CrossRef]
108. Brunel, A.-S.; Reynes, J.; Tuaillon, E.; Rubbo, P.-A.; Lortholary, O.; Montes, B.; Le Moing, V.; Makinson, A. Thalidomide for steroid-dependent immune reconstitution inflammatory syndromes during AIDS. *AIDS* **2012**, *26*, 2110–2112. [CrossRef]
109. Kaplan, J.E.; Benson, C.; Holmes, K.K.; Brooks, J.T.; Pau, A.; Masur, H. Guidelines for prevention and treatment of opportunistic infections in HIV-infected adults and adolescents: Recommendations from CDC, the National Institutes of Health, and the HIV Medicine Association of the Infectious Diseases Society of America. *MMR Recomm. Rep.* **2009**, *58*, 1–207.
110. Bergman, P.W.; Björkhem-Bergman, L. Is there a role for statins in fungal infections? *Expert Rev. Anti-Infect. Ther.* **2014**, *11*, 1391–1400. [CrossRef]
111. Sun, H.Y.; Singh, N. Potential role of statins for the management of immune reconstitution syndrome. *Med. Hypotheses* **2011**, *76*, 307–310. [CrossRef] [PubMed]
112. Tleyjeh, I.M.; Kashour, T.; Hakim, F.A.; Zimmerman, V.A.; Erwin, P.J.; Sutton, A.J.; Ibrahim, T. Statins for the prevention and treatment of infections: A systematic review and meta-analysis. *Arch. Intern. Med.* **2009**, *169*, 1658–1667. [CrossRef] [PubMed]
113. Zorzou, M.P.; Chini, M.; Lioni, A.; Tsekes, G.; Nitsotolis, T.; Tierris, I.; Panagiotou, N.; Rontogianni, D.; Harhalakis, N.; Lazanas, M. Successful treatment of immune reconstitution inflammatory syndrome-related hemophagocytic syndrome in an HIV patient with primary effusion lymphoma. *Hematol. Rep.* **2016**, *8*, 1–4. [CrossRef] [PubMed]
114. Calic, Z.; Cappelen-Smith, C.; Hodgkinson, S.J.; McDougall, A.; Cuganesan, R.; Brew, B.J. Treatment of progressive multifocal leukoencephalopathy immune reconstitution inflammatory syndrome with intravenous immunoglobulin in a patient with multiple sclerosis treated with fingolimod after discontinuation of natalizumab. *J. Clin. Neurosci.* **2015**, *22*, 598–600. [CrossRef] [PubMed]
115. Müller, M.; Wandel, S.; Colebunders, R.; Attia, S.; Furrer, H.; Egger, M. Immune reconstitution inflammatory syndrome in patients starting antiretroviral therapy for HIV infection: A systematic review and meta-analysis. *Lancet Infect. Dis.* **2010**, *10*, 251–261. [CrossRef]
116. Manabe, Y.C.; Campbell, J.D.; Sydnor, E.; Moore, R.D. Immune reconstitution inflammatory syndrome: Risk factors and treatment implications. *J. Acquir. Immune Defic. Syndr.* **2007**, *46*, 456–462. [CrossRef] [PubMed]

117. Chang, C.C.; Lim, A.; Omarjee, S.; Levitz, S.M.; Gosnell, B.I.; Spelman, T.; Elliott, J.H.; Carr, W.H.; Moosa, M.-Y.S.; Ndung'u, T.; et al. Cryptococcosis-IRIS is associated with lower *Cryptococcus*-specific IFN-γ responses before antiretroviral therapy but not higher T-cell responses during therapy. *J. Infect. Dis.* **2013**, *208*, 898–906. [CrossRef]
118. Chang, C.C.; Dorasamy, A.A.; Gosnell, B.I.; Elliott, J.H.; Spelman, T.; Omarjee, S.; Naranbhai, V.; Coovadia, Y.; Ndung'u, T.; Moosa, M.-Y.S.; et al. Clinical and mycological predictors of cryptococcosis-associated immune reconstitution inflammatory syndrome. *AIDS* **2013**, *27*, 2089–2099. [CrossRef]
119. Yoon, H.A.; Nakouzi, A.; Chang, C.C.; Kuniholm, M.H.; Carreño, L.J.; Wang, T.; Ndung'u, T.; Lewin, S.R.; French, M.A.; Pirofski, L.-A. Association between plasma antibody responses and risk for Cryptococcus-associated immune reconstitution inflammatory syndrome. *J. Infect. Dis.* **2018**, *17*, 873–880. [CrossRef]
120. Boulware, D.R.; Meya, D.B.; Bergemann, T.L.; Wiesner, D.L.; Rhein, J.; Musubire, A.; Lee, S.J.; Kambugu, A.; Janoff, E.N.; Bohjanen, P.R. Clinical features and serum biomarkers in HIV immune reconstitution inflammatory syndrome after cryptococcal meningitis: A prospective cohort study. *PLoS Med.* **2010**, *7*, e1000384. [CrossRef]
121. Boulware, D.R.; Bonham, S.C.; Meya, D.B.; Wiesner, D.L.; Park, G.S.; Kambugu, A.; Janoff, E.N.; Bohjanen, P.R. Paucity of initial cerebrospinal fluid inflammation in cryptococcal meningitis is associated with subsequent immune reconstitution inflammatory syndrome. *J. Infect. Dis.* **2010**, *202*, 962–970. [CrossRef] [PubMed]
122. Chang, C.C.; Omarjee, S.; Lim, A.; Spelman, T.; Gosnell, B.I.; Carr, W.H.; Elliott, J.H.; Moosa, M.-Y.S.; Ndung'u, T.; French, M.A.; Lewin, S.R. Chemokine levels and chemokine receptor expression in the blood and the cerebrospinal fluid of HIV-infected patients with cryptococcal meningitis and cryptococcosis-associated immune reconstitution inflammatory syndrome. *J. Infect. Dis.* **2013**, *208*, 1604–1612. [CrossRef] [PubMed]
123. Wilkinson, R.J.; Walker, N.F.; Scriven, J.; Meintjes, G. Immune reconstitution inflammatory syndrome in HIV-infected patients. *HIV* **2015**, *7*, 49–64. [CrossRef] [PubMed]
124. Bicanic, T.; Meintjes, G.; Rebe, K.; Williams, A.; Loyse, A.; Wood, R.; Hayes, M.; Jaffar, S.; Harrison, T. Immune reconstitution inflammatory syndrome in HIV-associated cryptococcal meningitis: A prospective study. *J. Acquir. Immune Defic. Syndr.* **2009**, *51*, 130–134. [CrossRef] [PubMed]
125. Shelburne, S.A.; Darcourt, J.; White, A.C.; Greenberg, S.B.; Hamill, R.J.; Atmar, R.L.; Visnegarwala, F. The role of immune reconstitution inflammatory syndrome in AIDS-related *Cryptococcus neoformans* disease in the era of highly active antiretroviral therapy. *Clin. Infect. Dis.* **2005**, *40*, 1049–1052. [CrossRef] [PubMed]
126. Vitoria, M.; Ford, N.; Clayden, P.; Pozniak, A.L.; Hill, A.M. When could new antiretrovirals be recommended for national treatment programmes in low-income and middle-income countries. *Curr. Opin. HIV AIDS* **2017**, *12*, 414–422. [CrossRef] [PubMed]
127. Psichogiou, M.; Basoulis, D.; Tsikala-Vafea, M.; Vlachos, S.; Kapelios, C.J.; Daikos, G.L. Integrase Strand Transfer inhibitors and the emergence of Immune Reconstitution Inflammatory Syndrome (IRIS). *CHR* **2018**, *15*, 1–6. [CrossRef]
128. Dutertre, M.; Cuzin, L.; Demonchy, E.; Puglièse, P.; Joly, V.; Valantin, M.-A.; Cotte, L.; Huleux, T.; Delobel, P.; Martin-Blondel, G. Initiation of antiretroviral therapy containing integrase inhibitors increases the risk of IRIS requiring hospitalization. *J. Acquir. Immune Defic. Syndr.* **2017**, *76*, e23–e26. [CrossRef]
129. Chandesris, M.-O.; Kelaidi, C.; Méchaï, F.; Bougnoux, M.-E.; Brousse, N.; Viard, J.-P.; Poirée, S.; Lecuit, M.; Hermine, O.; Lortholary, O. Granulocyte Colony Stimulating Factor-induced exacerbation of fungus-related Immune Restoration Inflammatory Syndrome: A case of chronic disseminated candidiasis exacerbation. *J. Microbiol. Immunol. Infect.* **2010**, *43*, 339–343. [CrossRef]
130. Blanc, F.-X.; Sok, T.; Laureillard, D.; Borand, L.; Rekacewicz, C.; Nerrienet, E.; Madec, Y.; Marcy, O.; Chan, S.; Prak, N.; et al. Earlier versus later start of antiretroviral therapy in HIV-infected adults with tuberculosis. *N. Engl. J. Med.* **2011**, *365*, 1471–1481. [CrossRef]
131. Torok, M.E.; Yen, N.T.B.; Chau, T.T.H.; Mai, N.T.H.; Phu, N.H.; Mai, P.P.; Dung, N.T.; Chau, N.V.V.; Bang, N.D.; Tien, N.A.; et al. Timing of Initiation of antiretroviral therapy in human immunodeficiency virus (HIV)-associated tuberculous meningitis. *Clin. Infect. Dis.* **2011**, *52*, 1374–1383. [CrossRef] [PubMed]
132. Zolopa, A.R.; Andersen, J.; Komarow, L.; Sanne, I.; Sanchez, A.; Hogg, E.; Suckow, C.; Powderly, W. Early antiretroviral therapy reduces AIDS progression/death in individuals with acute opportunistic infections: A multicenter randomized strategy trial. *PLoS ONE* **2009**, *4*, e5575. [CrossRef] [PubMed]

133. Makadzange, A.T.; Ndhlovu, C.E.; Takarinda, K.; Reid, M.; Kurangwa, M.; Gona, P.; Hakim, J.G. Early versus delayed initiation of antiretroviral therapy for concurrent HIV infection and cryptococcal meningitis in sub-saharan Africa. *Clin. Infect. Dis.* **2010**, *50*, 1532–1538. [CrossRef] [PubMed]
134. Bisson, G.P.; Molefi, M.; Bellamy, S.; Thakur, R.; Steenhoff, A.; Tamuhla, N.; Rantleru, T.; Tsimako, I.; Gluckman, S.; Ravimohan, S.; et al. Early versus delayed antiretroviral therapy and cerebrospinal fluid fungal clearance in adults with HIV and cryptococcal meningitis. *Clin. Infect. Dis.* **2013**, *56*, 1165–1173. [CrossRef] [PubMed]
135. Boulware, D.R.; Meya, D.B.; Muzoora, C.; Rolfes, M.A.; Huppler Hullsiek, K.; Musubire, A.; Taseera, K.; Nabeta, H.W.; Schutz, C.; Williams, D.A.; et al. Timing of antiretroviral therapy after diagnosis of cryptococcal meningitis. *N. Engl. J. Med.* **2014**, *370*, 2487–2498. [CrossRef] [PubMed]
136. Scriven, J.E.; Graham, L.M.; Schutz, C.; Scriba, T.J.; Wilkinson, K.A.; Wilkinson, R.J.; Boulware, D.R.; Urban, B.C.; Meintjes, G.; Lalloo, D.G. The CSF Immune Response in HIV-1-Associated Cryptococcal Meningitis: Macrophage Activation, Correlates of Disease Severity, and Effect of Antiretroviral Therapy. *J. Acquir. Imm. Defic. Syndr.* **2017**, *75*, 299–307. [CrossRef]
137. Southern African HIV Clinicians Society, T. Guideline for the prevention, diagnosis and management of cryptococcal meningitis among HIV-infected persons: 2013 update. *S. Afr. J. HIV Med.* **2013**, *14*, 76–86. [CrossRef]
138. Abassi, M.; Boulware, D.R.; Rhein, J. Cryptococcal Meningitis: Diagnosis and Management Update. *Curr. Trop. Med. Rep.* **2015**, *2*, 90–99. [CrossRef]
139. Singh, N. Hypercalcemia Related to Immune Reconstitution in Organ Transplant Recipients with Granulomatous Opportunistic Infections. *Transplantation* **2006**, *82*, 986. [CrossRef]

5

Antifungal Resistance: Specific Focus on Multidrug Resistance in *Candida auris* and Secondary Azole Resistance in *Aspergillus fumigatus*

Sevtap Arikan-Akdagli [1,*], Mahmoud Ghannoum [2] and Jacques F. Meis [3,4]

1 Department of Medical Microbiology, Mycology Laboratory, Hacettepe University Medical School, TR-06100 Ankara, Turkey
2 Center for Medical Mycology, Department of Dermatology, University Hospitals Cleveland Medical Center, Case Western Reserve University, Cleveland, OH 44106, USA; mag3@case.edu
3 Department of Medical Microbiology and Infectious Diseases, Canisius Wilhelmina Hospital (CWZ), 6532 Nijmegen, The Netherlands; jacques.meis@gmail.com
4 Centre of Expertise in Mycology Radboudumc/CWZ, 6532 Nijmegen, The Netherlands
* Correspondence: sarikanakdagli@gmail.com

Abstract: Antifungal resistance is a topic of concern, particularly for specific fungal species and drugs. Among these are the multidrug-resistant *Candida auris* and azole-resistant *Aspergillus fumigatus*. While the knowledge on molecular mechanisms of resistance is now accumulating, further data are also available for the clinical implications and the extent of correlation of in vitro resistance to clinical outcomes. This review article summarizes the epidemiology of *C. auris* infections, animal models focusing on the activity of novel antifungal compounds in *C. auris* infections, virulence factors, and the mechanisms of antifungal resistance for this multi-resistant *Candida* species. Regarding *A. fumigatus*, the significance of azoles in the treatment of *A. fumigatus* infections, reference methods available for the detection of resistance in vitro, molecular mechanisms of secondary azole resistance, routes of acquisition, and clinical implications of in vitro resistance are covered to provide guidance for the current status of azole resistance in *A. fumigatus*.

Keywords: *Candida auris*; *Aspergillus fumigatus*; antifungal resistance; multidrug resistance; mechanisms of antifungal resistance

---

1. *Candida auris*

1.1. *Epidemiology and Risk Factors for Candida auris Infection*

Nosocomial infections with resistant *Candida* species are increasing and candidemia is becoming a public health concern in Europe, the Americas, and Asia. This is associated with increasing numbers of immunocompromised individuals, the rampant empirical use of broad-spectrum antibiotics and fluconazole, and the widespread use of implanted medical devices. Invasive non-*albicans* candidiasis was mainly reported, until recently, due to *C. glabrata*, *C. parapsilosis*, *C. tropicalis*, and *Pichia kudriavzevii* (*C. krusei*). *C. parapsilosis* is common among newborns, while *C. glabrata* is more prevalent among older adults and patients with cancer. *C. tropicalis*, on the other hand, is more commonly seen in patients with leukemia and neutropenia. *C. parapsilosis*, a skin colonizer, is a common pathogen in intravascular catheter-related infections. *Pichia kudriavzevii*, in turn, is found more often among patients with leukemia and associated neutropenia, who receive fluconazole prophylaxis [1]. A new species, *C. auris*, associated with resistance to several antifungal drugs and difficulty in identification, has been observed to be emerging in the last decade. This yeast was first described in East Asia in 2009, after being isolated from a Japanese patient with otitis externa and three Korean patients with candidemia [2,3]. These observations did not attract much attention from the medical community at the time until clonal outbreaks were observed in several Indian hospitals [4,5]. Shortly after these seminal publications, reports followed from Kuwait, South Africa, and Venezuela [6–10]. *C. auris*, which was never heard of prior to the first publication in 2009, became an emerging global health threat with outbreaks occurring in many health facilities. It is highly likely that *C. auris* was an underreported infection in the first years after 2009 due to difficulties in identification [11–16]. At present, infected and colonized patients have been identified in Australia [17], Austria [18], Belgium [19], Canada [20], China [21–23], Colombia [24,25], Egypt (unpublished), France [19], Germany [19], India [4,26–29], Iran (unpublished), Israel [30,31], Kenya [15], Kuwait [7,9,10], Korea [3,32], Malaysia [33], the Netherlands [15], Norway [19], Oman [34,35], Pakistan [36], Panama [37], Russia [15], Saudi Arabia [38], Singapore [39], South Africa [8,40], Spain [41], Switzerland [42], Thailand [15], United Kingdom [43–46], United States [36,47], United Arab Emirates [48], and Venezuela [6]. More than 4000 cases of infection and colonization, the majority from India and South Africa, have been recorded to date, but it is highly likely that we are observing only the tip of the iceberg.

C. auris is a novel *Candida* species in the *Candida haemulonii* species complex, which causes a wide range of infections, especially in debilitated patients residing in intensive care units (ICUs). A large 18-month prospective study in Indian ICUs recorded 1400 candidemia cases; *C. auris* was identified as the fifth most common cause found in 19 out of 27 ICUs, with a prevalence of 5.3% [27]. In some tertiary care Indian hospitals, *C. auris* is the second most common cause of candidemia after *C. tropicalis* [49]. A tertiary medical center in South America reported *C. auris* as the sixth most common cause of nosocomial bloodstream infections between March 2012 and July 2013 [6]. The mode of spread within the hospital setting is through person to person transmission and via contaminated surfaces and/or equipment. During outbreaks, *C. auris* can contaminate the room of colonized or infected patients [50]. It is therefore of utmost importance to quickly identify contaminated surfaces and screen specimens of patients. Real-time detection and identification of *C. auris* is the target of several molecular kits [51–59]. The survival of *C. auris* for weeks, even months, within the hospital confirms the importance of infection prevention programs [60–62]. Transmission from patient to patient has been documented to lead to skin colonization by *C. auris* and increased risk for candidemia. The hospital environment represents a reservoir that contributes to the nosocomial transmission of *C. auris* similar to that seen with multi-resistant bacterial pathogens [63,64]. Risk factors for infection with *C. auris* are related to immunosuppression, hospitalization in intensive care units over prolonged periods, use of central venous and urinary catheters, and empirical use of antibiotics or antifungals. Adults are mainly affected, but in an outbreak situation in Venezuela 13/18 cases were pediatric patients [6]. As observed in many other studies, all isolates were initially mis-identified as *Candida haemulonii*, a commonly reported mistake [65–67]. Sequencing of the internal transcribed spacer (ITS) region and MALDI-TOF analysis were necessary to identify isolates of the outbreak involved as *C. auris*. The predisposing risk factors for *C. auris* infection are similar to other opportunistic *Candida* species [1]; that is, immunocompromised patients (diabetes mellitus, malignancy, chronic renal disease, neutropenia, HIV), concomitant bacteremia, broad spectrum antibacterial or antifungal therapy within 90 days, surgery within 90 days, presence of central venous catheters or urinary catheters, ICU stay, and parenteral nutrition (PN) administration confer an increased risk of acquiring *C. auris*. A case-control study in an Indian center was conducted to determine specific risk factors predisposing to *C. auris* candidemia [29]. Patients with *C. auris* (n = 74) and non-*auris* (n = 1087) fungemia cases were analyzed. Multivariate analysis showed that patients with respiratory diseases, vascular surgery, and prolonged exposure to fluconazole were more likely to develop ICU-onset *C. auris* fungemia. In describing the epidemiology of *C. auris* infections, the Center for Disease Control (CDC) used whole genome sequencing of 54 isolates collected from India, Pakistan, South Africa, Japan, and Venezuela [36]. Four distinct geographical clades were observed, suggesting emergence at the same time on three continents. Similar geographic clustering was observed with Amplified Fragment Length

Polymorphism(AFLP) and proteomic analysis of *C. auris* isolates from three different continents—Asia, Africa, and Latin America [68]. A recent Whole Genome Sequencing (WGS) and single-nucleotide polymorphism (SNP) analysis of *C. auris* strains isolated in the USA showed multiple introductions of *C. auris* isolates belonging to the four clades, and spread among healthcare facilities [47]. Most *C. auris* strains (>60–90%) are resistant to fluconazole, 10–30% exhibit a high minimum inhibitory concentration (MIC) for amphotericin B, and <5% can be considered resistant to echinocandins [28,69]. Given the recent unprecedented worldwide spread and multidrug resistance, *C. auris* is included in the world's 10 most feared fungi [70].

1.2. Virulence Factors of C. auris

To determine the virulence properties of *C. auris* relative to *C. albicans*, a set of clinical strains were investigated regarding the ability to germinate, adhere, and produce extracellular enzymes [71]. *C. auris* strains failed to germinate but, in contrast and as expected, *C. albicans* germinated profusely. Similarly, *C. auris* exhibited a significantly reduced ability to adhere to silicon elastomer disks relative to *C. albicans*. Moreover, the *C. auris* isolates produced phospholipase and proteinase in a strain-dependent manner (37.5% of the *C. auris* strains possessed phospholipase activity, while 64% evaluated secreted proteinase activity). The last virulence factor evaluated was the ability of *C. auris* to form biofilms. Our data showed that the formed biofilms were mainly composed of yeast cells, while biofilms formed by *C. albicans* had a heterogeneous architecture of biofilms comprised of yeast and hyphae morphology embedded within the extracellular matrix. Furthermore, *C. auris* biofilms had a limited amount of extracellular matrix relative to *C. albicans* and its biofilm thickness was significantly less than the biofilms formed by *C. albicans*. Taken together, these data show that *C. auris* is relatively less pathogenic than *C. albicans*.

1.3. C. auris Animal Models and Activity of Experimental Antifungals

To gain insight into the in vivo virulence of *C. auris*, an immunosuppressed murine model was developed [72,73]. Once the model was established it was used to evaluate the efficacy of two experimental antifungals (rezafungin and APX001A). The data showed that rezafungin had a significantly reduced CFUs/g kidneys fungal burden compared with vehicle- or amphotericin B-treated groups. Furthermore, treatment with rezafungin resulted in a significantly lower CFUs/g tissue fungal burden compared to micafungin-treated animals [72].

Evaluation of the efficacy of APX001 using the optimized immunocompromised mouse model showed that treatment with this experimental drug resulted in a significant increase in animal survival (between 80 and 100% survival in the three treatment groups). In contrast, treatment with anidulafungin led to only a 50% survival rate. In addition, APX001 treatment led to a significant reduction in CFUs/g of kidneys, lung, and brain tissue compared to the vehicle-treated group [73]. In an immunocompetent murine model, virulence was also highest for *C. albicans*, closely followed by *C. auris*, *C. glabrata*, and *C. haemulonii*, respectively [74].

1.4. Resistance of C. auris

Besides being antifungal-resistant, *C. auris* is thermotolerant, grows well up to 42 °C, and is salt-tolerant (up to 10%). These characteristics can be used to design selective media for the detection of *C. auris* for screening purposes which have been used successfully in outbreak investigations [75]. Concerning resistance to antifungal agents, *C. auris* has demonstrated extensive resistance to azoles and amphotericin B [24,28]. The ATP-binding cassette (ABC) transporter activity was significantly higher in *C. auris* than in *C. glabrata* [31]. Several genes show encoding of ABC transporters and the important families of *C. auris* major facilitator superfamily (MFS) genes [76]. An Indian study with a large number of isolates showed that 41% of *C. auris* from India showed resistance to two antifungal classes and 4% to three antifungal agents [28]. Molecular mechanisms responsible for antifungal resistance point to efflux pumps and mutations in the lanosterol 14-alpha-demethylase (*ERG11*) gene to explain the high rate of resistance to fluconazole [28,31]. The latter study demonstrated that 90% of *C. auris* isolates were resistant to fluconazole (MICs 32 to ≥64 mg/L). *ERG11* sequences of resistant *C. auris* exhibited substitutions of the Y132 and K143 amino acids in 77% of the fluconazole-resistant strains. No substitutions at these positions were observed in isolates with low fluconazole MICs (1–2 mg/L), suggesting that these substitutions confer the fluconazole resistance phenotype similar to that described for *C. albicans* [77].

Another study, in a murine model, showed that micafungin was superior compared to fluconazole or amphotericin B, with greater fungicidal activity [78]. These findings make echinocandins the drugs of choice to treat *C. auris* infections and clinical trials are on their way to explore the therapeutic potential of new drugs.

The combination of antifungals such as voriconazole and echinocandins has been shown to be promising in vitro against resistant *C. auris* [79]. Although some studies show variable susceptibility of *C. auris* to the echinocandin class [80], the good news is that there are new drugs in development with excellent activity against *C. auris* [71–73,81–85]. SCY-078, a novel orally bioavailable 1,3-β-D-glucan synthesis inhibitor, has been shown to exhibit both in vitro and in vivo activity against *C. auris*, including some echinocandin-resistant isolates. VT-1598 is another new azole drug with broad activity including *C. auris* isolates (MIC range 0.03–8 mg/L) [86,87].

The cleaning and terminal disinfection of rooms where *C. auris*-colonized patients have been problematic [61,88]. Moore et al. [89] showed that chlorine-based disinfectants and iodine-based skin antiseptics were effective against *C. auris* and reduced environmental contamination and skin colonization. Chlorhexidine-based products may also be effective. Abdolrasouli and collaborators [90] demonstrated that *C. auris* isolates were inhibited by chlorhexidine gluconate at 0.125–1.5% and by iodinated povidone at a concentration of 0.07–1.25%.

2. *Aspergillus fumigatus*

2.1. *Azole Resistance in A. fumigatus*

Aspergillus remains significant as one of the causative agents of invasive infections in immunocompromised individuals and frequently constitutes the most common mold genus isolated in this setting. While voriconazole is the primary drug of choice in the treatment of invasive aspergillosis, the emergence of azole resistance in *Aspergillus* has been a concern since the first report of secondary resistance of *A. fumigatus* to itraconazole in 1997 [91,92]. Antifungal drugs which exert activity against *Aspergillus* spp. are amphotericin B, triazoles, and echinocandins. Furthermore, triazoles are of particular significance due to the availability of oral formulations. Based on this, triazoles constitute significant therapeutic options for patients with chronic pulmonary aspergillosis and allergic bronchopulmonary aspergillosis who require long-term therapy [93] and azole resistance in *A. fumigatus* is thus a concern in this respect as well.

Secondary azole resistance in *A. fumigatus* has been reported from many countries and centers in six continents at extensively varying rates. Similar to those for strains isolated from clinical samples, resistance rates detected for environmental strains are also diverse [94–101]. The ISHAM/ECMM *Aspergillus* Resistance Surveillance Working Group aims to facilitate surveillance studies to determine resistance epidemiology in countries where data are currently lacking and provide further insight in terms of clinical implications [102].

While secondary azole resistance in *A. fumigatus* draws remarkable attention, the awareness and knowledge on primary antifungal resistance in *Aspergillus* strains are also increasing. Among the species which are relatively common causes of invasive infections and exhibit primary resistance or reduced susceptibility to one or more antifungal drugs are *Aspergillus lentulus* (resistance to azoles and amphotericin B and varied susceptibility to caspofungin), *Aspergillus flavus* (reduced susceptibility to amphotericin B and varied susceptibility to caspofungin), *Aspergillus alliaceus* (reduced susceptibility to amphotericin B and caspofungin), and *Aspergillus terreus* (resistance to amphotericin B) [96].

2.2. Detection of Antifungal Resistance In Vitro by Reference Methods

Reference CLSI [103] and EUCAST [104,105] microdilution susceptibility testing methods are available for testing antifungal drugs against *Aspergillus* and recommended for routine use [106,107]. A disk diffusion method of CLSI for testing non-dermatophyte molds and thus applying also to *Aspergillus* is also available [108]. Epidemiological cut-off values have been determined for the interpretation of the results obtained by the CLSI method [109–112], while both epidemiological cut-off values and clinical breakpoints are available for interpreting EUCAST minimum inhibitory concentration values (MIC, mg/L) for some drugs and species [113]. The official reading method for amphotericin B and azole MICs against *Aspergillus* is visual reading for both CLSI and EUCAST methodologies. A spectrophotometric reading alternative for EUCAST amphotericin B and azole MICs at 5% growth cut-off (vs. complete inhibition of growth visually) proved to be a reliable alternative [105].

An agar screening method for the detection of secondary azole resistance in *A. fumigatus* strains has also been validated recently by a multicenter study undertaken by EUCAST [114]. This method uses (in-house or commercially available) 4-well agar plates containing itraconazole (4 mg/L), voriconazole (2 mg/L), and posaconazole (0.5 mg/L); the fourth well serves as the growth control well without any antifungal drug. The ranges of 80–100% and 97–100% were obtained, respectively, for interobserver agreement rate and overall sensitivity. The inter-plate (in-house vs. commercial) agreement rate was high. Similarly, the sensitivity for simulated mixed samples of wild-type and mutant strains and the overall specificity rates also proved to be acceptably high (83–100% and 95–100%, respectively). Based on these data, the assay was validated and is now available as a reference method as documented in EUCAST E.DEF 10.1 [115]. It is an easy and reliable method recommended to be used for routine laboratory work-up, to be followed by reference MIC testing for confirmation in case of the detection of a resistant strain [106].

2.3. Molecular Mechanisms Involved in Secondary Azole Resistance and the Resulting Azole Susceptibility Profiles

Point mutations in the *cyp51A* gene associated with amino acid changes of M220, G54, G138, G448S, as well as L98H are the most common mechanisms of secondary azole resistance in *A. fumigatus*. Extra copies of the *cyp51A* gene (e.g., tandem repeats of a 34- or 46-bp sequence in the promoter of the *cyp51A* gene) may also accompany specific amino acid changes. The typical examples of this combined pattern are TR34/L98H and TR46/Y121F/T289A [116]. A tandem repeat of 53 bp without any accompanying amino acid change has also been described [117,118]. In addition, non-*cyp51* mutations and increased expression of efflux pumps may play a role in the development of secondary azole resistance. On the other hand, the mechanism remains unknown for a number of isolates. The expected azole susceptibility profiles in relation to the associated amino acid changes and/or tandem repeats are summarized in Table 1 [95,116].

Table 1. Expected azole susceptibility profiles with respect to the detected resistance mechanism(s).

Associated Amino Acid Change/Tandem Repeat	Resistance	Reduced Susceptibility	Variable Susceptibility Profile
G54	ITC, POS		
G138	ITC, POS		
G448S	VRC	ITC, POS	
M220	ITC	VRC	POS
TR34/L98H *	ITC, VRC, POS, ISV		
TR46/Y121F/T289A	VRC		ITC, POS
TR53	ITC, VRC	POS	

ISV: isavuconazole; ITC: itraconazole; POS: posaconazole; VRC: voriconazole; *: Isolates with TR34/L98H/S297T/F495I changes may have lower minimum inhibitory concentrations (MICs) of voriconazole in the wild-type range. The S297T mutation might be a compensatory mutation in these cases [119,120].

2.4. *Acquisition of Secondary Azole Resistance*

There are two mechanisms that play a role in the development of secondary azole resistance in *A. fumigatus*. First is the (long-term) azole therapy in an individual patient with chronic pulmonary lung disease mostly in existence of a pulmonary cavity, and second is the direct acquisition of a resistant strain from the environment. The latter develops due to the use of azole fungicides (penconazole, difenoconazole, tetraconazole, and tebuconazole) in the environment in agriculture for plant protection [98,121]. The molecular mechanisms leading to resistance also differ in general for these two routes of acquisition. In the patient-acquired route, M220, G54, and G138 changes are more common while TR34/L98H and TR46/Y121F/T289A patterns are mostly (but not always) observed following environmental acquisition [95,116].

2.5. *Clinical Implications and Current Recommendations for Treatment of Aspergillosis due to Azole-Resistant A. fumigatus*

While high azole MICs [122,123] or the existence of *cyp51A* mutations [124] were found to be correlated with clinical failure in some studies, other investigators were not able to detect any correlation between MICs and survival rates [125]. This may also emphasize the influence of host factors as well as several others on clinical outcomes in invasive fungal infections observed in immunocompromised individuals. The low rates of resistance, i.e., the low number of infections due to azole-resistant strains included in the analysis, may also render it more difficult to detect any possibly existing in vitro–in vivo correlation. "Strong" or "Moderate" recommendations for the treatment of documented azole-resistant aspergillosis, as included in the recently published ESCMID-ECMM-ERS Guideline [106], are liposomal amphotericin B monotherapy (Strength of Recommendation (SoR) and Quality of Evidence (QoE): AIIu) and voriconazole and anidulafungin combination (BIII), respectively. Other options with a "Marginal" level of recommendation (CIII for all noted alternatives) include amphotericin B lipid complex monotherapy, posaconazole and caspofungin combination, caspofungin or micafungin monotherapy. The expert opinion, on the other hand, recommends a modification in primary therapeutic choice of voriconazole in case of local environmental resistance rates of >10%. Voriconazole and echinocandin combination or liposomal amphotericin B monotherapy is recommended for initial therapy under these settings [126].

3. Concluding Remark

The emerging field of molecular mechanisms of antifungal resistance has been an underestimated area of global public health concern, but significant progress has been made lately in *A. fumigatus* and *C. auris*, although research challenges remain formidable.

Author Contributions: S.A.-A., M.G. and J.F.M. prepared the manuscript.

References

1. Pappas, P.G.; Lionakis, M.S.; Arendrup, M.C.; Ostrosky-Zeichner, L.; Kullberg, B.J. Invasive candidiasis. *Nat. Rev. Dis. Primers* **2018**, *4*, 18026. [CrossRef] [PubMed]
2. Satoh, K.; Makimura, K.; Hasumi, Y.; Nishiyama, Y.; Uchida, K.; Yamaguchi, H. *Candida auris* sp. nov., a novel ascomycetous yeast isolated from the external ear canal of an inpatient in a Japanese hospital. *Microbiol. Immunol.* **2009**, *53*, 41–44. [CrossRef] [PubMed]
3. Lee, W.G.; Shin, J.H.; Uh, Y.; Kang, M.G.; Kim, S.H.; Park, K.H.; Jang, H.C. First three reported cases of nosocomial fungemia caused by *Candida auris*. *J. Clin. Microbiol.* **2011**, *49*, 3139–3142. [CrossRef] [PubMed]

4. Chowdhary, A.; Sharma, C.; Duggal, S.; Agarwal, K.; Prakash, A.; Singh, P.K.; Jain, S.; Kathuria, S.; Randhawa, H.S.; Hagen, F.; et al. New clonal strain of *Candida auris*, Delhi, India. *Emerg. Infect. Dis.* **2013**, *19*, 1670–1673. [CrossRef] [PubMed]
5. Chowdhary, A.; Sharma, C.; Meis, J.F. *Candida auris*: A rapidly emerging cause of hospital-acquired multidrug-resistant fungal infections globally. *PLoS Pathog.* **2017**, *13*, e1006290. [CrossRef] [PubMed]
6. Calvo, B.; Melo, A.S.; Perozo-Mena, A.; Hernandez, M.; Francisco, E.C.; Hagen, F.; Meis, J.F.; Colombo, A.L. First report of *Candida auris* in America: Clinical and microbiological aspects of 18 episodes of candidemia. *J. Infect.* **2016**, *73*, 369–374. [CrossRef] [PubMed]
7. Emara, M.; Ahmad, S.; Khan, Z.; Joseph, L.; Al-Obaid, I.; Purohit, P.; Bafna, R. *Candida auris* candidemia in Kuwait, 2014. *Emerg. Infect. Dis.* **2015**, *21*, 1091–1092. [CrossRef]
8. Magobo, R.E.; Corcoran, C.; Seetharam, S.; Govender, N.P. *Candida auris*-associated candidemia, South Africa. *Emerg. Infect. Dis.* **2014**, *20*, 1250–1251. [CrossRef]
9. Khan, Z.; Ahmad, S.; Al-Sweih, N.; Joseph, L.; Alfouzan, W.; Asadzadeh, M. Increasing prevalence, molecular characterization and antifungal drug susceptibility of serial *Candida auris* isolates in Kuwait. *PLoS ONE* **2018**, *13*, e0195743. [CrossRef]
10. Khan, Z.; Ahmad, S.; Benwan, K.; Purohit, P.; Al-Obaid, I.; Bafna, R.; Emara, M.; Mokaddas, E.; Abdullah, A.A.; Al-Obaid, K.; et al. Invasive *Candida auris* infections in Kuwait hospitals: epidemiology, antifungal treatment and outcome. *Infection* **2018**, *46*, 641–650. [CrossRef]
11. Bidaud, A.L.; Chowdhary, A.; Dannaoui, E. *Candida auris*: An emerging drug resistant yeast-A mini-review. *J. Mycol Med.* **2018**, *28*, 568–573. [CrossRef] [PubMed]
12. Clancy, C.J.; Nguyen, M.H. Emergence of *Candida auris*: An international call to arms. *Clin. Infect. Dis.* **2017**, *64*, 141–143. [CrossRef] [PubMed]
13. Forsberg, K.; Woodworth, K.; Walters, M.; Berkow, E.L.; Jackson, B.; Chiller, T.; Vallabhaneni, S. *Candida auris*: The recent emergence of a multidrug-resistant fungal pathogen. *Med. Mycol.* **2018**. [CrossRef] [PubMed]
14. Jeffery-Smith, A.; Taori, S.K.; Schelenz, S.; Jeffery, K.; Johnson, E.M.; Borman, A.; Candida auris Incident Management, T.; Manuel, R.; Brown, C.S. *Candida auris*: a Review of the literature. *Clin. Microbiol. Rev.* **2018**, *31*, e00029-17. [CrossRef] [PubMed]
15. Saris, K.; Meis, J.F.; Voss, A. *Candida auris*. *Curr Opin Infect. Dis.* **2018**, *31*, 334–340. [CrossRef] [PubMed]
16. Tsay, S.; Kallen, A.; Jackson, B.R.; Chiller, T.M.; Vallabhaneni, S. Approach to the investigation and management of patients with *Candida auris*, an emerging multidrug-resistant yeast. *Clin. Infect. Dis.* **2018**, *66*, 306–311. [CrossRef]
17. Heath, C.H.; Dyer, J.R.; Pang, S.; Coombs, G.W.; Gardam, D.J. *Candida auris* sternal osteomyelitis diagnosis in man from Kenya visiting Australia, 2015. *Emerg. Infect. Dis.* **2019**, *25*. (in press).
18. Pekard-Amenitsch, S.; Schriebl, A.; Posawetz, W.; Willinger, B.; Kolli, B.; Buzina, W. Isolation of *Candida auris* from Ear of Otherwise Healthy Patient, Austria, 2018. *Emerg. Infect. Dis.* **2018**, *24*, 1596–1597. [CrossRef]
19. Kohlenberg, A.; Struelens, M.J.; Monnet, D.L.; Plachouras, D.; The Candida Auris Survey Collaborative, G. *Candida auris*: epidemiological situation, laboratory capacity and preparedness in European Union and European Economic Area countries, 2013 to 2017. *Euro Surveill* **2018**, *23*. [CrossRef]
20. Schwartz, I.S.; Hammond, G.W. First reported case of multidrug-resistant *Candida auris* in Canada. *Can. Commun Dis. Rep.* **2017**, *43*, 150–153. [CrossRef]
21. Chen, Y.; Zhao, J.; Han, L.; Qi, L.; Fan, W.; Liu, J.; Wang, Z.; Xia, X.; Chen, J.; Zhang, L. Emergency of fungemia cases caused by fluconazole-resistant *Candida auris* in Beijing, China. *J. Infect.* **2018**. [CrossRef]
22. Tian, S.; Rong, C.; Nian, H.; Li, F.; Chu, Y.; Cheng, S.; Shang, H. First cases and risk factors of super yeast *Candida auris* infection or colonization from Shenyang, China. *Emerg. Microbes Infect.* **2018**, *7*, 128. [CrossRef] [PubMed]
23. Wang, X.; Bing, J.; Zheng, Q.; Zhang, F.; Liu, J.; Yue, H.; Tao, L.; Du, H.; Wang, Y.; Wang, H.; et al. The first isolate of *Candida auris* in China: clinical and biological aspects. *Emerg. Microbes Infect.* **2018**, *7*, 93. [CrossRef] [PubMed]
24. Escandon, P.; Chow, N.A.; Caceres, D.H.; Gade, L.; Berkow, E.L.; Armstrong, P.; Rivera, S.; Misas, E.; Duarte, C.; Moulton-Meissner, H.; et al. Molecular epidemiology of *Candida auris* in Colombia reveals a highly-related, country-wide colonization with regional patterns in Amphotericin B resistance. *Clin. Infect. Dis.* **2018**. [CrossRef] [PubMed]

25. Morales-Lopez, S.E.; Parra-Giraldo, C.M.; Ceballos-Garzon, A.; Martinez, H.P.; Rodriguez, G.J.; Alvarez-Moreno, C.A.; Rodriguez, J.Y. Invasive infections with multidrug-resistant yeast *Candida auris*, Colombia. *Emerg. Infect. Dis.* **2017**, *23*, 162–164. [CrossRef] [PubMed]
26. Biswal, M.; Rudramurthy, S.M.; Jain, N.; Shamanth, A.S.; Sharma, D.; Jain, K.; Yaddanapudi, L.N.; Chakrabarti, A. Controlling a possible outbreak of *Candida auris* infection: lessons learnt from multiple interventions. *J. Hosp. Infect.* **2017**, *97*, 363–370. [CrossRef] [PubMed]
27. Chakrabarti, A.; Sood, P.; Rudramurthy, S.M.; Chen, S.; Kaur, H.; Capoor, M.; Chhina, D.; Rao, R.; Eshwara, V.K.; Xess, I.; et al. Incidence, characteristics and outcome of ICU-acquired candidemia in India. *Intensive Care Med.* **2015**, *41*, 285–295. [CrossRef] [PubMed]
28. Chowdhary, A.; Prakash, A.; Sharma, C.; Kordalewska, M.; Kumar, A.; Sarma, S.; Tarai, B.; Singh, A.; Upadhyaya, G.; Upadhyay, S.; et al. A multicentre study of antifungal susceptibility patterns among 350 *Candida auris* isolates (2009–17) in India: role of the ERG11 and FKS1 genes in azole and echinocandin resistance. *J. Antimicrob. Chemother.* **2018**, *73*, 891–899. [CrossRef]
29. Rudramurthy, S.M.; Chakrabarti, A.; Paul, R.A.; Sood, P.; Kaur, H.; Capoor, M.R.; Kindo, A.J.; Marak, R.S.K.; Arora, A.; Sardana, R.; et al. *Candida auris* candidaemia in Indian ICUs: analysis of risk factors. *J. Antimicrob. Chemother.* **2017**, *72*, 1794–1801. [CrossRef]
30. Belkin, A.; Gazit, Z.; Keller, N.; Ben-Ami, R.; Wieder-Finesod, A.; Novikov, A.; Rahav, G.; Brosh-Nissimov, T. *Candida auris* infection leading to nosocomial transmission, Israel, 2017. *Emerg. Infect. Dis.* **2018**, *24*, 801–804. [CrossRef]
31. Ben-Ami, R.; Berman, J.; Novikov, A.; Bash, E.; Shachor-Meyouhas, Y.; Zakin, S.; Maor, Y.; Tarabia, J.; Schechner, V.; Adler, A.; et al. Multidrug-resistant *Candida haemulonii* and *Candida auris*, Tel Aviv, Israel. *Emerg. Infect. Dis.* **2017**, *23*. [CrossRef]
32. Choi, H.I.; An, J.; Hwang, J.J.; Moon, S.Y.; Son, J.S. Otomastoiditis caused by *Candida auris*: Case report and literature review. *Mycoses* **2017**, *60*, 488–492. [CrossRef] [PubMed]
33. Mohd Tap, R.; Lim, T.C.; Kamarudin, N.A.; Ginsapu, S.J.; Abd Razak, M.F.; Ahmad, N.; Amran, F. A fatal case of *Candida auris* and *Candida tropicalis* candidemia in neutropenic patient. *Mycopathologia* **2018**, *183*, 559–564. [CrossRef]
34. Al-Siyabi, T.; Al Busaidi, I.; Balkhair, A.; Al-Muharrmi, Z.; Al-Salti, M.; Al'Adawi, B. First report of *Candida auris* in Oman: Clinical and microbiological description of five candidemia cases. *J. Infect.* **2017**, *75*, 373–376. [CrossRef] [PubMed]
35. Mohsin, J.; Hagen, F.; Al-Balushi, Z.A.M.; de Hoog, G.S.; Chowdhary, A.; Meis, J.F.; Al-Hatmi, A.M.S. The first cases of *Candida auris* candidaemia in Oman. *Mycoses* **2017**, *60*, 569–575. [CrossRef] [PubMed]
36. Lockhart, S.R.; Etienne, K.A.; Vallabhaneni, S.; Farooqi, J.; Chowdhary, A.; Govender, N.P.; Colombo, A.L.; Calvo, B.; Cuomo, C.A.; Desjardins, C.A.; et al. Simultaneous emergence of multidrug-resistant *Candida auris* on three continents confirmed by whole-genome sequencing and epidemiological analyses. *Clin. Infect. Dis.* **2017**, *64*, 134–140. [CrossRef] [PubMed]
37. Araúz, A.B.; Caceres, D.H.; Santiago, E.; Armstrong, P.; Arosemena, S.; Ramos, C.; Espinosa-Bode, A.; Borace, J.; Hayer, L.; Cedeno, I.; et al. Isolation of *Candida auris* from nine patients in Central America: Importance of accurate diagnosis and susceptibility testing. *Mycoses* **2018**, *61*, 44–47. [CrossRef] [PubMed]
38. Abdalhamid, B.; Almaghrabi, R.; Althawadi, S.; Omrani, A. First report of *Candida auris* infections from Saudi Arabia. *J. Infect. Public Health* **2018**, *11*, 598–599. [CrossRef] [PubMed]
39. Tan, Y.E.; Tan, A.L. Arrival of *Candida auris* fungus in Singapore: Report of the first three cases. *Ann. Acad Med. Singapore* **2018**, *47*, 260–262.
40. Govender, N.P.; Magobo, R.E.; Mpembe, R.; Mhlanga, M.; Matlapeng, P.; Corcoran, C.; Govind, C.; Lowman, W.; Senekal, M.; Thomas, J. *Candida auris* in South Africa, 2012–2016. *Emerg. Infect. Dis.* **2018**, *24*, 2036–2040. [CrossRef]
41. Ruiz-Gaitan, A.; Moret, A.M.; Tasias-Pitarch, M.; Aleixandre-Lopez, A.I.; Martinez-Morel, H.; Calabuig, E.; Salavert-Lleti, M.; Ramirez, P.; Lopez-Hontangas, J.L.; Hagen, F.; et al. An outbreak due to *Candida auris* with prolonged colonisation and candidaemia in a tertiary care European hospital. *Mycoses* **2018**, *61*, 498–505. [CrossRef]
42. Riat, A.; Neofytos, D.; Coste, A.; Harbarth, S.; Bizzini, A.; Grandbastien, B.; Pugin, J.; Lamoth, F. First case of *Candida auris* in Switzerland: discussion about preventive strategies. *Swiss Med. Wkly.* **2018**, *148*, w14622. [PubMed]

43. Borman, A.M.; Szekely, A.; Johnson, E.M. Comparative pathogenicity of United Kingdom isolates of the emerging pathogen *Candida auris* and other key pathogenic *Candida* species. *mSphere* **2016**, *1*. [CrossRef] [PubMed]
44. Schelenz, S.; Hagen, F.; Rhodes, J.L.; Abdolrasouli, A.; Chowdhary, A.; Hall, A.; Ryan, L.; Shackleton, J.; Trimlett, R.; Meis, J.F.; et al. First hospital outbreak of the globally emerging *Candida auris* in a European hospital. *Antimicrob. Resist. Infect. Control.* **2016**, *5*, 35. [CrossRef] [PubMed]
45. Eyre, D.W.; Sheppard, A.E.; Madder, H.; Moir, I.; Moroney, R.; Quan, T.P.; Griffiths, D.; George, S.; Butcher, L.; Morgan, M.; et al. A *Candida auris* outbreak and its Control in an intensive care setting. *N. Engl. J. Med.* **2018**, *379*, 1322–1331. [CrossRef] [PubMed]
46. Rhodes, J.; Abdolrasouli, A.; Farrer, R.A.; Cuomo, C.A.; Aanensen, D.M.; Armstrong-James, D.; Fisher, M.C.; Schelenz, S. Genomic epidemiology of the UK outbreak of the emerging human fungal pathogen *Candida auris*. *Emerg. Microbes Infect.* **2018**, *7*, 43. [CrossRef] [PubMed]
47. Chow, N.A.; Gade, L.; Tsay, S.V.; Forsberg, K.; Greenko, J.A.; Southwick, K.L.; Barrett, P.M.; Kerins, J.L.; Lockhart, S.R.; Chiller, T.M.; et al. Multiple introductions and subsequent transmission of multidrug-resistant *Candida auris* in the USA: a molecular epidemiological survey. *Lancet Infect. Dis.* **2018**, *18*, 1377–1384. [CrossRef]
48. Alatoom, A.; Sartawi, M.; Lawlor, K.; AbdelWareth, L.; Thomsen, J.; Nusair, A.; Mirza, I. Persistent candidemia despite appropriate fungal therapy: First case of *Candida auris* from the United Arab Emirates. *Int. J. Infect. Dis.* **2018**, *70*, 36–37. [CrossRef] [PubMed]
49. Mathur, P.; Hasan, F.; Singh, P.K.; Malhotra, R.; Walia, K.; Chowdhary, A. Five-year profile of candidaemia at an Indian trauma centre: High rates of *Candida auris* blood stream infections. *Mycoses* **2018**. [CrossRef] [PubMed]
50. Piedrahita, C.T.; Cadnum, J.L.; Jencson, A.L.; Shaikh, A.A.; Ghannoum, M.A.; Donskey, C.J. Environmental surfaces in healthcare facilities are a potential source for transmission of *Candida auris* and other *Candida* species. *Infect. Control. Hosp. Epidemiol.* **2017**, *38*, 1107–1109. [CrossRef] [PubMed]
51. Yamamoto, M.; Alshahni, M.M.; Tamura, T.; Satoh, K.; Iguchi, S.; Kikuchi, K.; Mimaki, M.; Makimura, K. Rapid detection of *Candida auris* based on loop-mediated isothermal amplification (LAMP). *J. Clin. Microbiol.* **2018**, *56*. [CrossRef]
52. Kordalewska, M.; Zhao, Y.; Lockhart, S.R.; Chowdhary, A.; Berrio, I.; Perlin, D.S. Rapid and accurate molecular identification of the emerging multidrug-resistant pathogen *Candida auris*. *J. Clin. Microbiol.* **2017**, *55*, 2445–2452. [CrossRef] [PubMed]
53. Leach, L.; Zhu, Y.; Chaturvedi, S. Development and validation of a real-time PCR assay for rapid detection of *Candida auris* from surveillance samples. *J. Clin. Microbiol.* **2018**, *56*. [CrossRef] [PubMed]
54. Martinez-Murcia, A.; Navarro, A.; Bru, G.; Chowdhary, A.; Hagen, F.; Meis, J.F. Internal validation of GPS() MONODOSE CanAur dtec-qPCR kit following the UNE/EN ISO/IEC 17025:2005 for detection of the emerging yeast *Candida auris*. *Mycoses* **2018**, *61*, 877–884. [CrossRef] [PubMed]
55. Ruiz-Gaitan, A.C.; Fernandez-Pereira, J.; Valentin, E.; Tormo-Mas, M.A.; Eraso, E.; Peman, J.; de Groot, P.W.J. Molecular identification of *Candida auris* by PCR amplification of species-specific GPI protein-encoding genes. *Int. J. Med. Microbiol.* **2018**, *308*, 812–818. [CrossRef] [PubMed]
56. Sexton, D.J.; Kordalewska, M.; Bentz, M.L.; Welsh, R.M.; Perlin, D.S.; Litvintseva, A.P. Direct detection of emergent fungal pathogen *Candida auris* in clinical skin swabs by SYBR Green qPCR assay. *J. Clin. Microbiol.* **2018**. [CrossRef] [PubMed]
57. Sexton, D.J.; Bentz, M.L.; Welsh, R.M.; Litvintseva, A.P. Evaluation of a new T2 Magnetic Resonance assay for rapid detection of emergent fungal pathogen *Candida auris* on clinical skin swab samples. *Mycoses* **2018**, *61*, 786–790. [CrossRef] [PubMed]
58. Theill, L.; Dudiuk, C.; Morales-Lopez, S.; Berrio, I.; Rodriguez, J.Y.; Marin, A.; Gamarra, S.; Garcia-Effron, G. Single-tube classical PCR for *Candida auris* and *Candida haemulonii* identification. *Rev. Iberoam Micol.* **2018**, *35*, 110–112. [CrossRef] [PubMed]
59. Hou, X.; Lee, A.; Jimenez-Ortigosa, C.; Kordalewska, M.; Perlin, D.S.; Zhao, Y. Rapid detection of ERG11-associated azole resistance and FKS-associated echinocandin resistance in *Candida auris*. *Antimicrob. Agents Chemother.* **2018**. [CrossRef]

60. Cadnum, J.L.; Shaikh, A.A.; Piedrahita, C.T.; Jencson, A.L.; Larkin, E.L.; Ghannoum, M.A.; Donskey, C.J. Relative resistance of the emerging fungal pathogen *Candida auris* and other *Candida* species to killing by ultraviolet light. *Infect. Control. Hosp. Epidemiol* **2018**, *39*, 94–96. [CrossRef]
61. Kean, R.; Sherry, L.; Townsend, E.; McKloud, E.; Short, B.; Akinbobola, A.; Mackay, W.G.; Williams, C.; Jones, B.L.; Ramage, G. Surface disinfection challenges for *Candida auris*: an in-vitro study. *J. Hosp. Infect.* **2018**, *98*, 433–436. [CrossRef]
62. Welsh, R.M.; Bentz, M.L.; Shams, A.; Houston, H.; Lyons, A.; Rose, L.J.; Litvintseva, A.P. Survival, persistence, and isolation of the emerging multidrug-resistant pathogenic yeast *Candida auris* on a plastic health care surface. *J. Clin. Microbiol.* **2017**, *55*, 2996–3005. [CrossRef] [PubMed]
63. Chowdhary, A.; Voss, A.; Meis, J.F. Multidrug-resistant *Candida auris*: 'new kid on the block' in hospital-associated infections? *J. Hosp. Infect.* **2016**, *94*, 209–212. [CrossRef] [PubMed]
64. Meis, J.F.; Chowdhary, A. *Candida auris*: a global fungal public health threat. *Lancet Infect. Dis.* **2018**, *18*, 1298–1299. [CrossRef]
65. Kathuria, S.; Singh, P.K.; Sharma, C.; Prakash, A.; Masih, A.; Kumar, A.; Meis, J.F.; Chowdhary, A. Multidrug-resistant *Candida auris* misidentified as *Candida haemulonii:* Characterization by matrix-assisted laser desorption ionization-time of flight mass spectrometry and DNA sequencing and its antifungal susceptibility profile variability by Vitek 2, CLSI broth microdilution, and Etest method. *J. Clin. Microbiol.* **2015**, *53*, 1823–1830. [PubMed]
66. Kumar, A.; Prakash, A.; Singh, A.; Kumar, H.; Hagen, F.; Meis, J.F.; Chowdhary, A. *Candida haemulonii* species complex: an emerging species in India and its genetic diversity assessed with multilocus sequence and amplified fragment-length polymorphism analyses. *Emerg. Microbes Infect.* **2016**, *5*, e49. [CrossRef] [PubMed]
67. Mizusawa, M.; Miller, H.; Green, R.; Lee, R.; Durante, M.; Perkins, R.; Hewitt, C.; Simner, P.J.; Carroll, K.C.; Hayden, R.T.; et al. Can multidrug-resistant *Candida auris* be reliably identified in clinical microbiology laboratories? *J. Clin. Microbiol.* **2017**, *55*, 638–640. [CrossRef] [PubMed]
68. Prakash, A.; Sharma, C.; Singh, A.; Kumar Singh, P.; Kumar, A.; Hagen, F.; Govender, N.P.; Colombo, A.L.; Meis, J.F.; Chowdhary, A. Evidence of genotypic diversity among *Candida auris* isolates by multilocus sequence typing, matrix-assisted laser desorption ionization time-of-flight mass spectrometry and amplified fragment length polymorphism. *Clin. Microbiol. Infect.* **2016**, *22*, e271–e279. [CrossRef]
69. Arendrup, M.C.; Prakash, A.; Meletiadis, J.; Sharma, C.; Chowdhary, A. Comparison of EUCAST and CLSI reference microdilution MICs of eight antifungal compounds for *Candida auris* and associated tentative epidemiological cutoff values. *Antimicrob. Agents Chemother.* **2017**, *61*. [CrossRef]
70. Hyde, K.D.; Al-Hatmi, A.M.S.; Andersen, B.; Boekhout, T.; Buzina, W.; Dawson, T.L.; Eastwood, D.C.; Jones, E.B.G.; de Hoog, S.; Kang, Y.; et al. The world's ten most feared fungi. *Fungal Diversity* **2018**. [CrossRef]
71. Larkin, E.; Hager, C.; Chandra, J.; Mukherjee, P.K.; Retuerto, M.; Salem, I.; Long, L.; Isham, N.; Kovanda, L.; Borroto-Esoda, K.; et al. The emerging pathogen *Candida auris*: Growth phenotype, virulence factors, activity of antifungals, and effect of SCY-078, a novel glucan synthesis inhibitor, on growth morphology and biofilm formation. *Antimicrob. Agents Chemother.* **2017**, *61*. [CrossRef]
72. Hager, C.L.; Larkin, E.L.; Long, L.A.; Ghannoum, M.A. Evaluation of the efficacy of rezafungin, a novel echinocandin, in the treatment of disseminated *Candida auris* infection using an immunocompromised mouse model. *J. Antimicrob. Chemother.* **2018**, *73*, 2085–2088. [CrossRef]
73. Hager, C.L.; Larkin, E.L.; Long, L.; Zohra Abidi, F.; Shaw, K.J.; Ghannoum, M.A. In vitro and in vivo evaluation of the antifungal activity of APX001A/APX001 against *Candida auris*. *Antimicrob. Agents Chemother.* **2018**, *62*. [CrossRef] [PubMed]
74. Fakhim, H.; Vaezi, A.; Dannaoui, E.; Chowdhary, A.; Nasiry, D.; Faeli, L.; Meis, J.F.; Badali, H. Comparative virulence of *Candida auris* with *Candida haemulonii*, *Candida glabrata* and *Candida albicans* in a murine model. *Mycoses* **2018**, *61*, 377–382. [CrossRef] [PubMed]
75. Adams, E.; Quinn, M.; Tsay, S.; Poirot, E.; Chaturvedi, S.; Southwick, K.; Greenko, J.; Fernandez, R.; Kallen, A.; Vallabhaneni, S.; et al. *Candida auris* in Healthcare Facilities, New York, USA, 2013–2017. *Emerg. Infect. Dis.* **2018**, *24*, 1816–1824. [CrossRef] [PubMed]
76. Chatterjee, S.; Alampalli, S.V.; Nageshan, R.K.; Chettiar, S.T.; Joshi, S.; Tatu, U.S. Draft genome of a commonly misdiagnosed multidrug resistant pathogen *Candida auris*. *BMC Genomics* **2015**, *16*, 686. [CrossRef] [PubMed]

77. Healey, K.R.; Kordalewska, M.; Jimenez Ortigosa, C.; Singh, A.; Berrio, I.; Chowdhary, A.; Perlin, D.S. Limited ERG11 mutations identified in isolates of *Candida auris* directly contribute to reduced azole susceptibility. *Antimicrob. Agents Chemother.* **2018**, *62*, e01427-18. [CrossRef] [PubMed]
78. Lepak, A.J.; Zhao, M.; Berkow, E.L.; Lockhart, S.R.; Andes, D.R. Pharmacodynamic optimization for treatment of invasive *Candida auris* infection. *Antimicrob. Agents Chemother.* **2017**, *61*. [CrossRef] [PubMed]
79. Fakhim, H.; Chowdhary, A.; Prakash, A.; Vaezi, A.; Dannaoui, E.; Meis, J.F.; Badali, H. In vitro interactions of echinocandins with triazoles against multidrug-resistant *Candida auris*. *Antimicrob. Agents Chemother.* **2017**, *61*. [CrossRef]
80. Kordalewska, M.; Lee, A.; Park, S.; Berrio, I.; Chowdhary, A.; Zhao, Y.; Perlin, D.S. Understanding echinocandin resistance in the emerging pathogen *Candida auris*. *Antimicrob. Agents Chemother.* **2018**, *62*. [CrossRef]
81. Arendrup, M.C.; Chowdhary, A.; Astvad, K.M.T.; Jorgensen, K.M. APX001A in vitro activity against contemporary blood isolates and *Candida auris* determined by the EUCAST reference method. *Antimicrob. Agents Chemother.* **2018**, *62*. [CrossRef]
82. Berkow, E.L.; Angulo, D.; Lockhart, S.R. In vitro activity of a novel glucan synthase inhibitor, SCY-078, against clinical isolates of *Candida auris*. *Antimicrob. Agents Chemother.* **2017**, *61*. [CrossRef] [PubMed]
83. Berkow, E.L.; Lockhart, S.R. Activity of novel antifungal compound APX001A against a large collection of *Candida auris*. *J. Antimicrob. Chemother.* **2018**, *73*, 3060–3062. [CrossRef] [PubMed]
84. Berkow, E.L.; Lockhart, S.R. Activity of CD101, a long-acting echinocandin, against clinical isolates of *Candida auris*. *Diagn Microbiol. Infect. Dis.* **2018**, *90*, 196–197. [CrossRef] [PubMed]
85. Lepak, A.J.; Zhao, M.; Andes, D.R. Pharmacodynamic evaluation of rezafungin (CD101) against *Candida auris* in the neutropenic mouse invasive candidiasis model. *Antimicrob. Agents Chemother.* **2018**, *62*. [CrossRef] [PubMed]
86. Wiederhold, N.P.; Patterson, H.P.; Tran, B.H.; Yates, C.M.; Schotzinger, R.J.; Garvey, E.P. Fungal-specific Cyp51 inhibitor VT-1598 demonstrates in vitro activity against Candida and Cryptococcus species, endemic fungi, including Coccidioides species, Aspergillus species and Rhizopus arrhizus. *J. Antimicrob. Chemother.* **2018**, *73*, 404–408. [CrossRef] [PubMed]
87. Break, T.J.; Desai, J.V.; Healey, K.R.; Natarajan, M.; Ferre, E.M.N.; Henderson, C.; Zelazny, A.; Siebenlist, U.; Yates, C.M.; Cohen, O.J.; et al. VT-1598 inhibits the in vitro growth of mucosal *Candida* strains and protects against fluconazole-susceptible and -resistant oral candidiasis in IL-17 signalling-deficient mice. *J. Antimicrob. Chemother.* **2018**, *73*, 2089–2094. [CrossRef] [PubMed]
88. Ku, T.S.N.; Walraven, C.J.; Lee, S.A. *Candida auris*: Disinfectants and implications for infection control. *Front. Microbiol.* **2018**, *9*, 726. [CrossRef]
89. Moore, G.; Schelenz, S.; Borman, A.M.; Johnson, E.M.; Brown, C.S. Yeasticidal activity of chemical disinfectants and antiseptics against *Candida auris*. *J. Hosp. Infect.* **2017**, *97*, 371–375. [CrossRef] [PubMed]
90. Abdolrasouli, A.; Armstrong-James, D.; Ryan, L.; Schelenz, S. In vitro efficacy of disinfectants utilised for skin decolonisation and environmental decontamination during a hospital outbreak with *Candida auris*. *Mycoses* **2017**, *60*, 758–763. [CrossRef]
91. Denning, D.W.; Venkateswarlu, K.; Oakley, K.L.; Anderson, M.J.; Manning, N.J.; Stevens, D.A.; Warnock, D.W.; Kelly, S.L. Itraconazole resistance in *Aspergillus fumigatus*. *Antimicrob. Agents Chemother.* **1997**, *41*, 1364–1368. [CrossRef]
92. Verweij, P.E.; Chowdhary, A.; Melchers, W.J.; Meis, J.F. Azole resistance in *Aspergillus fumigatus*: Can we retain the clinical use of mold-active antifungal azoles? *Clin. Infect. Dis.* **2016**, *62*, 362–368. [CrossRef] [PubMed]
93. Denning, D.W.; Perlin, D.S. Azole resistance in *Aspergillus*: a growing public health menace. *Future Microbiol.* **2011**, *6*, 1229–1232. [CrossRef] [PubMed]
94. van der Linden, J.W.; Arendrup, M.C.; Warris, A.; Lagrou, K.; Pelloux, H.; Hauser, P.M.; Chryssanthou, E.; Mellado, E.; Kidd, S.E.; Tortorano, A.M.; et al. Prospective multicenter international surveillance of azole resistance in *Aspergillus fumigatus*. *Emerg. Infect. Dis.* **2015**, *21*, 1041–1044. [CrossRef] [PubMed]
95. Meis, J.F.; Chowdhary, A.; Rhodes, J.L.; Fisher, M.C.; Verweij, P.E. Clinical implications of globally emerging azole resistance in *Aspergillus fumigatus*. *Philos Trans. R Soc. Lond B Biol. Sci.* **2016**, *371*. [CrossRef] [PubMed]
96. Goncalves, S.S.; Souza, A.C.; Chowdhary, A.; Meis, J.F.; Colombo, A.L. Epidemiology and molecular mechanisms of antifungal resistance in *Candida* and *Aspergillus*. *Mycoses* **2016**. [CrossRef]

97. Mortensen, K.L.; Mellado, E.; Lass-Florl, C.; Rodriguez-Tudela, J.L.; Johansen, H.K.; Arendrup, M.C. Environmental study of azole-resistant *Aspergillus fumigatus* and other aspergilli in Austria, Denmark, and Spain. *Antimicrob. Agents Chemother.* **2010**, *54*, 4545–4549. [CrossRef] [PubMed]
98. Snelders, E.; Huis In 't Veld, R.A.; Rijs, A.J.; Kema, G.H.; Melchers, W.J.; Verweij, P.E. Possible environmental origin of resistance of *Aspergillus fumigatus* to medical triazoles. *Appl. Environ. Microbiol.* **2009**, *75*, 4053–4057. [CrossRef]
99. Badali, H.; Vaezi, A.; Haghani, I.; Yazdanparast, S.A.; Hedayati, M.T.; Mousavi, B.; Ansari, S.; Hagen, F.; Meis, J.F.; Chowdhary, A. Environmental study of azole-resistant *Aspergillus fumigatus* with TR34/L98H mutations in the *cyp51A* gene in Iran. *Mycoses* **2013**, *56*, 659–663. [CrossRef]
100. Ozmerdiven, G.E.; Ak, S.; Ener, B.; Agca, H.; Cilo, B.D.; Tunca, B.; Akalin, H. First determination of azole resistance in *Aspergillus fumigatus* strains carrying the TR34/L98H mutations in Turkey. *J. Infect. Chemother.* **2015**, *21*, 581–586. [CrossRef]
101. Koehler, P.; Hamprecht, A.; Bader, O.; Bekeredjian-Ding, I.; Buchheidt, D.; Doelken, G.; Elias, J.; Haase, G.; Hahn-Ast, C.; Karthaus, M.; et al. Epidemiology of invasive aspergillosis and azole resistance in patients with acute leukaemia: the SEPIA Study. *Int J. Antimicrob. Agents* **2017**, *49*, 218–223. [CrossRef]
102. Resendiz Sharpe, A.; Lagrou, K.; Meis, J.F.; Chowdhary, A.; Lockhart, S.R.; Verweij, P.E.; ISHAM ECMM Aspergillus Resistance Surveillance Working Group. Triazole resistance surveillance in *Aspergillus fumigatus*. *Med. Mycol.* **2018**, *56*, 83–92. [CrossRef]
103. CLSI. *CLSI Document M38-A2. Reference Method for Broth Dilution Antifungal Susceptibility Testing of Filamentous Fungi; Approved Standard-Second Edition*; Clinical and Laboratory Standards Institute: Wayne, PA, USA, 2008.
104. Arendrup, M.C.; Meletiadis, J.; Mouton, J.W.; Lagrou, K.; Hamal, P.; Guinea, J.; Subcommittee on AFST of the ESCMID for EUCAST. EUCAST Definitive Document E.DEF 9.3.1 Method for the Determination of Broth Dilution Minimum Inhibitory Concentrations of Antifungal Agents for Conidia Forming Moulds. Available online: http://www.eucast.org/ast_of_fungi/methodsinantifungalsusceptibilitytesting/susceptibility_testing_of_moulds/ (accessed on 1 November 2018).
105. Meletiadis, J.; Leth Mortensen, K.; Verweij, P.E.; Mouton, J.W.; Arendrup, M.C. Spectrophotometric reading of EUCAST antifungal susceptibility testing of *Aspergillus fumigatus*. *Clin. Microbiol. Infect.* **2017**, *23*, 98–103. [CrossRef] [PubMed]
106. Ullmann, A.J.; Aguado, J.M.; Arikan-Akdagli, S.; Denning, D.W.; Groll, A.H.; Lagrou, K.; Lass-Flörl, C.; Lewis, R.E.; Munoz, P.; Verweij, P.E.; et al. Diagnosis and management of *Aspergillus* diseases: executive summary of the 2017 ESCMID-ECMM-ERS guideline. *Clin. Microbiol. Infect.* **2018**, *24*, e1–e38. [CrossRef] [PubMed]
107. Patterson, T.F.; Thompson, G.R., 3rd; Denning, D.W.; Fishman, J.A.; Hadley, S.; Herbrecht, R.; Kontoyiannis, D.P.; Marr, K.A.; Morrison, V.A.; Nguyen, M.H.; et al. Practice guidelines for the diagnosis and management of aspergillosis: 2016 Update by the Infectious Diseases Society of America. *Clin. Infect. Dis.* **2016**, *63*, e1–e60. [CrossRef] [PubMed]
108. CLSI. *CLSI Document M51-A. Method for Antifungal Disk Diffusion Susceptibility Testing of Nondermatophyte Filamentous Fungi; Approved Guideline*; Clinical and Laboratory Standards Institute: Wayne, PA, USA, 2010.
109. Espinel-Ingroff, A.; Chowdhary, A.; Gonzalez, G.M.; Lass-Florl, C.; Martin-Mazuelos, E.; Meis, J.; Pelaez, T.; Pfaller, M.A.; Turnidge, J. Multicenter study of isavuconazole MIC distributions and epidemiological cutoff values for *Aspergillus* spp. for the CLSI M38-A2 broth microdilution method. *Antimicrob. Agents Chemother.* **2013**, *57*, 3823–3828. [CrossRef] [PubMed]
110. Espinel-Ingroff, A.; Cuenca-Estrella, M.; Fothergill, A.; Fuller, J.; Ghannoum, M.; Johnson, E.; Pelaez, T.; Pfaller, M.A.; Turnidge, J. Wild-type MIC distributions and epidemiological cutoff values for amphotericin B and *Aspergillus* spp. for the CLSI broth microdilution method (M38-A2 document). *Antimicrob. Agents Chemother.* **2011**, *55*, 5150–5154. [CrossRef]
111. Espinel-Ingroff, A.; Diekema, D.J.; Fothergill, A.; Johnson, E.; Pelaez, T.; Pfaller, M.A.; Rinaldi, M.G.; Canton, E.; Turnidge, J. Wild-type MIC distributions and epidemiological cutoff values for the triazoles and six *Aspergillus* spp. for the CLSI broth microdilution method (M38-A2 document). *J. Clin. Microbiol.* **2010**, *48*, 3251–3257. [CrossRef]
112. CLSI. *CLSI Document M59. Epidemiological Cutoff Values for Antifungal Susceptibility Testing*, 1st ed.; Clinical and Laboratory Standards Institute: Wayne, PA, USA, 2016.
113. EUCAST. Available online: http://www.eucast.org/ (accessed on 1 November 2018).

114. Arendrup, M.C.; Verweij, P.E.; Mouton, J.W.; Lagrou, K.; Meletiadis, J. Multicentre validation of 4-well azole agar plates as a screening method for detection of clinically relevant azole-resistant *Aspergillus fumigatus*. *J. Antimicrob. Chemother.* **2017**, *72*, 3325–3333. [CrossRef]
115. Guinea, J.; Verweij, P.E.; Meletiadis, J.; Mouton, J.W.; Barchiesi, F.; Arendrup, M.C.; Subcommittee on Antifungal Susceptibility Testing of the ESCMID European Committee for Antimicrobial Susceptibility Testing (EUCAST), EUCAST-AFST; Arendrup, M.C.; Arikan-Akdagli, S.; Barchiesi, F.; et al. How to: EUCAST recommendations on the screening procedure E.Def 10.1 for the detection of azole resistance in *Aspergillus fumigatus* isolates using four well azole-containing agar plates. *Clin. Microbiol. Infect.* **2018**. [CrossRef]
116. Chowdhary, A.; Sharma, C.; Meis, J.F. Azole-resistant aspergillosis: Epidemiology, molecular mechanisms, and treatment. *J. Infect. Dis.* **2017**, *216*, S436–S444. [CrossRef]
117. Alvarez-Moreno, C.; Lavergne, R.A.; Hagen, F.; Morio, F.; Meis, J.F.; Le Pape, P. Azole-resistant *Aspergillus fumigatus* harboring TR34/L98H, TR46/Y121F/T289A and TR53 mutations related to flower fields in Colombia. *Sci Rep.* **2017**, *7*, 45631. [CrossRef] [PubMed]
118. Hodiamont, C.J.; Dolman, K.M.; Ten Berge, I.J.; Melchers, W.J.; Verweij, P.E.; Pajkrt, D. Multiple-azole-resistant *Aspergillus fumigatus* osteomyelitis in a patient with chronic granulomatous disease successfully treated with long-term oral posaconazole and surgery. *Med. Mycol.* **2009**, *47*, 217–220. [CrossRef] [PubMed]
119. Abdolrasouli, A.; Rhodes, J.; Beale, M.A.; Hagen, F.; Rogers, T.R.; Chowdhary, A.; Meis, J.F.; Armstrong-James, D.; Fisher, M.C. Genomic context of azole resistance mutations in *Aspergillus fumigatus* determined using whole-genome sequencing. *MBio* **2015**, *6*, e00536. [CrossRef]
120. Deng, S.; Zhang, L.; Ji, Y.; Verweij, P.E.; Tsui, K.M.; Hagen, F.; Houbraken, J.; Meis, J.F.; Abliz, P.; Wang, X.; et al. Triazole phenotypes and genotypic characterization of clinical *Aspergillus fumigatus* isolates in China. *Emerg. Microbes Infect.* **2017**, *6*, e109. [CrossRef] [PubMed]
121. Snelders, E.; van der Lee, H.A.; Kuijpers, J.; Rijs, A.J.; Varga, J.; Samson, R.A.; Mellado, E.; Donders, A.R.; Melchers, W.J.; Verweij, P.E. Emergence of azole resistance in *Aspergillus fumigatus* and spread of a single resistance mechanism. *PLoS Med.* **2008**, *5*, e219. [CrossRef] [PubMed]
122. van der Linden, J.W.; Snelders, E.; Kampinga, G.A.; Rijnders, B.J.; Mattsson, E.; Debets-Ossenkopp, Y.J.; Kuijper, E.J.; Van Tiel, F.H.; Melchers, W.J.; Verweij, P.E. Clinical implications of azole resistance in *Aspergillus fumigatus*, The Netherlands, 2007–2009. *Emerg. Infect. Dis.* **2011**, *17*, 1846–1854. [CrossRef] [PubMed]
123. Lestrade, P.P.; Bentvelsen, R.G.; Schauwvlieghe, A.; Schalekamp, S.; van der Velden, W.; Kuiper, E.J.; van Paassen, J.; van der Hoven, B.; van der Lee, H.A.; Melchers, W.J.G.; et al. Voriconazole resistance and mortality in invasive aspergillosis: A multicenter retrospective cohort study. *Clin. Infect. Dis.* **2018**. [CrossRef]
124. Chong, G.M.; van der Beek, M.T.; von dem Borne, P.A.; Boelens, J.; Steel, E.; Kampinga, G.A.; Span, L.F.; Lagrou, K.; Maertens, J.A.; Dingemans, G.J.; et al. PCR-based detection of *Aspergillus fumigatus Cyp51A* mutations on bronchoalveolar lavage: a multicentre validation of the AsperGenius assay(R) in 201 patients with haematological disease suspected for invasive aspergillosis. *J. Antimicrob. Chemother.* **2016**, *71*, 3528–3535. [CrossRef]
125. Heo, S.T.; Tatara, A.M.; Jimenez-Ortigosa, C.; Jiang, Y.; Lewis, R.E.; Tarrand, J.; Tverdek, F.; Albert, N.D.; Verweij, P.E.; Meis, J.F.; et al. Changes in in vitro susceptibility patterns of *Aspergillus* to triazoles and correlation with aspergillosis outcome in a tertiary care cancer center, 1999–2015. *Clin. Infect. Dis.* **2017**, *65*, 216–225. [CrossRef]
126. Verweij, P.E.; Ananda-Rajah, M.; Andes, D.; Arendrup, M.C.; Bruggemann, R.J.; Chowdhary, A.; Cornely, O.A.; Denning, D.W.; Groll, A.H.; Izumikawa, K.; et al. International expert opinion on the management of infection caused by azole-resistant *Aspergillus fumigatus*. *Drug Resist. Updates* **2015**, *21–22*, 30–40. [CrossRef]

6

Genome-Wide Identification of circRNAs in Pathogenic Basidiomycetous Yeast *Cryptococcus neoformans* Suggests Conserved circRNA Host Genes over Kingdoms

Liang Huo †, Ping Zhang †, Chenxi Li, Kashif Rahim, Xiaoran Hao, Biyun Xiang and Xudong Zhu *

Beijing Key Laboratory of Genetic Engineering Drug and Biotechnology, Institute of Biochemistry and Molecular Biology, College of Life Sciences, Beijing Normal University (CLS-BNU), Beijing 100875, China; cryptoleon@gmail.com (L.H.); zp1516@163.com (P.Z.); lcx1219@163.com (C.L.); kashifbangash073@gmail.com (K.R.); hxrr_563@163.com (X.H.); xby6024@126.com (B.X.)

* Correspondence: zhu11187@bnu.edu.cn

† These authors contributed equally to this work.

Abstract: Circular RNAs (circRNAs), a novel class of ubiquitous and intriguing noncoding RNA, have been found in a number of eukaryotes but not yet basidiomycetes. In this study, we identified 73 circRNAs from 39.28 million filtered RNA reads from the basidiomycete *Cryptococcus neoformans* JEC21 using next-generation sequencing (NGS) and the bioinformatics tool circular RNA identification (CIRI). Furthermore, mapping of newly found circRNAs to the genome showed that 73.97% of the circRNAs originated from exonic regions, whereas 20.55% were from intergenic regions and 5.48% were from intronic regions. Enrichment analysis of circRNA host genes was conducted based on the Gene Ontology and Kyoto Encyclopedia of Genes and Genomes pathway databases. The results reveal that host genes are mainly responsible for primary metabolism and, interestingly, ribosomal protein production. Furthermore, we uncovered a high-level circRNA that was a transcript from the guanosine triphosphate (GTP)ase gene *CNM01190* (gene ID: 3255052) in our yeast. Coincidentally, *YPT5*, *CNM01190*'s ortholog of the GTPase in *Schizosaccharomyces pombe*, protists, and humans, has already been proven to generate circRNAs. Additionally, overexpression of RNA debranching enzyme *DBR1* had varied influence on the expression of circRNAs, indicating that multiple circRNA biosynthesis pathways exist in *C. neoformans*. Our study provides evidence for the existence of stable circRNAs in the opportunistic human pathogen *C. neoformans* and raises a question regarding their role related to pathogenesis in this yeast.

Keywords: *Cryptococcus neoformans*; next-generation sequencing (NGS); circRNAs; RNA debranching enzyme; GTPase-encoding gene

---

1. Introduction

Circular RNAs (circRNAs), characterized by a closed loop structure, have been a hot topic of research in RNA biology since their wildly diverse and multiple functions were confirmed [1,2]. The fact that the 3′ and 5′ ends of those RNAs are joined by covalent bonds makes them lack polyadenylated tails and 5′–3′ polarity [3]. As a result, circRNAs are considered more stable than linear RNA molecules and more resistant to degradation by RNase R, which is an efficient 3′ to 5′ exoribonuclease [4].

Although the first case of circRNAs was reported in plant-based virus as early as 1976 [5], circRNAs have been discarded as "junk-RNA developed by messenger RNA (mRNA) splicing" and ignored by most research groups [6]. This situation remained for decades, until abundant circRNAs were uncovered in a variety of normal and malignant human cells in 2012 [7] and circRNAs were demonstrated as efficient "microRNA sponges" in 2013 [8]. With the development of high-throughput sequencing technology and RNA circularization prediction algorithms, such as circular RNA identification (CIRI) [9], circular (CIRC) explorer [10], and known and novel isoform explorer (KNIFE) [11], an increasing number of circRNAs have been detected in protists, yeasts, plants, flies, and mammals [12,13].

The mechanism of circRNA biogenesis is intricate, regulated by multiple factors, and varying among different species. In general, the circularization of RNAs can be accomplished through at least four disparate paths: spliceosome-dependent [14], intron-pairing-driven [15], protein factors-associated [16], and lariat-driven paths [17]. Recent studies also reveal distinctly crucial functions of circRNAs, such as microRNA (miRNA) sponge, post-transcription regulation, rolling circle translation, and creation of circRNA-derived pseudogenes [6,18,19]. However, the mechanism has not been illustrated thoroughly and it deserves to be investigated further.

The basidiomycetous yeast *Cryptococcus neoformans* is an opportunistic human pathogen that has been life-threatening to immunodeficient groups such as human immunodeficiency virus (HIV)-infected patients [20]. Efforts have been made by laboratories worldwide to understand the fundamentals of its pathogenic progress and its virulence determinants. Considering the fact that knowledge about circRNA molecules is limited, it may be necessary to define the potential role of circRNA in *C. neoformans*. Unfortunately, circRNAs have not been reported in this fungus, nor in the whole group of basidiomycetes. Thus, here we attempted to identify circRNAs from *C. neoformans*, and subsequently analyzed the features and conducted functional annotation of those circRNAs. We identified in this study 73 unique circRNAs in this basidiomycetous yeast. Interestingly, we also found the existence of small guanosine triphosphatase (GTPase)-encoding genes, which are conserved circRNA-host genes in yeasts and some other eukaryotic organisms. Finally, we demonstrate the influence of an RNA debranching enzyme, Dbr1, on the expression of circRNAs.

2. Materials and Methods

2.1. Strains and Media

The strain *C. neoformans* var. *neoformans* JEC21 (serotype D, MATα) was used for circRNA analysis in this study. Yeast extract–peptone–dextrose (YPD) medium (2% glucose, 2% peptone, 1% yeast extract, pH 6.0) was used for routine growth of *C. neoformans*.

2.2. RNA Isolation and Quality Control

JEC21 was cultured in 5 mL liquid YPD medium for 18 h at 30 °C. Fresh yeast cells were collected by centrifugation, and approximately 0.1 g of yeast cells was washed by wash buffer (0.1 M ethylenediaminetetraacetic acid (EDTA), 0.5 M sodium chloride) three times at 4 °C. Fungal capsule was broken by Bullet Blender Storm 24 (Next Advance, Troy, NY, USA) for 2 min. Total RNA was extracted using the RNAiso (Takara, Shiga, Japan) according to the protocol supplied with the reagent. RNA concentration was measured by POLARstar Omega (BMG Labtech, Offenburg, Germany), and RNA quality was tested by Agilent 2100 (Agilent Technologies, Santa Clara, CA, USA). The quality control threshold was set as follows: A260/A280 ratio > 1.8, A260/A230 ratio > 1.8, RNA integrity number value > 7.0.

2.3. Deep RNA Sequencing and In Silico Discovery of Circular RNAs

Construction of a RNA library, as well as deep RNA sequencing, was accomplished by a commercial service (Genewiz, Suzhou, China). Briefly, Ribominus^{TM} transcriptome isolation kit (Thermo Fisher Scientific, Waltham, MA, USA) was used to remove ribosome RNA in the total RNA. RNase R (Takara) treatment was performed according to the manufacturer's protocol to remove linear RNA in the RNA samples. KAPA Stranded mRNA-seq Kit (Kapa Biosystems, Wilmington,

MA, USA) was utilized for the generation of RNA-sequencing (RNA-seq) libraries according to the manufacturer's protocol. Next-generation sequencing was then conducted on a HighSeqTM 2500 system (Illumina, San Diego, CA, USA). To remove the low-quality reads in the raw paired-end data, such as the primer/adaptor sequences and non-ATGC reads, IlluQC_PRLL.pl v 2.3.3 software [21] was used to perform quality check with the parameter set as 20. The reads with more than or equal to the specified quality score (20 in this study) are filtered as high-quality reads. Subsequently, clean data were aligned to the *C. neoformans* JEC21 genome (Cryptococcus_neoformans.GCA_000091045.1.dna.toplevel.fa, release 37) using Burrows–Wheeler aligner (BWA) (version 0.6) software with default settings [22]. The 19Mb genome sequence of *C. neoformans* JEC21 consists of 14 chromosomes with different lengths changing from 762 kilobase (kb) pairs to 2.3 megabase (Mb) pairs.

The CIRI algorithm (version 1.2) was the tool to identify circRNAs in *C. neoformans* JEC21 [9]. CIRI was performed with default options, with the computer command: CIRI_v1.2.pl -I input.sam -O output_circRNAs.txt –F genome.fa -P -A Ensembl_Cn37.gtf. Counts of identified circRNA reads were normalized by read length, and the number of reads mapping (spliced reads per billion mapping) was determined after CIRI prediction [23].

2.4. Gene Ontology Category and Kyoto Encyclopedia of Genes and Genomes Pathway Analysis

The circRNA host genes were functionally analyzed according to gene ontology (GO) by the database for annotation, visualization, and integrated discovery (DAVID) 6.7 web server (https://david.ncifcrf.gov) with the default options [24]. The KOBAS 2.0 web server was used to uncover the Kyoto Encyclopedia of Genes and Genomes (KEGG) biological pathways of circRNA host genes with the default settings [25].

2.5. Validation of Circular RNAs

To confirm the existence of certain circRNAs of interest, e.g., circCNYPT5, we adopted an approach of outward polymerase chain reaction (PCR) with a pair of primers designed for outward amplification. Briefly, total RNA was extracted with RNAiso reagent (Takara) as described in Section 2.2. complementary DNA (cDNA) synthesis was performed with the FastQuant RT Kit with genomic DNase (gDNase) (Tiangen Biotech, Beijing, China). The 50 μL amplification reaction system contained 0.5 μL Takara Ex Taq, 5 μL 10× Ex Taq Buffer, 4 μL deoxyribonucleotide triphosphates (dNTPs), 2 μL/2 μL forward/reverse primers, and 36.5 μL double distilled water (ddH_2O). The PCR program was set as follows: 98 °C for 2 min, 32 cycles at 98 °C for 10 s, 55 °C for 20 s, and 72 °C for 30 s; the final elongation step was run at 72 °C for 5 min. PCR products with expected length (~250 base pairs (bp)) were separated by 0.8% agarose gel electrophoresis and purified with TIANgel midi purification kit (Tiangen Biotech) according to the manufacturer's instruction. Sanger sequencing was employed to confirm the existence of the back-splicing junction sites (Genewiz).

2.6. Other Online Database and Software

The annotation and nomenclature of *C. neoformans* JEC21 genes in this article were referred to the Ensemble Fungi database (http://fungi.ensembl.org). The multiple alignments of amino acid sequences were conducted by the Clustal Omega web server [26] with default settings.

2.7. Construction of DBR1 Gene Overexpression Vector

To investigate the regulation of circRNAs by *DBR1*, we overexpressed the gene in the wild-type JEC21 strain. The whole *DBR1* gene, including an 800-bp flanking sequence, was obtained by PCR with the protocol described in Section 2.5, except the elongation time for each cycle was 2 min. The pBS-HYG plasmid was linearized with the restriction enzyme Hind III. Then the In-Fusion® HD cloning kit (Takara) was employed to ligate the linearized plasmid and *DBR1* fragment. Subsequently, recombinant plasmid pBS-HYG-DBR1 was linearized by Xba I enzyme and transformed into the wild-type *C. neoformans* JEC21 cells. To select positive transformants, cells were screened on YPD plates containing 100 μg/mL hygromycin. Genomic DNA of two randomly selected clones, OE-1 and OE-2, was extracted and used in subsequent experiments. PCR was performed to confirm the existence of pBS-HYG-DBR1 in the genome of selected transformants using the same protocol as described in Section 2.5.

2.8. Quantitative and Semiquantitative Reverse Transcription Polymerase Chain Reaction

Total RNA of JEC21, OE-1, and OE-2 was extracted as described in Section 2.2. Reverse transcription (RT) of total RNA was conducted by Fast Quant RT kit with gDNase (Tiangen Biotech). Briefly, 1 μL total RNA, 2 μL 5× *g* DNA buffer, and 7 μL ddH_2O were incubated at 42 °C for 10 min, then 2 μL 10× Fast RT Buffer, 1 μL RT enzyme mix, 2 μL Fast Quant RT primer mix, and 5 RNase-Free ddH_2O were added to previous tubes and incubated at 42 °C for 15 min. The reaction was stopped by incubating at 95 °C for 10 s. For *DBR1* mRNA quantification, LightCycler 480 II and corresponding LC 480 SYBR Green I Master (Roche, Basel, Switzerland) were employed. The PCR reaction system included 10 μL 2× Master Mix, 1 μL forward/reverse primers (10 μm), 1 μL cDNA, and 7 μL ddH_2O. Each reaction was performed in triplicate. Non-RT RNA was used as a template in negative control and actin mRNA served as reference. Specificity of primers was validated by checking the melting curves. The $2^{-\Delta\Delta Ct}$ method was employed to calculate expression levels of target genes in this study. Semiquantitative reverse transcription PCR was performed using the PCR protocol described in Section 2.5, except only 25 circles were applied.

3. Results

3.1. Genomewide Identification of Circular RNAs

To investigate circRNAs on a genome-wide level, we isolated total RNAs from the *C. neoformans* JEC21 strain. After eliminating ribosome RNAs (rRNAs) and treating with RNase R, the total RNA was utilized to construct libraries for deep sequencing by the Illumina HighSeq 2500 platform. The sequencing data reached 6.26 Giga nucleotides (Gnt) raw bases in total, covering 41.70 million paired-end individual reads sized above 150 nt. After trimming adaptors and filtering low-quality reads, we obtained 39.28 million clean reads (Table 1).

Table 1. RNA-sequencing data of *Cryptococcus neoformans* JEC1.

Sample Name	Raw Reads	Filtered Reads	Raw Base	Filtered Base	Q20 (%) [1]
Cn JEC21	41,703,834	39,280,024	6.26 Gnt	6.16 Gnt	98.52

[1] Q20 refers to the percentage of nucleotides with Phred quality score > 20, which means base accuracy is 99%. Gnt: Giga nucleotides.

Clean reads were then mapped to the *C. neoformans* JEC21 genome by BWA software. The mapped reads were input to CIRI, a published circRNA identifier, to identify the candidates of circRNAs. To reduce false-positive candidates, the circRNAs that had more than one back-splicing junction read were considered. After a two-step filtration, 73 individual circRNAs containing high-confident back-splicing junctions were obtained. The number of reads for the 73 unique circRNAs was counted to 820. Only 20 of the 73 circRNAs (27.4%) had more than four back-splicing junction reads. The 10 with the highest junction reads are listed (Table 2) and detailed information on all predicted circRNAs is available (Supplementary Table S2). The above data show that the absolute number of unique cryptococcal circRNAs is low compared to that of circRNAs in higher eukaryotes, such as animals or plants. Specifically, researchers have detected 3001 circRNAs from human cells [27] and 5372 circRNAs from soybeans [28]. However, when referring to the relative expression levels using the ratio of circRNAs number to genome size (Mb), the results changed in which the relative expression of *C. neoformans* circRNAs (~3.74) is much higher than that of human (~1.00), but a little lower than soybean (~4.88).

Table 2. Detailed information on the 10 circRNAs with the highest back-splicing reads.

circRNA ID	Chr	RNA Size	circRNA Start Loci	CircRNA End Loci	Junction Reads [1]
12:174494-175325	12	831	174494	175325	410
13:359406-359654	13	248	359406	359654	67
7:1027082-1027487	7	405	1027082	1027487	29
13:603431-604144	13	713	603431	604144	28
4:1303545-1304160	4	615	1303545	1304160	24
12:174265-175325	12	1060	174265	175325	23
12:174461-175325	12	864	174461	175325	22
11:62574-63095	11	521	62574	63095	11
13:89597-90783	13	1186	89597	90783	8
2:661847-663003	2	1156	661847	663003	7

[1] Junction reads means counts of back-splicing reads. Chr: Chromosome.

We sorted the unique circRNAs into three groups according to the positioning of their two ends on chromosomes (exonic, intronic, and intergenic regions). Among them, 54 (73.97%) of the 73 circRNAs were generated from exons of protein-coding open reading frames (ORFs) and 15 (20.55%) were intergenic circRNAs. Only four (5.48%) had intronic junctions. Besides unique circRNAs, we also calculated the total reads of each type of circRNA. Our data show that 38.17, 1.46, and 60.37% of the total 820 reads were distributed to exonic, intronic, and intergenic circRNAs, respectively (Figure 1). However, exons, introns and intergenic sequences occupy 54.14, 11.97, and 33.89%, respectively, of the whole *C. neoformans* genome [20]. Thus, these results reveal that intergenic circRNAs have higher mean reads than exonic circRNAs, although the latter consists of the majority of unique circRNAs.

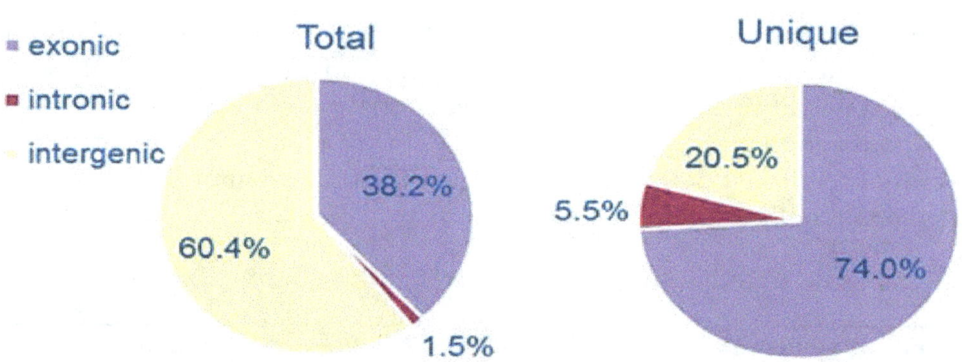

Figure 1. Percentages of three groups of circular RNAs. The circRNAs were classified as exonic, intronic, and intergenic according to the back-splicing junction position on chromosomes. Total circRNAs, calculated as back-splicing junction reads, are shown in the left panel, while unique circRNAs are shown in the right panel.

3.2. Properties of Cryptococcal Circular RNAs

In order to determine the properties of cryptococcal circRNAs, we performed a set of counting calculations for unique and total circRNAs respectively. Firstly, chromosomal distribution for unique and total circRNAs was examined. According to our analysis, 461 total reads were located on chromosome 12. The reason is simple: the highest-expressed circRNA, circ12:174494-175325 (410 reads), was found on Chr12. Correspondingly, chromosome 8 contains the least amount of total back-splicing junction reads, which is only four (Figure 2a, upper panel). The distribution of unique circRNAs among the 14 chromosomes is also displayed in Figure 2a, bottom panel. We found that chromosome 8 contains the least amount of unique circRNAs, two, and chromosomes 1 and 4 contain 10 each.

Secondly, we examined the size distribution of cryptococcal circRNAs. For unique circRNAs, the length was mostly (72.60%) between 201 and 800 nt (Figure 2b). Only a few unique circRNAs were <200 nt (1.37%) or >1400 nt (6.85%). As for total reads, the length concentrated on 801–1000 nt as the size of circ12:174494-175325, which possesses the most reads, is 831 nt. Also, only two reads in total circRNAs were found <200 nt (0.24%, totally) and 17 were >1400 nt (2.07%, totally). Finally, we normalized the expression of each unique circRNA to spliced reads per billion mapping (SRPBM), in order to analyze their expressional features. SRPBM of most circRNAs (63.01%) was <50, while only two circRNAs (2.74%) had SRPBM >500 (Figure 2c).

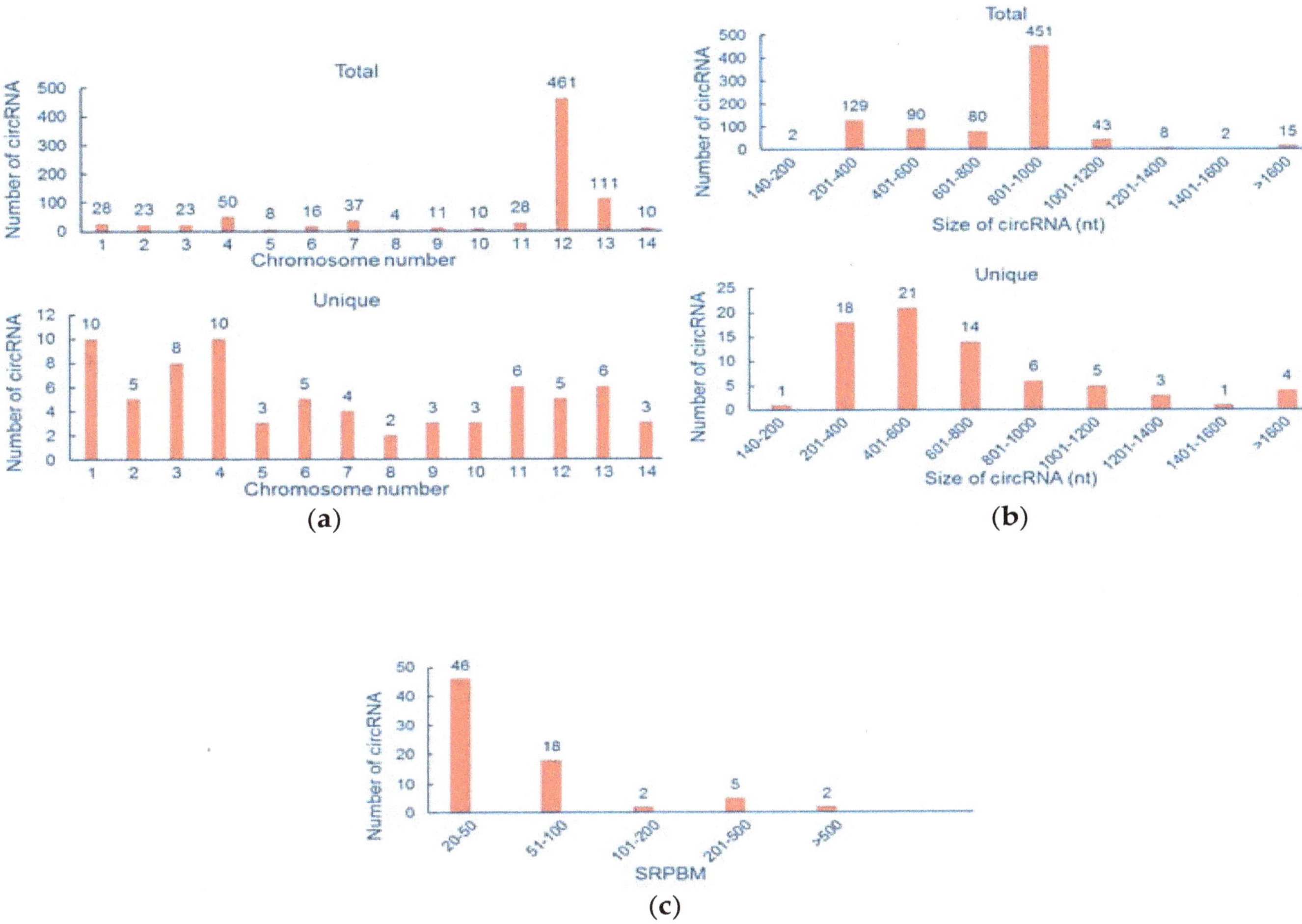

Figure 2. Counting calculations of circRNAs in *C. neoformans*. (**a**) Chromosome distribution of unique circRNAs (bottom panel) and total reads (upper panel). (**b**) Size distribution of unique circRNAs (bottom panel) and total reads (upper panel). (**c**) Expression level distribution of unique circRNAs. SRPBM: spliced reads per billion mapping.

3.3. Functional Analysis of circRNA Host Genes

To investigate the function of circRNA host genes, we performed GO analysis and KEGG pathway analysis. GO analysis suggested that circRNA host genes mainly encode proteins of the large ribosomal subunit, cell surface proteins, and plasma membrane proteins (p-value < 0.05). For GO molecular function analysis, circRNA host genes were associated with beta-glucosidase activity and structural constituents of ribosome (p-value < 0.05). For the GO biological process, those genes were enriched in translation, glucan catabolic process, arginine transport, and fungal cell wall organization (p-value < 0.05) (Figure 3). As for distribution in KEGG pathways, the results show that circRNA host genes were significantly (p-value < 0.05) enriched in two pathways: The ribosome biogenesis and starch-sucrose metabolism pathways (Table 3).

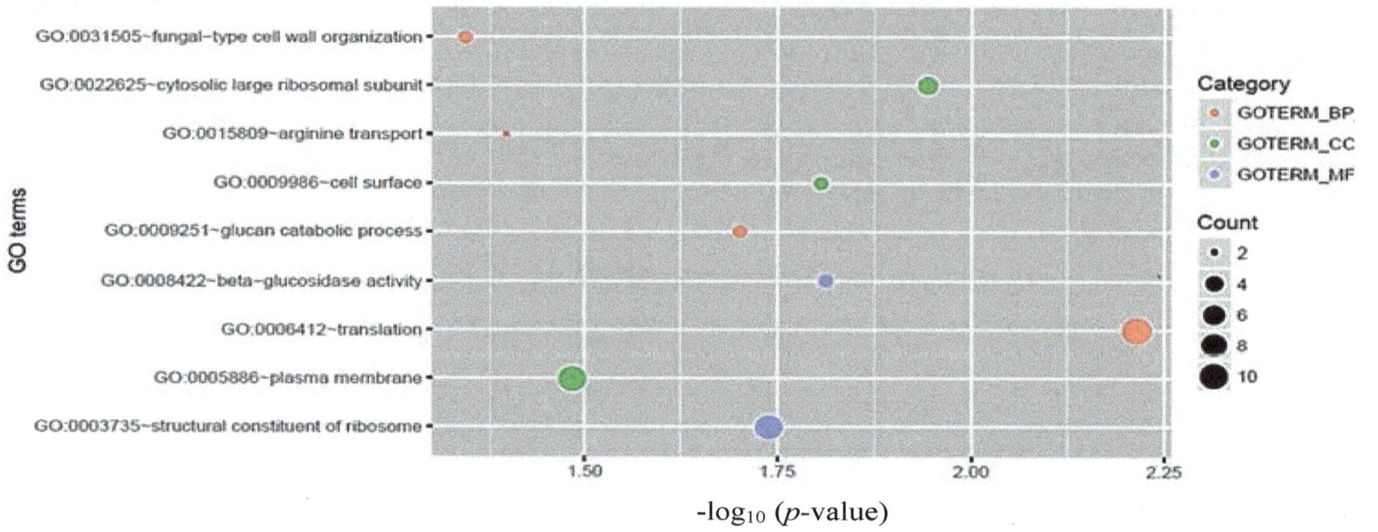

Figure 3. Gene Ontology (GO) category analysis of circRNA host genes in *C. neoformans*. GO terms with the threshold of p-value < 0.05 are listed. GO terms were classified in three categories: Biological process (BP), cellular component (CC), and molecular function (MF).

Table 3. Kyoto Encyclopedia of Genes and Genomes pathway enrichment analysis of circRNA-host genes in *C. neoformans*.

Pathway ID [1]	Description	Gene Count	p-Value
cne03010	Ribosome	6	0.023
cne00500	Starch and sucrose metabolism	3	0.031

[1] Pathway with the threshold of p-value < 0.05 is listed.

3.4. Small Guanosine Triphosphatase-Encoding Orthologs Are Conserved circRNA Hosts

In order to validate the existence of circRNAs, we performed verification by PCR amplification with a pair of outward-designed primers and a cDNA template. In total, primers and PCR reaction systems for six potential circRNAs were designed, including the circ13:359406-359654 whose expression was the highest among all exonic circRNAs (Supplementary Table S1). Consequently, only two specific bands were obtained, respectively, for circ13:359406-359654 and circ7:1027082-1027487. To further confirm the results, we successfully got the PCR band with expected length (248 bp) for circ13:359406-359654 (Figure 4a). Not surprisingly, we failed to observe a corresponding band at the exact level in the control reaction, in which genomic DNA was used as a template. Subsequent Sanger sequencing confirmed that it contained the predicted back-splicing junction site (Figure 4b).

According to genomic distribution data, circ13:359406-359654 was derived from the 5′ end of the gene *CNM01190* (National Center for Biotechnology Information [NCBI] ID: 3255052). By virtue of splicing information stored in the Ensemble Fungi database, we found that the gene *CNM01190* has two splice variants, which encode either a short version (174 aminoacides (aa)) or a long version (252 aa) of protein (Figure 4c). Through a conserved domain basic local alignment search tool (BLAST) search [29], we found that the long variant product encoded by *CNM01190* belongs to the Rab-related GTPase family, which is exemplified by *YPT5* in *Schizosaccharomyces pombe*. Given this, we named the cryptococcal circRNA circCNYPT5. We then used Clustal Omega to compare amino acid sequences of *YPT5* and *CNM01190* long version and found that their identity rate was as high as 57.62% (Figure 4d). Surprisingly, *YPT5* has also been reported to generate circRNAs in *S. pombe*, residing at the exonic regions instead of the 5′-untranslated region (5′-UTR) [17,30]. Therefore, we also performed DNA sequence alignments between the two homologous genes with the BLAST algorithm available at the

NCBI website, but no significant similarity was found. In general, our data suggest a conservation of circRNA host genes in yeasts.

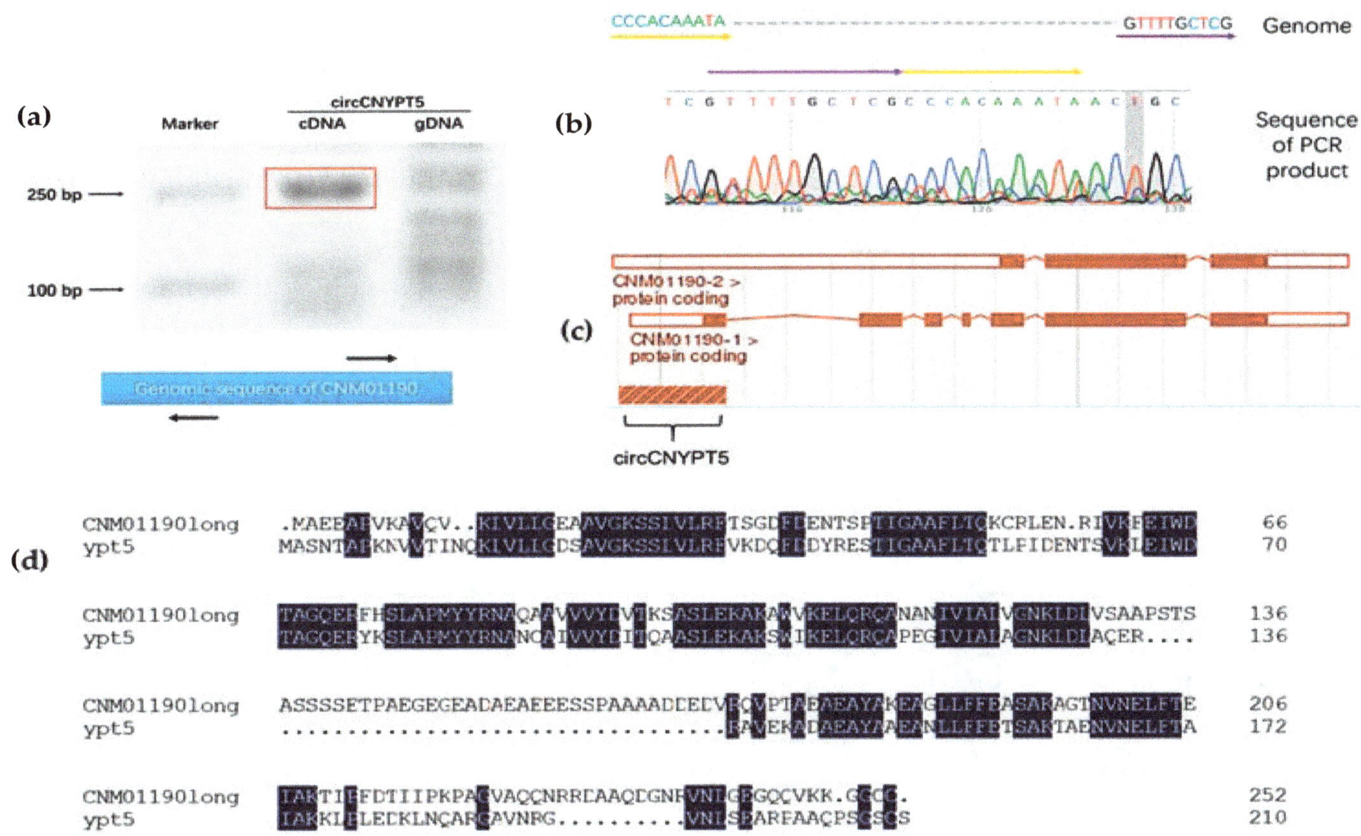

Figure 4. Small GTPase-encoding genes are conserved in circRNA origination among yeasts. (**a**) The upper panel shows that circCNYPT5 can be amplified using outward polymerase chain reactions (PCRs). By contrast, PCR using a genomic DNA template was unable to produce a corresponding band at the same level. Primers in the amplification (black arrows) are shown in the bottom panel. (**b**) Sanger sequencing confirmed the back-splicing junction in PCR products. The 5′ (yellow arrow) and 3′ (purple arrow) were found connected according to sequencing data. (**c**) circCNYPT5 is derived from the 5′ region of *CNM01190*, which has two splice variants. (**d**) Multiple alignments of amino acid sequences showed a high identity between proteins encoded by *CNM01190* in *C. neoformans* and *YPT5* in *Schizosaccharomyces pombe*. Identical amino acids between the two proteins are highlighted in dark blue.

3.5. DBR1 Expression Level Is Negatively Associated with circDPEPS but Not circCNYPT5

According to the lariat-driven model, circRNAs are derived from exon-containing lariat precursors. Inhibiting Dbr1 protein, which degrades lariat, could lead to increased circRMA levels. The expression level of global circRNAs in the *DBR1Δ* mutant strain increased by three- to four-fold over the level in the wild-type (WT) *S. pombe* [31]. To investigate the function of *DBR1* in circRNA regulation in *C. neoformans*, we tried to knock out the counterpart *DBR1* gene in *C. neoformans* JEC21 with the latest clustered regularly interspaced short palindromic repeats (CRISPR)-Cas9 editing system [32,33]. Unfortunately, we failed to get any *DBR1* knockout strain, which implies that the *DBR1* gene might be essential in serotype D strains. As a solution, we overexpressed the *DBR1* gene in JEC21. The overexpression (OE) vector pBS-HYG-DBR1 was detected in transformants OE-1 and OE-2, but not WT, through amplification of a hygromycin-resistant fragment (Figure 5a). Quantitative reverse-transcription (RT) PCR showed that *DBR1* mRNA increased up to 4.89- and 3.76-fold in OE-1 and OE-2, respectively, compared to WT (Figure 5b).

We speculated that overexpression of *DBR1* could reduce circRNA levels in *C. neoformans*. Thus, we analyzed the expression levels of circCNYPT5 in OE-1, OE-2, and WT by semiquantitative RT-PCR. To our surprise, no significant difference in circCNYPT5 expression level was found between WT and overexpression strains according to the electrophoretogram (Olympus, Tokyo, Japan). On the other hand, another highly expressed circular RNA, circDPEPS, which is derived from the whole sequence of gene *CNG03660* (putatively encoding DNA polymerase epsilon p12 subunit, gene ID: 3258898), showed a dramatically decreased level in both overexpression strains (Figure 5c). One possible explanation for these divergent results is that circDPEPS might be processed through an exon-containing lariat precursor, while the generation of circCNYPT5 might rely on a lariat-independent mechanism. On the other hand, these two circRNAs might both be regulated by the *DBR1* gene which plays an important role upstream, but the different downstream action elements may contribute to the wildly different results, which requires further investigation.

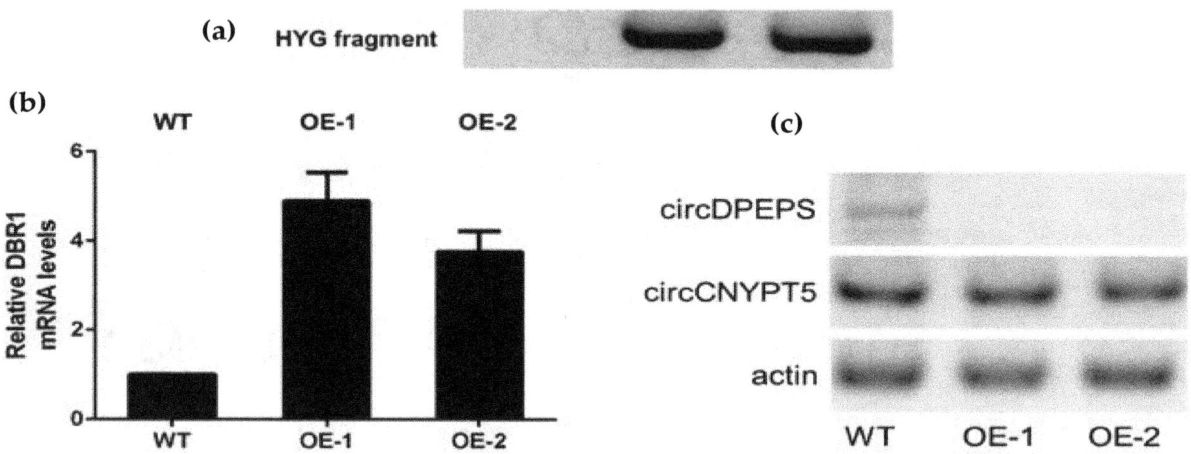

Figure 5. Overexpression (OE) of *DBR1* has a diverse influence on circDPEPS and circCNYPT5. (**a**) PCR was performed to confirm that *DBR1* overexpression of plasmid pBS-HYG-DBR1 was transformed into two transformants, OE-1 and OE-2 (lane 2 and lane 3). JEC21 (wild-type, WT) was used as control. (**b**) Quantitative reverse-transcription (RT) PCR analysis showed that *DBR1* expression level increased up to 4.89- and 3.76-fold in OE-1 and OE-2 compared to WT. Error bars show standard error of the mean. (**c**) Semiquantitative RT-PCR analysis shows that the circDPEPS level declined significantly in the OE strains, while circCNYPT5 remained at a similar level in all three strains. Actin-encoding gene *ACT1* mRNA was used as an internal control.

4. Discussion

In the present study, we report the results of a genomewide screening for circRNAs in the basidiomycetous yeast *C. neoformans* serotype D JEC21 using RNA-seq with bioinformatics analysis. A total of 73 unique circRNAs—including 54 exonic, 4 intronic, and 15 intergenic circRNAs—were identified by the CIRI algorithm. Considering the number of exonic circRNAs and intronic circRNAs, we got 58 predicted circRNA host genes, which was near the number obtained from *S. pombe* (42 genes) [30], but notably less than higher eukaryotes [27,28,34]. The reason might be that different biosynthesis paths are adopted in various organisms. For instance, neural circular RNAs were generated in a spliceosome-dependent manner [35], whereas lariat precursors, which are byproducts in an exon-skipping event, are required for the production of circRNAs in *S. pombe* [17].

Furthermore, we conducted an analysis of the functions of circRNA host genes by GO and KEGG pathways. According to the top-rank rule in GO annotation, we found that circRNA host genes are enriched in encoding structural proteins of the ribosome, plasma membrane, and cell wall, all of which are important in routine growth of the yeast. In addition, we found that the ribosome and starch–sucrose metabolism pathways are the most enriched pathways in the KEGG analysis.

However, the relationship between circRNAs and their host genes still remains elusive due to the limitations of the mutagenesis strategy in the study of circRNAs. CircRNA biosynthesis can compete with pre-mRNA splicing in some cases [36]. On the other hand, some circular intronic RNAs (ciRNAs), such as Ci-ankrd52, are able to promote the transcription of corresponding genes [37]. Additionally, circRNAs in plants like rice and tomato usually exhibit developmental specificity [38,39], while soybean circRNAs show mainly tissue specificity [28].

Interestingly, we found that Rab GTPase-encoding orthologs are conserved circRNA hosts in *C. neoformans* and *S. pombe*. In fact, previous studies reported GTPase-derived circRNAs in protists [30] and humans [40]. Given the low occurrence of unique circRNAs in yeasts, these results may have meaningful implication as to their biogenesis and the function of circRNAs. In our yeast, the host gene, *CNM01190* (NCBI ID: 3255052), has two alternative splicing products that putatively encode 174-aa and 252-aa proteins separately. The circCNYPT5 was derived from the 5′-UTR region of the gene and the first exon in the longer variant. Whether the formation of circCNYPT5 is associated with the alternative splicing process is an intriguing question. The long version of *CNM01190* encodes a member of the small GTPase family. Many of the members of the family have been shown to play vital roles in pathogenesis, thermotolerance, mating, and septin localization in *C. neoformans* [41–43]. Thus, circCNYPT5 that originated from the 5′-UTR region of the gene could presumably act as a profound regulator of the transcription of the *YPT5* gene. Biogenesis of circRNAs within the conserved host ortholog genes across the eukaryotic domain of life raises a question for further investigation.

Finally, we showed that the RNA lariat debranching enzyme (*DBR1*) has variable influence on different circRNA expression in *C. neoformans*. *DBR1* was demonstrated to play key roles in circRNA biogenesis by the lariat-driven pathway in fission yeast [17]. Whether cryptococcal *DBR1* mediates circRNAs biosynthesis in a fission yeast style is still unknown. We failed to knock out *DBR1* in the *C. neoformans* JEC21 serotype D strain, although it could be deleted in the serotype A H99 strain [44]. This phenomenon suggests diverse functions of this gene. Overexpression of *DBR1* in the JEC21 strain decreased circDPEPS levels but had no effect on circCNYPT5 levels. We also attempted to detect other potential circRNAs with PCR amplification but failed, maybe due to the background disturbance from rRNA and linear RNA which were removed from the RNA samples in the RNA-seq. Our data indicate that circCNYPT5 is not processed through an exon-containing lariat precursor. As to the biogenesis of circCNYPT5, the intron-driven model may not be applicable in this case, as no intronic secondary structure was predictable by Mfold software [45]. Whether circCNYPT5 is produced through a spliceosome-dependent path or a protein factors-associated path needs to be investigated. Consistent with our research, a recent RNA-seq study revealed an approximately three- to four-fold increase in circRNAs when *DBR1* was mutated in *S. pombe* [31]. However, researchers also found that the effect of *DBR1* deletion on particular genes seems to have statistical significance [17]. As for circDPEPS, it might be produced through a classic lariat-precursor pathway. However, there is still the possibility that this circRNA derives from other pathways. For instance, the *DBR1* gene may have an indirect influence on circDPEPS expression due to the multiple functions of *DBR1*. It is noteworthy that, according to recent work on *C. neoformans* serotype A H99, *DBR1* is indispensable in the biosynthesis of some transposon-derived small interference RNAs (siRNAs) [44]. In sum, the exact cryptococcal circRNA biosynthesis pathway, along with the comprehensive function of *DBR1* in *C. neoformans*, may need further investigation.

5. Conclusions

In the present study, we identified 73 unique circular RNAs from basidiomycetous yeast *C. neoformans* using RNA-seq and bioinformatics tools such as CIRI. The function of circRNA host genes enriches in primary metabolism, especially translation and carbohydrate metabolism. In addition, we found that the small GTPase ortholog genes are conserved hosts of circRNAs among eukaryotic organisms. Primary analysis revealed that the cryptococcal *DBR1* gene has a differential impact on the generation of different circRNAs. Our study on the identification of circRNAs opens an avenue to understanding their biological function in the pathogenesis of this pathogen.

Acknowledgments: This work was partially funded by a grant from the National Science Foundation of China (#31470251).

Author Contributions: X.Z. conceived and designed the experiments; L.H., P.Z., and C.L. performed the experiments and conducted bioinformatics; K.R. and X.H. participated in analysis of the data; B.X. contributed reagents and materials; L.H. and P.Z. wrote the paper.

References

1. Salzman, J. Circular RNA expression: Its potential regulation and function. *Trends. Genet.* **2016**, *32*, 309–316. [CrossRef] [PubMed]
2. Jeck, W.R.; Sharpless, N.E. Detecting and characterizing circular RNAs. *Nat. Biotechnol.* **2014**, *32*, 453–461. [CrossRef] [PubMed]
3. Chen, L.L.; Yang, L. Regulation of circRNA biogenesis. *RNA Biol.* **2015**, *12*, 381–388. [CrossRef] [PubMed]
4. Suzuki, H.; Zuo, Y.; Wang, J.; Zhang, M.Q.; Malhotra, A.; Mayeda, A. Characterization of RNase R-digested cellular RNA source that consists of lariat and circular RNAs from pre-mRNA splicing. *Nucleic Acids Res.* **2006**, *34*, e63. [CrossRef] [PubMed]
5. Sanger, H.L.; Klotz, G.; Riesner, D.; Gross, H.J.; Kleinschmidt, A.K. Viroids are single-stranded covalently closed circular RNA molecules existing as highly base-paired rod-like structures. *Proc. Natl. Acad. Sci. USA* **1976**, *73*, 3852–3856. [CrossRef] [PubMed]
6. Liu, J.; Liu, T.; Wang, X.; He, A. Circles reshaping the RNA world: From waste to treasure. *Mol. Cancer* **2017**, *16*, 58. [CrossRef] [PubMed]
7. Salzman, J.; Gawad, C.; Wang, P.L.; Lacayo, N.; Brown, P.O. Circular RNAs are the predominant transcript isoform from hundreds of human genes in diverse cell types. *PLoS ONE* **2012**, *7*, e30733. [CrossRef] [PubMed]
8. Hansen, T.B.; Jensen, T.I.; Clausen, B.H.; Bramsen, J.B.; Finsen, B.; Damgaard, C.K.; Kjems, J. Natural RNA circles function as efficient microRNA sponges. *Nature* **2013**, *495*, 384–388. [CrossRef] [PubMed]
9. Gao, Y.; Wang, J.; Zhao, F. Ciri: An efficient and unbiased algorithm for de novo circular RNA identification. *Genome Biol.* **2015**, *16*, 4. [CrossRef] [PubMed]
10. Zhang, X.O.; Wang, H.B.; Zhang, Y.; Lu, X.; Chen, L.L.; Yang, L. Complementary sequence-mediated exon circularization. *Cell* **2014**, *159*, 134–147. [CrossRef] [PubMed]
11. Szabo, L.; Morey, R.; Palpant, N.J.; Wang, P.L.; Afari, N.; Jiang, C.; Parast, M.M.; Murry, C.E.; Laurent, L.C.; Salzman, J. Statistically based splicing detection reveals neural enrichment and tissue-specific induction of circular RNA during human fetal development. *Genome Biol.* **2015**, *16*, 126. [CrossRef] [PubMed]
12. Zhao, Y.; Alexandrov, P.N.; Jaber, V.; Lukiw, W.J. Deficiency in the ubiquitin conjugating enzyme UBE2A in Alzheimer's Disease (AD) is linked to deficits in a natural circular miRNA-7 sponge (circRNA; ciRS-7). *Genes* **2016**, *7*, 116. [CrossRef] [PubMed]
13. Chen, L.L. The biogenesis and emerging roles of circular RNAs. *Nat. Rev. Mol. Cell Biol.* **2016**, *17*, 205–211. [CrossRef] [PubMed]
14. Lasda, E.; Parker, R. Circular RNAs: Diversity of form and function. *RNA* **2014**, *20*, 1829–1842. [CrossRef] [PubMed]
15. Liang, D.; Wilusz, J.E. Short intronic repeat sequences facilitate circular RNA production. *Genes Dev.* **2014**, *28*, 2233–2247. [CrossRef] [PubMed]
16. Conn, S.J.; Pillman, K.A.; Toubia, J.; Conn, V.M.; Salmanidis, M.; Phillips, C.A.; Roslan, S.; Schreiber, A.W.; Gregory, P.A.; Goodall, G.J. The RNA binding protein quaking regulates formation of circRNAs. *Cell* **2015**, *160*, 1125–1134. [CrossRef] [PubMed]
17. Barrett, S.P.; Wang, P.L.; Salzman, J. Circular RNA biosynthesis can proceed through an exon-containing lariat precursor. *eLife* **2015**, *4*, e07540. [CrossRef] [PubMed]

18. Huang, S.; Yang, B.; Chen, B.J.; Bliim, N.; Ueberham, U.; Arendt, T.; Janitz, M. The emerging role of circular RNAs in transcriptome regulation. *Genomics* **2017**, *109*, 401–407. [CrossRef] [PubMed]
19. Granados-Riveron, J.T.; Aquino-Jarquin, G. The complexity of the translation ability of circRNAs. *Biochim. Biophys. Acta* **2016**, *1859*, 1245–1251. [CrossRef] [PubMed]
20. Loftus, B.J.; Fung, E.; Roncaglia, P.; Rowley, D.; Amedeo, P.; Bruno, D.; Vamathevan, J.; Miranda, M.; Anderson, I.J.; Fraser, J.A.; et al. The genome of the basidiomycetous yeast and human pathogen *Cryptococcus neoformans*. *Science* **2005**, *307*, 1321–1324. [CrossRef] [PubMed]
21. Patel, R.K.; Jain, M. NGS QC toolkit: a toolkit for quality control of next generation sequencing data. *PLoS ONE* **2012**, *7*, e30619. [CrossRef] [PubMed]
22. Li, H.; Durbin, R. Fast and accurate long-read alignment with burrows-wheeler transform. *Bioinformatics* **2010**, *26*, 589–595. [CrossRef] [PubMed]
23. Li, Y.; Zheng, Q.; Bao, C.; Li, S.; Guo, W.; Zhao, J.; Chen, D.; Gu, J.; He, X.; Huang, S. Circular RNA is enriched and stable in exosomes: A promising biomarker for cancer diagnosis. *Cell Res.* **2015**, *25*, 981–984. [CrossRef] [PubMed]
24. Huang da, W.; Sherman, B.T.; Lempicki, R.A. Systematic and integrative analysis of large gene lists using DAVID bioinformatics resources. *Nat. Protoc.* **2009**, *4*, 44–57. [CrossRef] [PubMed]
25. Xie, C.; Mao, X.; Huang, J.; Ding, Y.; Wu, J.; Dong, S.; Kong, L.; Gao, G.; Li, C.Y.; Wei, L. KOABS 2.0: A web server for annotation and identification of enriched pathways and diseases. *Nucleic Acids Res.* **2011**, *39*, W316–W322. [CrossRef] [PubMed]
26. Sievers, F.; Wilm, A.; Dineen, D.; Gibson, T.J.; Karplus, K.; Li, W.; Lopez, R.; McWilliam, H.; Remmert, M.; Soding, J.; et al. Fast, scalable generation of high-quality protein multiple sequence alignments using clustal omega. *Mol. Syst. Biol.* **2011**, *7*, 539. [CrossRef] [PubMed]
27. Shen, Y.; Guo, X.; Wang, W. Identification and characterization of circular RNAs in zebrafish. *FEBS Lett.* **2017**, *591*, 213–220. [CrossRef] [PubMed]
28. Zhao, W.; Cheng, Y.; Zhang, C.; You, Q.; Shen, X.; Guo, W.; Jiao, Y. Genome-wide identification and characterization of circular RNAs by high throughput sequencing in soybean. *Sci. Rep.* **2017**, *7*, 5636. [CrossRef] [PubMed]
29. Johnson, M.; Zaretskaya, I.; Raytselis, Y.; Merezhuk, Y.; McGinnis, S.; Madden, T.L. NCBI BLAST: A better web interface. *Nucleic Acids Res.* **2008**, *36*, W5–W9. [CrossRef] [PubMed]
30. Wang, P.L.; Bao, Y.; Yee, M.C.; Barrett, S.P.; Hogan, G.J.; Olsen, M.N.; Dinneny, J.R.; Brown, P.O.; Salzman, J. Circular RNA is expressed across the eukaryotic tree of life. *PLoS ONE* **2014**, *9*, e90859. [CrossRef] [PubMed]
31. Bitton, D.A.; Atkinson, S.R.; Rallis, C.; Smith, G.C.; Ellis, D.A.; Chen, Y.Y.; Malecki, M.; Codlin, S.; Lemay, J.F.; Cotobal, C.; et al. Widespread exon skipping triggers degradation by nuclear RNA surveillance in fission yeast. *Genome Res.* **2015**, *25*, 884–896. [CrossRef] [PubMed]
32. Wang, Y.; Wei, D.; Zhu, X.; Pan, J.; Zhang, P.; Huo, L.; Zhu, X. A 'suicide' CRISPR-Cas9 system to promote gene deletion and restoration by electroporation in *Cryptococcus neoformans*. *Sci. Rep.* **2016**, *6*, 31145. [CrossRef] [PubMed]
33. Rahim, K.; Huo, L.; Li, C.; Zhang, P.; Basit, A.; Xiang, B.; Ting, B.; Hao, X.; Zhu, X. Identification of a basidiomycete-specific Vilse-like GTPase activating proteins (GAPs) and its roles in the production of virulence factors in *Cryptococcus neoformans*. *FEMS Yeast Res.* **2017**, *17*. [CrossRef] [PubMed]
34. Lu, T.; Cui, L.; Zhou, Y.; Zhu, C.; Fan, D.; Gong, H.; Zhao, Q.; Zhou, C.; Zhao, Y.; Lu, D.; et al. Transcriptome-wide investigation of circular RNAs in rice. *RNA* **2015**, *21*, 2076–2087. [CrossRef] [PubMed]
35. You, X.; Vlatkovic, I.; Babic, A.; Will, T.; Epstein, I.; Tushev, G.; Akbalik, G.; Wang, M.; Glock, C.; Quedenau, C.; et al. Neural circular RNAs are derived from synaptic genes and regulated by development and plasticity. *Nat. Neurosci.* **2015**, *18*, 603–610. [CrossRef] [PubMed]
36. Ashwal-Fluss, R.; Meyer, M.; Pamudurti, N.R.; Ivanov, A.; Bartok, O.; Hanan, M.; Evantal, N.; Memczak, S.; Rajewsky, N.; Kadener, S. CircRNA biosynthesis competes with pre-mRNA splicing. *Mol. Cell* **2014**, *56*, 55–66. [CrossRef] [PubMed]
37. Zhang, Y.; Zhang, X.O.; Chen, T.; Xiang, J.F.; Yin, Q.F.; Xing, Y.H.; Zhu, S.; Yang, L.; Chen, L.L. Circular intronic long noncoding RNAs. *Mol. Cell* **2013**, *51*, 792–806. [CrossRef] [PubMed]
38. Ye, C.Y.; Chen, L.; Liu, C.; Zhu, Q.H.; Fan, L. Widespread noncoding circular RNAs in plants. *New Phytol.* **2015**, *208*, 88–95. [CrossRef] [PubMed]

39. Tan, J.; Zhou, Z.; Niu, Y.; Sun, X.; Deng, Z. Identification and functional characterization of tomato circRNAs derived from genes involved in fruit pigment accumulation. *Sci. Rep.* **2017**, *7*, 8594. [CrossRef] [PubMed]
40. Siede, D.; Rapti, K.; Gorska, A.A.; Katus, H.A.; Altmuller, J.; Boeckel, J.N.; Meder, B.; Maack, C.; Volkers, M.; Muller, O.J.; et al. Identification of circular RNAs with host gene-independent expression in human model systems for cardiac differentiation and disease. *J. Mol. Cell Cardiol.* **2017**, *109*, 48–56. [CrossRef] [PubMed]
41. Ballou, E.R.; Selvig, K.; Narloch, J.L.; Nichols, C.B.; Alspaugh, J.A. Two Rac paralogs regulate polarized growth in the human fungal pathogen *Cryptococcus neoformans*. *Fungal Genet. Biol.* **2013**, *57*, 58–75. [CrossRef] [PubMed]
42. Ballou, E.R.; Nichols, C.B.; Miglia, K.J.; Kozubowski, L.; Alspaugh, J.A. Two *CDC42* paralogues modulate *Cryptococcus neoformans* thermotolerance and morphogenesis under host physiological conditions. *Mol. Microbiol.* **2010**, *75*, 763–780. [CrossRef] [PubMed]
43. Ballou, E.R.; Kozubowski, L.; Nichols, C.B.; Alspaugh, J.A. Ras1 acts through duplicated Cdc42 and Rac proteins to regulate morphogenesis and pathogenesis in the human fungal pathogen *Cryptococcus neoformans*. *PLoS Genet.* **2013**, *9*, e1003687. [CrossRef] [PubMed]
44. Dumesic, P.A.; Natarajan, P.; Chen, C.; Drinnenberg, I.A.; Schiller, B.J.; Thompson, J.; Moresco, J.J.; Yates, J.R., 3rd; Bartel, D.P.; Madhani, H.D. Stalled spliceosomes are a signal for RNAi-mediated genome defense. *Cell* **2013**, *152*, 957–968. [CrossRef] [PubMed]
45. Zuker, M. Mfold web server for nucleic acid folding and hybridization prediction. *Nucleic Acids Res.* **2003**, *31*, 3406–3415. [CrossRef] [PubMed]

7

Paracoccidioidomycosis in Immunocompromised Patients

João N. de Almeida Jr. [1], Paula M. Peçanha-Pietrobom [2] and Arnaldo L. Colombo [2,*]

[1] Central Laboratory Division, Hospital das Clínicas da Faculdade de Medicina da Universidade de São Paulo, CEP 05403-000 São Paulo, Brazil; jnaj99@gmail.com

[2] Department of Medicine, Division of Infectious Diseases, Escola Paulista de Medicina, Universidade Federal de São Paulo, CEP 04039-032 São Paulo, Brazil; paulampecanha@gmail.com

* Correspondence: arnaldolcolombo@gmail.com

Abstract: *Paracoccidioidomycosis* (PCM) is an endemic mycosis found in Latin America that causes systemic disease mostly in immunocompetent hosts. A small percentage of PCM occurs in immunocompromised patients where low clinical suspicion of the infection, late diagnosis, and uncertainties about its management are factors that negatively impact their outcomes. We conducted a literature review searching reports on PCM associated to HIV, cancer, maligned hemopathies, solid organ transplantation, and immunotherapies, in order to check for peculiarities in terms of natural history and challenges in the clinical management of PCM in this population. HIV patients with PCM usually had low T $CD4^+$ cell counts, pulmonary and lymph nodes involvement, and a poorer prognosis (≈50% mortality). Most of the patients with PCM and cancer had carcinoma of the respiratory tract. Among maligned hemopathies, PCM was more often related to lymphoma. In general, PCM prognosis in patients with malignant diseases was related to the cancer stage. PCM in transplant recipients was mostly associated with the late phase of kidney transplantation, with a high mortality rate (44%). Despite being uncommon, reactivation of latent PCM may take place in the setting of immunocompromised patients exhibiting clinical particularities and it carries higher mortality rates than normal hosts.

Keywords: paracoccidioidomycosis; HIV; cancer; lymphoma; kidney transplant; TNF inhibitors; literature review

---

1. Introduction

Paracoccidioidomycosis (PCM) is a systemic endemic mycosis caused by *Paracoccidioides brasiliensis* and *Paracoccidioides lutzii*, exhibiting geographic distribution restricted to Latin America, mainly Brazil, Argentina, Colombia and Venezuela [1].

The real burden of the disease is still not defined but incidence rates ranging from 0.7–3 and 9–40 cases/100,000 inhabitants have been reported in endemic and hyperendemic areas of Latin America, respectively [2,3]. The vast majority of cases are reported in normal hosts and continuous exposure to infecting propagules in rural areas is considered to be the main risk factor for this condition [1].

PCM may present in two clinical forms: (i) an acute/subacute form, usually reported in children (or adults < 30years old), with high fever, disseminated lymphadenopathy, hepatosplenomegaly, skin lesions with limited or absent lung involvement and eventually bone lesions, among other symptoms; (ii) a chronic form that represents >80% of all cases reported, presenting with exuberant lung involvement, skin, mucocutaneous lesions or both, and eventually, lesions of the central nervous system and other organs [4,5]. In both clinical forms, adrenal involvement may take place. The polarization between clinical forms is related to the pattern of the adaptive T cell immune response, with a Th2 and

Th9 response leading to an uncontrolled inflammatory process in the acute form, and a deficient Th1 mixed with a Th17 immune response leading to the chronic form of the disease [6,7]. Mortality rates of PCM in normal hosts is usually <5%, but sequelae are frequently documented and include chronic respiratory failure and Addison disease [5,8]. Diagnosis is mainly obtained by conventional methods, including direct examination, culture, histopathology, and detection of specific anti-*Paracoccidioides* antibodies (immunodiffusion or counterimmunoelectrophoresis). PCR-based methods and assays for specific antigen detection were developed by reference labs but are not available in the vast majority of the medical centers in Latin America [9].

Antifungal treatment of mild and moderate cases usually relies on itraconazole or the combination of sulfamethoxazole-trimethoprim. Severe and disseminated infections may require the use of amphotericin B formulations followed by consolidation therapy with itraconazole or sulfamethoxazole-trimethoprim. Patients are usually treated for 12–24 months, depending on clinical presentation [5].

All the aforementioned knowledge applies to PCM in the normal host, and data regarding PCM and immunocompromised patients are scarce and limited. Lack of its clinical suspicion, late diagnosis, and uncertainties about its management are factors that may negatively impact the outcomes of PCM in this population. The present paper describes the peculiarities in terms of natural history and challenges in the clinical management of PCM in patients with HIV, cancer, malignant hemopathies, solid organ transplantation, and immunobiological drugs.

2. Material and Methods

2.1. Search Strategy

We searched the Pubmed database for reports of PCM in immunocompromised patients that were published in the last 30 years. We made all efforts to identify papers addressing epidemiology, fungal diagnosis and antifungal therapy in five different scenarios: HIV, cancer, hematologic patients, solid organ transplant, and related to use of immunobiological agents such as TNF inhibitors and anti-CD20 blockers. Search terms included various combinations of the terms "paracoccidioidomycosis" or "*Paracoccidioides*" with one of the following: "HIV", "AIDS", "cancer", "leukemia", "lymphoma", "myelodysplastic syndrome", "aplastic anemia", "stem cell transplantation", "kidney transplantation", "liver transplantation", "heart transplantation", "lung transplantation"; "TNF inhibitor"; "infliximab"; "etanercept"; "adalimumab"; "anti-CD20"; "rituximab"; "natalizumab". We reviewed all articles retrieved from these search terms and relevant references cited in those articles. There were no language restrictions and only cases with proven or probable PCM were included, following criteria defined elsewhere [5].

Data on age, sex, underlying diseases, immunological status, risk factors (e.g., rural work, tobacco or alcohol consumption), immunosuppressive therapy, laboratorial diagnosis, details of antifungal induction, maintenance therapies, as well as relapse and outcome were recorded. The outcome was considered to be favorable if the patient met the cure criteria according to the Brazilian Guidelines for the Clinical Management of PCM [5]. Recurrence of clinical signs and symptoms, or radiology findings in the presence of any laboratory results suggesting active PCM, were used to define a relapse episode.

2.2. Statistical Analysis

Comparisons between groups were performed using Fisher's exact or chi-square tests when appropriate for the categorical variables (SPSS v.25, IBM, Armonk, NY, USA). p values of <0.05 were considered to be statistically significant.

3. Results and Discussion

3.1. *Paracoccidioidomycosis and HIV Infection*

The first two cases of PCM associated with HIV infection were reported in 1989 [10]. Since then, PCM/HIV coinfection occurrence has been reported as small case-series in endemic areas in Brazil [11–13], and in isolated cases reports in Colombia and Argentina [14,15]. Two retrospective case-control studies have been conducted up until the present date. In the first study published in 2009, Morejón, Machado and Martinez reported 53 cases of PCM and HIV coinfection in Brazil [16]. In the second controlled study, Almeida et al. 2016, reported thirty-one HIV-infected patients with PCM between 1993 and 2014 [17]. After compiling the data from these two case-control studies [16,17], two case-series reports [13,18], and 30 single case reports [10,14,19–35], we retrieved 136 cases of PCM and HIV coinfection reported in the last 30 years. They aged between 13 and 59 years, with a mean age of 35.9 years. Twenty-six (19%) were female, and only two were in the adult PCM form (6%). The higher proportion of females in the casuistic of immunocompromised patients with PCM compared to the usual gender distribution observed in normal adult hosts (over 6%) suggests that the hormonal protection described for normal hosts is mitigated in the setting of immunosuppression [5]. Most patients worked in the urban area (68%), which is different from the usual epidemiology of the disease. Thus, an ancient exposure and activation of a latent infection might have occurred on these coinfected patients.

In 56 cases, data regarding the awareness of the HIV status at the PCM diagnosis were provided, and only 31 (55%) patients were known to be HIV-infected at that time. Over 80% of the PCM-HIV coinfected patients for whom CD4+ cell counts were available had <200 cells/mm^3. This finding suggests that *Paracoccidioides* spp. may take advantage of the T-cell immunosuppression related to AIDS to shift from quiescent infection to systemic disease. Fever, generalized lymphadenopathy, splenomegaly, and skin lesions, which are generally reported in the acute form of the PCM disease, were more common in PCM-HIV coinfected patients than in the immunocompetent group (see Table 1, Figures 1 and 2).

Table 1. Comparison of clinical, laboratory and outcome data from adult patients with paracoccidioidomycosis coinfected and non-coinfected with HIV virus.

	PCM and HIV (%)	PCM (%)	*p* Value
Clinical Data			
Fever	82.7	35.4 **	<0.001
Lymphadenopathy	72.9 #	50.6 *	<0.001
Splenomegaly	22.6	4.7 *	<0.001
Skin Lesions	58.9	29.6 *	<0.001
Pneumopathy	70.3	63.8 *	0.15
Oral mucosa	29	50 *	<0.001
Laboratory data (positivity rates)			
Direct microscopy	57.4	44 **	0.052
Culture	42.2	25.3 *	<0.001
Histopathology	94.5	64.7 *	<0.001
Serology	74.6	97.2 *	<0.001
Outcomes			
Relapse rates	11	8.2 **	0.48
Mortality rates	35	7.9 **	<0.001

* Data extracted from the references: [2,4]; ** data extracted from the references [16,17]. # PCM coinfected patients usually present multiple lymph nodes involvement, in different anatomic sites.

Pulmonary disease was reported in most of the coinfected population despite the age of the patient, characterizing a mixed clinical form (juvenile–adult) exhibiting simultaneous lung involvement and disseminated infection of the reticuloendothelial system. This is a clinical presentation suggestive of an opportunistic manifestation of PCM in this specific population. This mixed clinical form, already reported by other authors, may be a consequence of the inefficient immune control of the primary lung foci followed by lymphohematogenous dissemination [36,37].

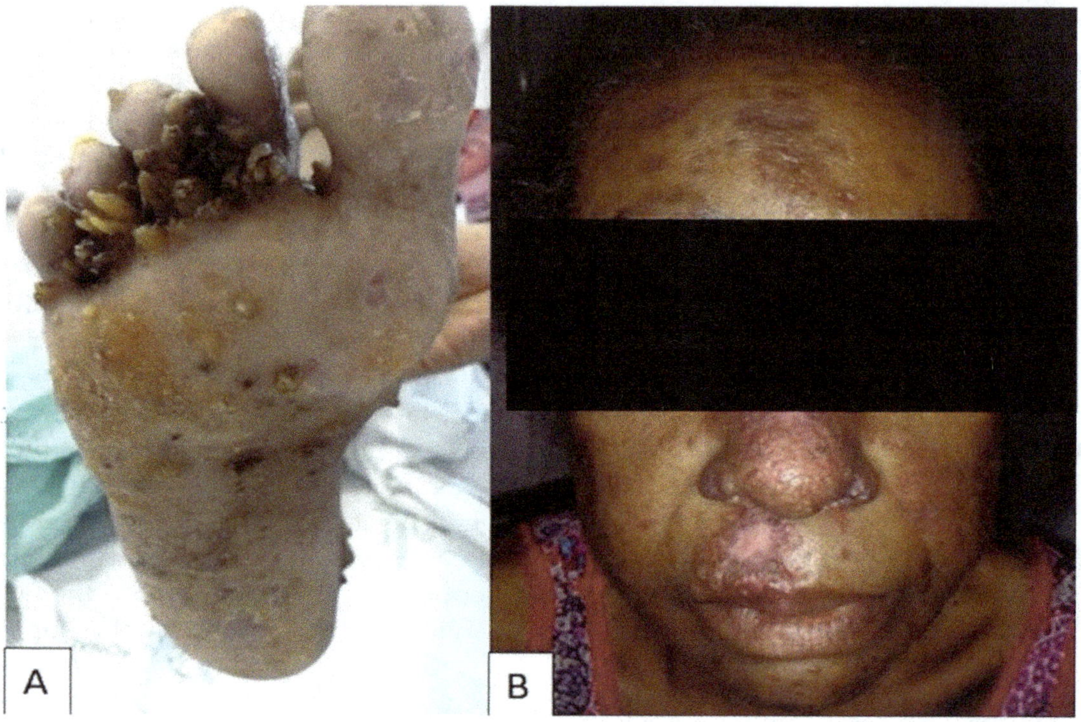

Figure 1. Skin involvement in PCM-HIV coinfection. (**A**) Verrucous lesions on the foot caused by hematogenous dissemination. (**B**) Papulonodular ulcerative lesions caused by hematogenous dissemination. Illustration provided by Prof. Paulo Mendes Peçanha from Infectious Disease Unit, Universidade Federal do Espírito Santo.

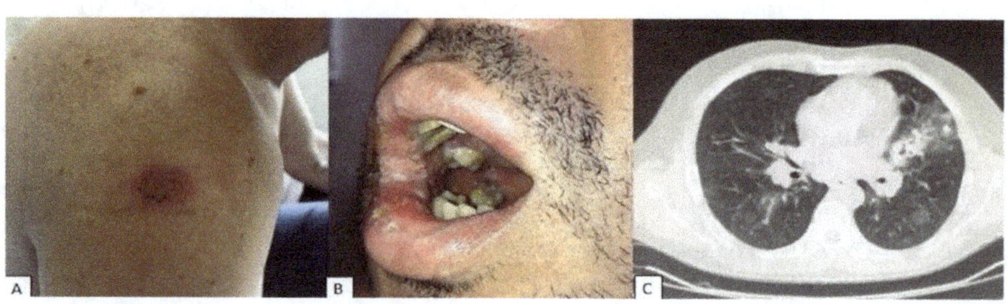

Figure 2. Clinical presentation of PCM-HIV coinfection. (**A**) Ulcerative lesions on the arm. (**B**) Moriform ulcerative perioral involvement. (**C**) Diffuse ground-glass opacities and consolidation in left superior lobe on chest computed tomography. Illustration provided by Dr. Adriana Maria Porro from the Dermatology Department, Escola Paulista de Medicina-Universidade Federal de São Paulo.

Coinfected patients presented more often with positive histopathology and culture results when compared to HIV-negative patients with PCM (see Table 1). These data reflect the higher fungal burden in the coinfected patients. In contrast, the detection of anti-*Paracoccidioides* serum antibody by quantitative double immunodiffusion test or counterimmunoelectrophoresis had lower positive rates in the PCM-HIV population (74.6% vs. 97.2%, $p < 0.001$). Therefore, in patients with AIDS, *Paracoccidioides* sp. negative serological results do not exclude the PCM diagnosis, which should be investigated with alternative microbiological tests and histopathological examination.

Two case reports described PCM in patients receiving cotrimoxazole prophylaxis [24,38]. Similarly, Morejón et al. described 10 out 25 coinfected patients that were diagnosed with PCM under cotrimoxazole prophylaxis. Consequently, PCM should not be ruled out in patients under trimethoprim–sulfamethoxazole prophylaxis.

The overall mortality rate was higher in the coinfected population (35% vs. 7.9%, $p < 0.001$, see Table 1), mainly as a consequence of the severe immunodepression seen in most of the patients. Information about the presence of any other (non-PCM) concomitant opportunistic infections was mentioned by the authors in only 65 (47.7%) of 136 patients. Of note, only 19 cases (29%) of the 65 patients where this information was available had other severe infections concomitantly with PCM. This means that the outcome of PCM in this population was not impacted by other severe conditions in 71% of the cases. Fungemia by *Paracoccidioides* seems to be a predictor of poor prognosis since all three patients with positive blood cultures died. The choice of the initial antifungal therapy did not influence the outcome. Amphotericin B deoxycholate (AMB) was used as primary therapy in 19 cases, and 9 patients died (47.3%). Of note, all these nine patients with a fatal outcome had concomitant severe opportunist infections. Among 18 cases in which cotrimoxazole or itraconazole was used as initial therapy, seven died (38.8%, $p = 0.7$). Otherwise, one could suggest that there was one imbalance in the clinical severity of patients exposed to amphotericin B and other drugs that may certainly influence the expected mortality in both groups.

3.2. Paracoccidioidomycosis and Solid Organ Malignancies

The relationship between PCM and solid cancer was first described more than 80 years ago [39]. Concomitant PCM and solid cancer are reported in 0.16 to 11% of the cases, according to some cohorts [39–41]. Most of the solid cancers are carcinomas (>80%) from the respiratory or digestive tract [42], and are related to the chronic form of PCM and its risk factors, such as male sex, rural workers with a history of smoking and alcohol intake [1,42]. Likewise, among the 36 cases that fulfilled the inclusion criteria (31 from two case series [42,43] and five from isolated case reports [44–48]), 26 (72%) were related to carcinomas of the upper and lower respiratory ($n = 16$, 44%) and digestive tracts, mainly the oropharynx and esophagus ($n = 7$, 19%). Carcinoma was diagnosed at the same anatomical site of the fungal lesion in twenty-one cases (58%). In thirteen cases (36%) PCM appeared before cancer, and in 19 patients (53%) cancer was diagnosed simultaneously with PCM. These findings have led researchers to raise the hypothesis that PCM may be an additive factor for cancer development due to chronic antigenic stimulation of the pathogenic yeasts on the epithelial cells [43].

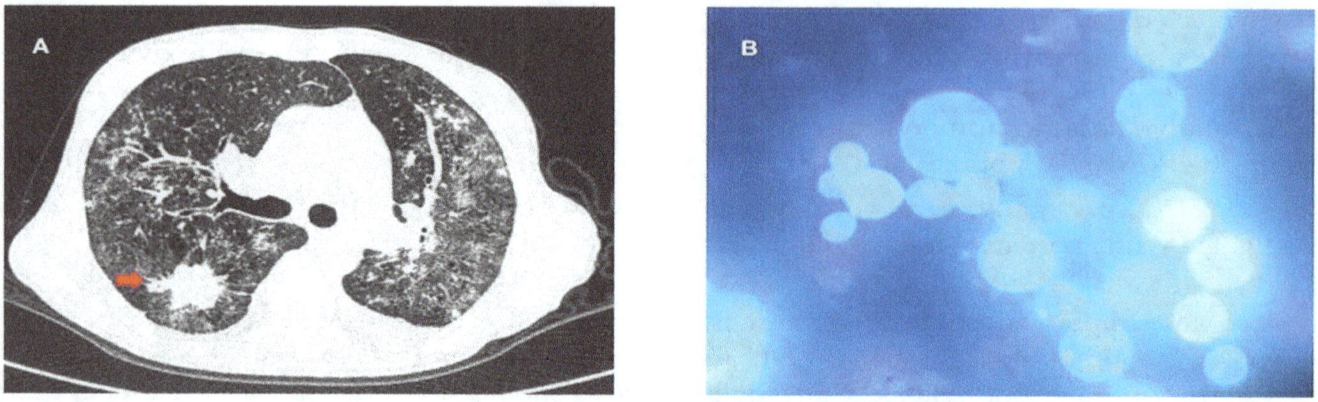

Figure 3. (**A**) Chest computed tomography scan showing spiculated nodule from adenocarcinoma (red arrow) and bilateral diffuse bronchoalveolar infiltrates from PCM. (**B**) Bronchoalveolar lavage with yeast cells with multiple daughter buds (Calcofluor white, 1000×). Figure **A** provided by Dr. Drielle Peixoto Bittencourt from Hospital do Cancer, Universidade de São Paulo; Figure **B** provided by the authors.

So far, we were not able to identify any particularity in terms of clinical presentation of PCM in patients with solid cancer. Serology was useful for PCM diagnosis in this population in only 50% of cases [43]. Figure 3 illustrates a case of concomitant pulmonary adenocarcinoma and PCM. In a retrospective analysis of 25 cases of PCM and cancer, Rodrigues et al. reported a mortality rate of 16%, a rate apparently higher than that associated to normal hosts [43,49].

3.3. Paracoccidioidomycosis and Hematologic Malignancies

Hematologic malignancies are rarely reported in patients with PCM, with an estimated prevalence of 0–3% [42]. A dozen cases were reported in the last 30 years, most of them were B cell lymphomas (either Hodgkin or non-Hodgkin) that were diagnosed after the PCM disease (1–8 years) [41–43,50]. Resende et al. reported four detailed cases of PCM and lymphoma, all of them had lymph nodes with PCM yeasts found in histopathology and positive serology [50]. The patients were treated for a long time, from 2 to 10 years, and two of them showed PCM recurrence. Two patients died due to complications related to the lymphoma [50]. The authors suggested that the chronic PCM antigenic stimulation may have had a role in the development of B cell lymphoma [50], but further investigation is necessary to confirm this hypothesis. The limited casuistic precludes any conclusion in terms of putative peculiarities of natural history or diagnostic tools for PCM in this specific setting.

3.4. Paracoccidioidomycosis and Solid Organ Transplant

Among the different solid organ transplant modalities, chronic PCM has been described predominantly in kidney transplant recipients. Nine cases of PCM in kidney transplant patients and a single episode in a liver transplant recipient fulfilled the inclusion criteria [51–55]. We excluded from the present series one episode of PCM mentioned in a report of a lung transplant recipient without any further details [56,57]. The patients had a median age of 55 years; three of them were rural workers before the transplantation, and three (60%) out of five cases with gender description were male. Seven cases developed PCM after one year of transplantation (range 1–14 years), none of them were having cotrimoxazole prophylaxis at diagnosis, and symptoms of PCM appeared 2 to 6 months before diagnosis. One case lacked a description of the time elapsed between transplant and PCM diagnosis [51]. Three (33%) of those reported cases had skin lesions, either combined with oral mucosal and lung infiltrates (two cases), or with lymphadenopathy (one case). One illustrative case is presented in Figure 4.

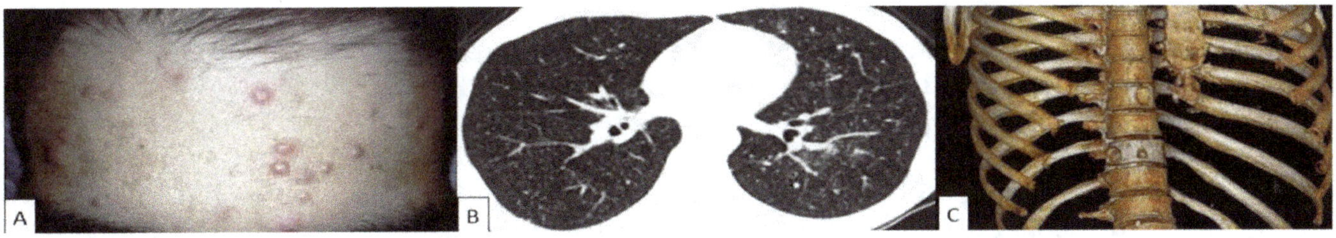

Figure 4. Disseminated paracoccidioidomycosis in a kidney transplant recipient. (**A**) Vesiculopapular lesions on the face. (**B**) Chest computerized tomography showing a miliary nodular pattern. (**C**) Chest computerized tomography and 3D reconstruction of the thoracic bone structure showing osteolytic vertebral lesions. Illustration provided by Dr. Daniel Wagner from Hospital do Rim, Universidade Federal de São Paulo.

Three reports provided information regarding immunosuppressive therapy, that consisted of corticosteroids and the combination of other immunosuppressants, such as cyclosporine and azathioprine [52], mycophenolate mofetil (MMF) and tacrolimus [53], and mesalazine and tacrolimus [54]. The diagnosis was mainly achieved through direct examination or histopathology of clinical samples. All patients required hospitalization, four were initially treated with AMB formulations, three out nine patients (33%) died due to the mycosis. Of note, a 57-year-old female patient developed acute respiratory failure due to PCM only two days after the kidney transplantation [55]. This particular patient lived in a rural area and was diagnosed with a solitary pulmonary nodule before the transplant, which was considered to be latent tuberculosis. The pre-transplant immunosuppression therapy consisted of anti-thymocyte globulin (ATG) and MMF. The patient was successfully treated with liposomal AMB (1 mg/Kg) for 14 days followed by itraconazole (200mg/day) for one year. ID serology tested in the acute phase of the disease and during clinical follow-up were both negative.

One case of severe disseminated PCM in a 3-year-old girl was reported 24 months after liver transplantation due to congenital biliary atresia [56]. She was initially treated with cotrimoxazole (200/40 mg, q12h), and due to a poor clinical response, AMB was also prescribed. Initial CIE serology was positive (titer 1/64), and after six months of cotrimoxazole (100/20 mg q12h) maintenance therapy, the patient was considered cured [56].

Prophylaxis with cotrimoxazole after transplantation explains the rarity of PCM in this scenario, as this drug is active against *P. brasiliensis*. Most of the reported cases occur after the first year of transplantation when immunosuppression is tapered and cotrimoxazole prophylaxis is no longer necessary. However, despite being rare, PCM in kidney transplant patients seems to have a poor prognosis, possibly related to its low clinical suspicion, difficult and late diagnosis (negative serological tests), and immunosuppression. Indeed, it has been demonstrated that immunosuppressed kidney transplant recipients have a persistent poor Th1 immune response to *Paracoccidioides* antigen gp43 [58].

Due to the rarity of PCM in organ transplant recipients, there is no formal recommendation for living donors and recipients that have lived in endemic areas to be routinely screened for PCM latent infection before transplant. Serological tests have poor value for the clinical management of PCM disease in kidney transplant recipients, and AMB lipid formulations have to be considered as initial therapy in severe cases [59].

3.5. Paracoccidioidomycosis and Immunotherapies

Only three cases of PCM disease related to immunobiological agents have been reported so far [60,61]. A 60-year-old man with rheumatoid arthritis and on immunosuppressive therapy, including methotrexate, leflunomide and adalimumab (40mg every 15 days), for 3 years, was hospitalized to investigate a chronic hip pain that was further diagnosed as an osteosarcoma. Chest CT-scan revealed an excavated pulmonary lesion on the lower left lobe and biopsy revealed granuloma and yeasts compatible with *P. brasiliensis*. Despite AMB induction therapy and adalimumab interruption, the patient developed sepsis after a hip surgery for tumor resection and died [60]. A 47-year old man with psoriatic spondyloarthritis and on infliximab therapy for 18 months developed fever and respiratory symptoms. CT-scan revealed a left inferior pulmonary lobe nodule and mediastinal lymphadenopathy. Lung biopsy histological analysis diagnosed PCM. Investigation of anti-*Paracoccidioides* antibodies by the immunodiffusion technique was negative. Infliximab was suspended and the patient was successfully treated with cotrimoxazole for 29 months. A 46-year old man with multiple sclerosis developed pulmonary PCM after 15 months of natalizumab therapy [62]. The diagnosis was made by lung biopsy and the patient was treated with itraconazole and natalizumab was discontinued.

In the USA, TNF inhibitors, mainly infliximab, have been related to histoplasmosis, with a median of 15 months after initiation of the immunobiological drug [63]. Likewise, the reported cases of PCM in patients undergoing TNF inhibitor therapy occurred more than one year after the introduction of the medication. These cases highlight the need to include PCM in the list of opportunistic infections in patients under long-term immunotherapy from endemic areas. Moreover, negative serology should not exclude the diagnosis of PCM in these patients and infection must be managed with interruption of the TNF blocker agent and prolonged antifungal therapy.

4. Conclusions

Despite being uncommon, PCM may be reported in patients with immunosuppression, including AIDS, cancer, patients with solid organ transplantations, or on immunobiological therapy. The vast majority of PCM in immunosuppressed patients has been reported in HIV patients, where this disease may exhibit simultaneously the clinical characteristics of chronic (lung involvement) and acute forms (generalized lymph adenomegaly and hepatosplenomegaly) of the disease. In this population, more disease relapses and higher mortality rates are reported than in non-immunocompromised hosts.

Lymphoma was the most common hematologic malignancy reported with PCM, and few cases of PCM have been reported in the late period after kidney transplantation. We were not able to identify any change in terms of the natural history of PCM documented in patients with cancer or solid organ transplant recipients.

Diagnosis of PCM may be challenging in immunosuppressed patients where serology usually has a low sensitivity and PCR-based methods or assays for antigen detection are not available in the vast majority of routine laboratories. Consequently, invasive procedures (e.g., biopsy) may be required to confirm the diagnosis [17,62]. Of note, in endemic areas, paracoccidioidomycosis should be included in the differential diagnosis of any patient with a disease associated with T-cell immunodeficiency who presents with pulmonary infiltrates with nodules, cavitation or chronic alveolar consolidation, as well as skin or mucocutaneous lesions with a chronic evolution.

Regarding specific therapy of patients with severe clinical forms of PCM, amphotericin B should be promptly initiated, followed by 12 to 24 months of treatment with itraconazole or sulfamethoxazole-trimethoprim. Treatment duration relies on the severity of clinical presentation, sites of infection, restoration of the host immune response, as well as the clinical and laboratorial response to therapy [5].

Finally, immunocompromised patients who travel to endemic areas of PCM should be counseled before traveling to avoid high-risk exposures. Once the transplant recipient returns from an endemic area, the clinician must instigate a complete diagnostic investigation if any sign or symptom of PCM appears, in order to treat it rapidly and to mitigate against morbidity and a poor outcome [59].

Author Contributions: J.N.d.A.J. and P.M.P.-P. reviewed the literature and were responsible for writing the first draft of the manuscript. A.L.C. designed the study strategy, wrote the introduction and conclusions, as well as reviewed the whole manuscript.

Acknowledgments: A.L.C. received grants from Conselho Nacional de Desenvolvimento Científico e Tecnológico, Brazil, (CNPq, Grant 307510/2015-8). We thank Paulo Mendes Peçanha from Infectious Disease Unit, Universidade Federal do Espírito Santo; Adriana Maria Porro from the Dermatology Department, Universidade Federal de São Paulo; Daniel Wagner from Hospital do Rim, Universidade Federal de São Paulo; Drielle Peixoto Bittencourt from Hospital do Cancer, University of São Paulo; that kindly provided us the photos.

References

1. Martinez, R. New Trends in Paracoccidioidomycosis Epidemiology. *J. Fungi* **2017**, *3*, 1. [CrossRef] [PubMed]
2. Bellissimo-Rodrigues, F.; Machado, A.A.; Martinez, R. Paracoccidioidomycosis epidemiological features of a 1,000-cases series from a hyperendemic area on the southeast of Brazil. *Am. J. Trop. Med. Hyg.* **2011**, *85*, 546–550. [CrossRef] [PubMed]
3. Vieira, G.D.; Alves, T.D.; Lima, S.M.; Camargo, L.M.; Sousa, C.M. Paracoccidioidomycosis in a western Brazilian Amazon State: Clinical-epidemiologic profile and spatial distribution of the disease. *Rev. Soc. Bras. Med. Trop.* **2014**, *47*, 63–68. [CrossRef] [PubMed]
4. Bellissimo-Rodrigues, F.; Bollela, V.R.; Da Fonseca, B.A.L.; Martinez, R. Endemic paracoccidioidomycosis: Relationship between clinical presentation and patients' demographic features. *Med. Mycol.* **2013**, *51*, 313–318. [CrossRef] [PubMed]
5. Shikanai-Yasuda, M.A.; Mendes, R.P.; Colombo, A.L.; de Queiroz-Telles, F.; Kono, A.S.G.; Paniago, A.M.M.; Nathan, A.; do Valle, A.C.F.; Bagagli, E.; Benard, G.; et al. Brazilian guidelines for the clinical management of paracoccidioidomycosis. *Rev. Soc. Brasil. Med. Trop.* **2017**, *50*, 715–740. [CrossRef] [PubMed]
6. De Castro, L.F.; Ferreira, M.C.; da Silva, R.M.; Blotta, M.H.; Longhi, L.N.A.; Mamoni, R.L. Characterization of the immune response in human paracoccidioidomycosis. *J. Infect.* **2013**, *67*, 470–485. [CrossRef] [PubMed]
7. De Oliveira, H.C.; Assato, P.A.; Marcos, C.M.; Scorzoni, L.; de Paula, E.; Silva, A.C.A.; Da Silva, J.D.F.; Singulani, J.D.; Alarcon, K.M.; Fusco-Almeida, A.M.; et al. Paracoccidioides-host Interaction: An Overview on Recent Advances in the Paracoccidioidomycosis. *Front. Microbiol.* **2015**, *6*, 1319. [CrossRef] [PubMed]
8. Colombo, A.L.; Tobón, A.; Restrepo, A.; Queiroz-Telles, F.; Nucci, M. Epidemiology of endemic systemic fungal infections in Latin America. *Med. Mycol.* **2011**, *49*, 785–798. [CrossRef] [PubMed]
9. Queiroz-Telles, F.; Fahal, A.H.; Falci, D.R.; Caceres, D.H.; Chiller, T.; Pasqualotto, A.C. Neglected endemic mycoses. *Lancet Infect. Dis.* **2017**, *17*, e367–e377. [CrossRef]
10. Pedro, R.D.; Aoki, F.H.; Boccato, R.S.; Branchini, M.L.; Gonçales Júnior, F.L.; Papaiordanou, P.M.; Ramos, M.D. Paracoccidioidomicose e infecção pelo virus da imunodeficiência humana. *Rev. Inst. Med. Trop São Paulo* **1989**, *31*, 119–125. [CrossRef]
11. Marques, S.A.; Conterno, L.O.; Sgarbi, L.P.; Villagra, A.M.; Sabongi, V.P.; Bagatin, E.; Gonçalves, V.L. Paracoccidioidomycosis associated with acquired immunodeficiency syndrome. Report of seven cases. *Rev. Inst. Med. Trop. Sao Paulo* **1995**, *37*, 261–265. [CrossRef]
12. Silva-Vergara, M.L.; Teixeira, A.C.; Curi, V.G.M.; Costa Júnior, J.C.; Vanunce, R.; Carmo, W.M.; Silva, M.R. Paracoccidioidomycosis associated with human immunodeficiency virus infection. Report of 10 cases. *Med. Mycol.* **2003**, *41*, 259–263. [CrossRef] [PubMed]
13. Paniago, A.M.M.; de Freitas, A.C.C.; Aguiar, E.S.A.; Aguiar, J.I.A.; da Cunha, R.V.; Castro, A.R.C.M.; Wanke, B. Paracoccidioidomycosis in patients with human immunodeficiency virus: Review of 12 cases observed in an endemic region in Brazil. *J. Infect.* **2005**, *51*, 248–252. [CrossRef] [PubMed]
14. Tobon, A.M.; Orozco, B.; Estrada, S.; Jaramillo, E.; de Bedout, C.; Arango, M.; Restrepo, A. Paracoccidioidomycosis and AIDS: Report of the first two Colombian cases. *Rev. Inst. Med. Trop. Sao Paulo* **1998**, *40*, 377–381. [CrossRef] [PubMed]
15. Corti, M.; Trione, N.; Risso, D.; Soto, I.; Villafañe, M.F.; Yampolsky, C.; Negroni, R. Disseminated paracoccidioidomycosis with a single brainstem lesion. A case report and literature review. *Neuroradiol. J.* **2010**, *23*, 454–458. [CrossRef] [PubMed]
16. Morejón, K.M.L.; Machado, A.A.; Martinez, R. Paracoccidioidomycosis in patients infected with and not infected with human immunodeficiency virus: A case-control study. *Am. J. Trop. Med. Hyg.* **2009**, *80*, 359–366. [CrossRef] [PubMed]

17. De Almeida, F.A.; Neves, F.F.; Mora, D.J.; Reis, T.A.D.; Sotini, D.M.; Ribeiro, B.D.M.; Andrade-Silva, L.E.; Nascentes, G.N.; Ferreira-Paim, K.; Silva-Vergara, M.L. Paracoccidioidomycosis in Brazilian Patients with and Without Human Immunodeficiency Virus Infection. *Am. J. Trop. Med. Hyg.* **2017**, *96*, 368–372. [CrossRef] [PubMed]
18. Macedo, P.M.; Almeida-Paes, R.; Almeida, M.D.; Coelho, R.A.; Andrade, H.B.; Ferreira, A.B.T.B.C.; Zancopé-Oliveira, R.M.; Valle, A.C.F. Paracoccidioidomycosis due to Paracoccidioides brasiliensis S1 plus HIV co-infection. *Mem. Inst. Oswaldo Cruz* **2018**, *113*, 167–172. [CrossRef]
19. Goldani, L.Z.; Martinez, R.; Landell, G.A.; Machado, A.A.; Coutinho, V. Paracoccidioidomycosis in a patient with acquired immunodeficiency syndrome. *Mycopathologia* **1989**, *105*, 71–74. [CrossRef]
20. Bakos, L.; Kronfeld, M.; Hampe, S.; Castro, I.; Zampese, M. Disseminated paracoccidioidomycosis with skin lesions in a patient with acquired immunodeficiency syndrome. *J. Am. Acad. Dermatol.* **1989**, *20*, 854–855. [CrossRef]
21. Benard, G.; Bueno, J.P.; Yamashiro-Kanashiro, E.H.; Shikanai-Yasuda, M.A.; Del Negro, G.M.; Melo, N.T.; Sato, M.N.; Amato Neto, V.; Shiroma, M.; Duarte, A.J. Paracoccidioidomycosis in a patient with HIV infection: Immunological study. *Trans. R. Soc. Trop. Med. Hyg.* **1990**, *84*, 151–152. [CrossRef]
22. De Lima, M.A.; Silva-Vergara, M.L.; Demachki, S.; dos Santos, J.A. Paracoccidioidomycosis in a patient with human immunodeficiency virus infection. A necropsy case. *Rev. Soc. Bras. Med. Trop.* **1995**, *28*, 279–284. [PubMed]
23. Silletti, R.P.; Glezerov, V.; Schwartz, I.S. Pulmonary paracoccidioidomycosis misdiagnosed as Pneumocystis pneumonia in an immunocompromised host. *J. Clin. Microbiol.* **1996**, *34*, 2328–2330. [PubMed]
24. Dos Santos, J.W.; Costa, J.M.; Cechella, M.; Michel, G.T.; de Figueiredo, C.W.; Londero, A.T. An unusual presentation of paracoccidioidomycosis in an AIDS patient: A case report. *Mycopathologia* **1998**, *142*, 139–142. [CrossRef] [PubMed]
25. Nobre, V.; Braga, E.; Rayes, A.; Serufo, J.C.; Godoy, P.; Nunes, N.; Antunes, C.M.; Lambertucci, J.R. Opportunistic infections in patients with AIDS admitted to an university hospital of the Southeast of Brazil. *Rev. Inst. Med. Trop. Sao Paulo* **2003**, *45*, 69–74. [CrossRef] [PubMed]
26. Corti, M.; Villafañe, M.F.; Negroni, R.; Palmieri, O. Disseminated paracoccidioidomycosis with peripleuritis in an AIDS patient. *Rev. Inst. Med. Trop. Sao Paulo* **2004**, *46*, 47–50. [CrossRef] [PubMed]
27. Caseiro, M.M.; Etzel, A.; Soares, M.C.B.; Costa, S.O.P. Septicemia caused by Paracoccidioides brasiliensis (Lutz, 1908) as the cause of death of an AIDS patient from Santos, São Paulo State, Brazil—A nonendemic area. *Rev. Inst. Med. Trop. Sao Paulo* **2005**, *47*, 209–211. [CrossRef] [PubMed]
28. Godoy, P.; Lelis, S.S.R.; Resende, U.M. Paracoccidioidomycosis and acquired immunodeficiency syndrome: Report of necropsy. *Rev. Soc. Bras. Med. Trop.* **2006**, *39*, 79–81. [CrossRef]
29. Castro, G.; Martinez, R. Images in clinical medicine. Disseminated paracoccidioidomycosis and coinfection with HIV. *N. Engl. J. Med.* **2006**, *355*, 2677. [CrossRef]
30. Brunaldi, M.O.; Rezende, R.E.F.; Zucoloto, S.; Garcia, S.B.; Módena, J.L.P.; Machado, A.A. Co-infection with paracoccidioidomycosis and human immunodeficiency virus: Report of a case with esophageal involvement. *Am. J. Trop. Med. Hyg.* **2010**, *82*, 1099–1101. [CrossRef]
31. De Freitas, R.S.; Dantas, K.C.; Garcia, R.S.P.; Magri, M.M.C.; de Andrade, H.F. Paracoccidioides brasiliensis causing a rib lesion in an adult AIDS patient. *Hum. Pathol.* **2010**, *41*, 1350–1354. [CrossRef] [PubMed]
32. Nunura, R.J.; Salazar, M.D.; Vásquez, L.T.; Endo, G.S.; Rodríguez, F.A.; Zerpa, L.R. Paracoccidioidomicosis and multidrug-resistant tuberculosis (TBC-MDR) in patient coinfected with HIV and hepatitis C. *Rev. Chilena Infectol.* **2010**, *27*, 551–555.
33. Lambertucci, J.R.; Vale, T.C.; Voieta, I. Images in infectious diseases. Concomitant progressive multifocal leukoencephalopathy and disseminated paracoccidioidomycosis in an AIDS patient. *Rev. Soc. Bras. Med. Trop.* **2010**, *43*, 758. [CrossRef] [PubMed]
34. Nogueira, L.M.C.; Santos, M.; Ferreira, L.C.; Talhari, C.; Rodrigues, R.R.; Talhari, S. AIDS-associated paracoccidioidomycosis in a patient with a CD4+ T-cell count of 4 cells/mm^3. *Anais Bras. Dermatol.* **2011**, *86*, S129–S132. [CrossRef]
35. Silva-Vergara, M.L.; Rocha, I.H.; Vasconcelos, R.R.; Maltos, A.L.; Neves, F.; Teixeira, L.; Mora, D.J. Central nervous system paracoccidioidomycosis in an AIDS patient: Case report. *Mycopathologia* **2014**, *177*, 137–141. [CrossRef] [PubMed]

36. Cimerman, S.; Bacha, H.A.; Ladeira, M.C.; Silveira, O.S.; Colombo, A.L. Paracoccidioidomycosis in a boy infected with HIV. *Mycoses* **1997**, *40*, 343–344. [CrossRef] [PubMed]
37. Benard, G.; Duarte, A.J. Paracoccidioidomycosis: A model for evaluation of the effects of human immunodeficiency virus infection on the natural history of endemic tropical diseases. *Clin. Infect. Dis.* **2000**, *31*, 1032–1039. [CrossRef] [PubMed]
38. Hadad, D.J.; Pieres, M.; Petry, T.C.; Orozco, S.F.; Melhem, M.; Paes, R.A.; Gianini, M.J. Paracoccidioides brasiliensis (Lutz, 1908) isolated by hemoculture in a patient with the acquired immunodeficiency syndrome (AIDS). *Rev. Inst. Med. Trop. Sao Paulo* **1992**, *34*, 565–567. [CrossRef]
39. Rabello Filho, E. Lupus eritematoso disseminado, blastomicose e epitelioma do lábio superior. *Anais Bras. Derm. Sif.* **1933**, *8*, 38–39.
40. Padilha-Gonçalves, A. Adenopatia na Micose de Lutz. Thesis, Escola de Medicina e Cirurgia do Rio de Janeiro, Rio de Janeiro, Brazil, 1971; p. 234.
41. Da Conceição, Y.T.M. Frequência da Associação em Estudo de Necropsias. Master's Thesis, Faculdade Medicina Universidade de São Paulo, São Paulo, Brazil, 1996; p. 102.
42. Shikanai-Yasuda, M.A.; Conceição, Y.M.T.; Kono, A.; Rivitti, E.; Campos, A.F.; Campos, S.V. Neoplasia and paracoccidioidomycosis. *Mycopathologia* **2008**, *165*, 303–312. [CrossRef]
43. Rodrigues, G.D.; Severo, C.B.; Oliveira, F.D.; Moreira, J.D.; Prolla, J.C.; Severo, L.C. Association between paracoccidioidomycosis and cancer. *J. Bras. Pneumol.* **2010**, *36*, 356–362. [CrossRef]
44. Maymó Argañaraz, M.; Luque, A.G.; Tosello, M.E.A.; Perez, J. Paracoccidioidomycosis and larynx carcinoma. *Mycoses* **2003**, *46*, 229–232. [CrossRef] [PubMed]
45. Marques, S.A.; Lastória, J.C.; Marques, M.E.A. Paracoccidioidomicose em paciente com carcinoma do colo uterino. *Anais Bras. Dermatol.* **2011**, *86*, 587–588. [CrossRef]
46. Porro, A.M.; Rotta, O. Cutaneous and pulmonary paracoccidioidomycosis in a patient with a malignant visceral tumor. *Anais Bras. Dermatol.* **2011**, *86*, 1220–1221. [CrossRef]
47. Azevedo, R.S.; Gouvêa, A.F.; Lopes, M.A.; Corrêa, M.B.; Jorge, J. Synchronous oral paracoccidioidomycosis and oral squamous cell carcinomas with submandibular enlargement. *Med. Mycol.* **2011**, *49*, 84–89. [CrossRef] [PubMed]
48. Tubino, P.V.A.; Sarmento, B.J.; dos Santos, V.M.; Borges, E.R.; da Silva, L.E.C.; Lima, R. Synchronous oral paracoccidioidomycosis and esophageal carcinoma. *Mycopathologia* **2012**, *174*, 157–161. [CrossRef] [PubMed]
49. Peçanha, P.M.; Ferreira, M.E.; Peçanha, M.A.; Schmidt, E.B.; de Araújo, M.L.; Zanotti, R.L.; Potratz, F.F.; Nunes, N.E.; Ferreira, C.U.; Delmaestro, D.; et al. Paracoccidioidomycosis: Epidemiological and Clinical Aspects in 546 Cases Studied in the State of Espírito Santo, Brazil. *Am. J. Trop. Med. Hyg.* **2017**, *97*, 836–844. [CrossRef]
50. Ruiz e Resende, L.S.; Yasuda, A.G.; Mendes, R.P.; Marques, S.A.; Niéro-Melo, L.; Defaveri, J.; Domingues, M.A.C. Paracoccidioidomycosis in patients with lymphoma and review of published literature. *Mycopathologia* **2015**, *179*, 285–291. [CrossRef]
51. Reis, M.A.; Costa, R.S.; Ferraz, A.S. Causes of death in renal transplant recipients: A study of 102 autopsies from 1968 to 1991. *J. R. Soc. Med.* **1995**, *88*, 24–27.
52. Zavascki, A.P.; Bienardt, J.C.; Severo, L.C. Paracoccidioidomycosis in organ transplant recipient: Case report. *Rev. Inst. Med. Trop. Sao Paulo* **2004**, *46*, 279–281. [CrossRef]
53. Pontes, A.M.; Borborema, J.; Correia, C.R.B.; de Almeida, W.L.; Maciel, R.F. A rare paracoccidioidomycosis diagnosis in a kidney transplant receptor: Case report. *Transplant. Proc.* **2015**, *47*, 1048–1050. [CrossRef] [PubMed]
54. Góes, H.F.; Durães, S.M.B.; Lima, C.; Souza, M.B.; Vilar, E.A.G.; Dalston, M.O. Paracoccidioidomycosis in a Renal Transplant Recipient. *Rev. Inst. Med. Trop. Sao Paulo* **2016**, *58*, 12. [CrossRef] [PubMed]
55. Radisic, M.V.; Linares, L.; Afeltra, J.; Pujato, N.; Vitale, R.G.; Bravo, M.; Dotta, A.C.; Casadei, D.H. Acute pulmonary involvement by paracoccidiodomycosis disease immediately after kidney transplantation: Case report and literature review. *Transpl. Infect. Dis.* **2017**, *19*, e12655. [CrossRef] [PubMed]
56. Lima, T.C.; Bezerra, R.O.F.; Siqueira, L.T.; Menezes, M.R.; Leite, C.; Porta, G.; Cerri, G.G. Paracoccidioidomycosis in a liver transplant recipient. *Rev. Soc. Bras. Med. Trop.* **2017**, *50*, 138–140. [CrossRef] [PubMed]
57. Campos, S.; Caramori, M.; Teixeira, R.; Afonso, J.; Carraro, R.; Strabelli, T.; Samano, M.; Pêgo-Fernandes, P.; Jatene, F. Bacterial and Fungal Pneumonias After Lung Transplantation. *Transpl. Proc.* **2008**, *40*, 822–824. [CrossRef] [PubMed]

58. Batista, M.V.; Sato, P.K.; Pierrotti, L.C.; de Paula, F.J.; Ferreira, G.F.; Ribeiro-David, D.S.; Nahas, W.C.; Duarte, M.I.S.; Shikanai-Yasuda, M.A. Recipient of kidney from donor with asymptomatic infection by Paracoccidioides brasiliensis. *Med. Mycol.* **2012**, *50*, 187–192. [CrossRef] [PubMed]
59. Abdala, E.; Miller, R.; Pasqualotto, A.C.; Muñoz, P.; Colombo, A.L.; Cuenca-Estrella, M. Endemic Fungal Infection Recommendations for Solid-Organ Transplant Recipients and Donors. *Transplantation* **2018**, *102*, S52–S59. [CrossRef] [PubMed]
60. Woyciechowsky, T.G.; Dalcin, D.C.; dos Santos, J.W.A.; Michel, G.T. Paracoccidioidomycosis induced by immunosuppressive drugs in a patient with rheumatoid arthritis and bone sarcoma: Case report and review of the literature. *Mycopathologia* **2011**, *172*, 77–81. [CrossRef]
61. Covre, L.C.P.; Hombre, P.M.; Falqueto, A.; Peçanha, P.M.; Valim, V. Pulmonary paracoccidioidomycosis: A case report of reactivation in a patient receiving biological therapy. *Rev. Soc. Bras. Med. Trop.* **2018**, *51*, 249–252. [CrossRef]
62. Almeida, K.J.; Barreto-Soares, R.V.; Campos-Sousa, R.N.; Campos-Sousa, M.G.; Bor-Seng-Shu, E. Pulmonary paracoccidioidomycosis associated with the use of natalizumab in multiple sclerosis. *Mult. Scler.* **2018**, *24*, 1002–1004. [CrossRef]
63. Vergidis, P.; Avery, R.K.; Wheat, L.J.; Dotson, J.L.; Assi, M.A.; Antoun, S.A.; Hamoud, K.A.; Burdette, S.D.; Freifeld, A.G.; McKinsey, D.S.; et al. Histoplasmosis complicating tumor necrosis factor-α blocker therapy: A retrospective analysis of 98 cases. *Clin. Infect. Dis.* **2015**, *61*, 409–417. [CrossRef] [PubMed]

8

Invasive Candidiasis in Infants and Children: Recent Advances in Epidemiology, Diagnosis and Treatment

Thomas J. Walsh [1,*], Aspasia Katragkou [2], Tempe Chen [3], Christine M. Salvatore [4] and Emmanuel Roilides [5]

1 Departments of Medicine, Pediatrics, and Microbiology & immunology, Weill Cornell Medicine of Cornell University and New York Presbyterian Hospital, New York, NY 10065, USA

2 Department of Pediatrics, Division of Pediatric Infectious Diseases, Nationwide Children's Hospital and The Ohio State University School of Medicine, Columbus, OH 43205, USA; Aspasia.Katragkou@nationwidechildrens.org

3 Pediatric Infectious Diseases, Department of Pediatrics, Miller Children's Hospital and University of California Irvine, Long Beach, CA 90806, USA; TChen@memorialcare.org

4 Department of Pediatrics, Division of Pediatric Infectious Diseases, Weill Cornell Medicine of Cornell University and New York Presbyterian Hospital, New York, NY 10065, USA; chs2032@med.cornell.edu

5 Infectious Diseases Section, 3rd Department of Pediatrics, Faculty of Medicine, Aristotle University School of Health Sciences and Hippokration General Hospital, 54642 Thessaloniki, Greece; roilides@med.auth.gr

* Correspondence: thw2003@med.cornell.edu

Abstract: This paper reviews recent advances in three selected areas of pediatric invasive candidiasis: epidemiology, diagnosis, and treatment. Although the epidemiological trends of pediatric invasive candidiasis illustrate a declining incidence, this infection still carries a heavy burden of mortality and morbidity that warrants a high index of clinical suspicion, the need for rapid diagnostic systems, and the early initiation of antifungal therapy. The development of non-culture-based technologies, such as the T2Candida system and (1→3)-β-D-glucan detection assay, offers the potential for early laboratory detection of candidemia and CNS candidiasis, respectively. Among the complications of disseminated candidiasis in infants and children, hematogenous disseminated *Candida* meningoencephalitis (HCME) is an important cause of neurological morbidity. Detection of (1→3)-β-D-glucan in cerebrospinal fluid serves as an early diagnostic indicator and an important biomarker of therapeutic response. The recently reported pharmacokinetic data of liposomal amphotericin B in children demonstrate dose–exposure relationships similar to those in adults. The recently completed randomized clinical trial of micafungin versus deoxycholate amphotericin B in the treatment of neonatal candidemia provides further safety data for an echinocandin in this clinical setting.

Keywords: candidemia; *Candida* meningoencephalitis; (1→3)-β-D-glucan; T2Candida; PCR; liposomal amphotericin B; micafungin; anidulafungin

---

1. Introduction

This paper reviews the recent advances in three selected areas of pediatric invasive candidiasis: epidemiology, diagnosis, and treatment, as presented in a lecture at the 20th Meeting of the International Immunocompromised Host Society. The paper reviews the nationwide secular trends of pediatric invasive candidiasis in the United States and Europe. Our review then further discusses new approaches to laboratory diagnosis and therapeutic monitoring while underscoring the continued need for bedside clinical evaluation. We then further review recent studies in pediatric antifungal pharmacology and therapeutics that provide new insights into safety, tolerability, pharmacokinetics, and efficacy for the management of invasive candidiasis.

2. Epidemiology

2.1. Secular Trends of Candidemia

Candidemia is the leading cause of invasive fungal infections in hospitalized children. Among the different populations of pediatric patients, the highest rates of candidemia have been recorded in neonates and infants <1 year of age [1–4]. However, candidemia in pediatric patients is associated with better therapeutic outcomes than in adults. For neonates and young infants, this improved outcome is associated with higher inpatient costs, in comparison with the costs associated with the treatment of adults. Additional comparative data pertaining to pediatric and adult secular trends are depicted at https://www.cdc.gov/fungal/diseases/candidiasis/invasive/statistics.html [5].

During the last decade, there has been a declining secular trend in the incidence of pediatric candidemia the United States and European Union [1–5]. The United States Centers for Diseases Control (CDC) initiated a population-based surveillance of four US metropolitan areas between 2009 and 2015 [5]. The overall incidence of candidemia in neonates decreased from 31.5 cases/100,000 births in 2009 to 10.7 and to 11.8 cases/100,000 births between 2012 and 2015, while the incidence in infants decreased from 52.1 cases/100,000 births in 2009 to 15.7 and to 17.5 between 2012 and 2015. The incidence of candidemia in non-infant children decreased similarly from 1.8 cases/100,000 births in 2009 to 0.8 cases/100,000 births in 2014.

Consistent with these data, there was a decline in the incidence of candidemia in patients who were <1 year in a population-based observational study conducted in Atlanta, Georgia, from approximately 60 per 100,000 person-years in 2008–2009, to less than 40 per 100,000 person-years in 2012–2013. Similarly, there was a decline of approximately 40 per 100,000 person-years in 2008–2009 to less than 20 per 100,000 person-years in 2012–2013. The secular trends in adults were relatively stable.

This decrease in the incidence of pediatric candidemia may be related to several factors regarding the care of central venous catheters [1,2]. These include hospital-wide implementation bundles, guiding insertion and the maintenance of central lines. These measures underscore the importance of using fully sterile barrier precautions, using chlorhexidine in the preparation of the skin during insertion of central lines, taking meticulous care of the catheter and its insertion site, and having daily discussions over the need for a central venous catheter.

2.2. Risk Factors

The risk factors for invasive candidiasis in neonates, particularly in prematurely born infants, warrant special consideration. In a study involving a prospective observational cohort of 1515 extremely low-birth-weight (ELBW) infants, which took place over three years at 19 centers of the US Eunice Kennedy Shriver National Institute of Child Health and Human Development (NICHD) Neonatal Research Network, Benjamin et al. quantified the risk factors predicting infection in high-risk premature infants [3]. Among the 1515 infants enrolled, 137 (9.0%) developed invasive candidiasis, documented by positive culture from one or more of the following sources: blood (n = 96); urine obtained by catheterization or suprapubic aspiration (n = 52); CSF (n = 9); other sterile body fluids (n = 10).

Among the different predictive models that have been developed for invasive candidiasis in neonates, a multivariable analysis of potentially modifiable risk factors associated with candidiasis identified the presence of an endotracheal tube, the presence of a central venous catheter, and a receipt of an intravenous lipid emulsion [3]. A second model predicted candidiasis at the time of blood cultures. Components of the history, physical exam, and initial laboratory evaluation that predicted candidiasis included vaginal delivery, week of gestational age, presence of *Candida*-like dermatitis observed during the physical exam, central venous catheter, lack of enteral feeding, hyperglycemia, number of days of antibiotic exposure in the week prior to culture, and thrombocytopenia [3]. The clinical prediction model had an area under the receiver operating characteristic curve of 0.79 and was superior to clinician judgment (0.70) in predicting neonatal invasive candidiasis.

In this groundbreaking study, invasive candidiasis was found to increase the risk of death in neonates; for example, 47 of 137 (34%) infants with candidiasis died, in comparison with 197 of 1378 (14%) patients without candidiasis ($p < 0.0001$) [3]. Mortality was the highest in the infants from whom *Candida* was isolated from multiple sources. For infant patients with positive urine and blood or positive urine and CSF, the rate of mortality was 16 of 28 (57%). Underscoring the significance of the recovery of *Candida* spp. from urine in neonates, mortality rate was similar in patients who had *Candida* spp. isolated only from blood and those with *Candida* isolated only from urine.

3. Diagnosis

3.1. Clinical Diagnosis

The bedside assessment of disseminated candidiasis begins with an understanding of the relative risks and a recognition of its clinical manifestations [6–10]. The clinical manifestations of invasive candidiasis include endophthalmitis (chorioretinal and vitreal lesions), hematogenous *Candida* meningoencephalitis (HCME) (seizures, intraventricular hemorrhages, developmental regression or delays, and CSF pleocytosis), endocarditis (murmurs, peripheral embolic manifestations, and congestive heart failure), hepatosplenic candidiasis (chronic disseminated candidiasis, persistent fever, left upper quadrant or right upper quadrant abdominal pain, and anorexia), acute disseminated candidiasis (multiple cutaneous lesions, diffuse myalgias, hypotension, and multiorgan failure), renal candidiasis (decreasing creatinine clearance, obstructive nephropathy, and renal bezoars), and osteoarticular infections (osteoarticular lesions that are unresponsive to empirical antibacterial therapy).

3.2. Laboratory Detection

Blood culture systems are relatively insensitive in the detection of deeply invasive candidiasis [11]. Non-culture-based methods, such as nucleic acid amplification systems, enzyme immunoassays for circulating mannans, and enzymatic systems for detection of (1→3)-β-D-glucan, are emerging as important laboratory tools for the diagnosis of invasive candidiasis [12–16].

3.3. T2Candida for Detection of Candidemia

The T2Candida system was recently licensed by the US FDA and was designated as superior to conventional blood culture systems for the detection of candidemia. In detecting the five most commonly recovered medically important *Candida* spp. (*Candida albicans*, *Candida tropicalis*, *Candida parapsilosis*, *Candida glabrata*, and *Candida krusei*), the T2Candida system utilizes a T2 magnetic resonance technology coupled with pathogen-derived nucleic acid amplification to identify the five target pathogens within 2 to 5 h from the time of initiation of the assay. Studies in adults have demonstrated a more rapid time to detection, in comparison with that of conventional blood cultures [15,16].

Little is known about the diagnostic utility of the T2Candida system in pediatric patients. In a study conducted at Children's Hospital of Philadelphia, whole blood from 15 children with candidemia was collected immediately following a blood culture draw [14]. Given the need for conserving the blood volume in this pediatric study, the amount of blood required by the system was reduced by pipetting whole blood directly onto the T2Candida cartridge. The specimens were subsequently run on the T2Dx Instrument (T2 Biosystems). The T2Candida biosystem correctly identified 15 positive and nine negative results within 3 to 5 h. The authors concluded that the T2Candida system was able to efficiently diagnose candidemia in pediatric patients while using low-volume blood specimens.

3.4. CSF (1→3)-β-D-Glucan as a Biomarker for Detection and Therapeutic Monitoring of Candida Infections of the Central Nervous System

HCME in pediatric patients is a life-threatening infection that is fraught with the potential of serious neurologic morbidity if not recognized and treated early [6,17]. HCME is observed in neonates, as well as in children with B-cell acute lymphoblastic leukemia, acute myelogenous leukemia, and primary immunodeficiencies. Associated with seizures, intraventricular hemorrhage, cortical blindness, and neurocognitive impairment, as well as the loss of developmental milestones, the early diagnosis of HCME is difficult, and its recurrence following the completion of antifungal therapy is common.

Petraitiene et al. originally demonstrated that CSF (1→3)-β-D-glucan levels correlated with CNS tissue infection in experimental HCME [18]. The expression of CSF and plasma (1→3)-β-D-glucan in the non-neutropenic rabbit model of experimental HCME treated with micafungin and with amphotericin B was predictive of the clinical features of this infection. Consistent with clinical observations regarding the difficulty in establishing a microbiological diagnosis, despite a well-established infection throughout CNS tissues, only 8% of CSF cultures were positive in untreated control animals. By comparison, all 25 CSF samples from these animals were found to be positive for (1→3)-β-D-glucan (755 to 7,750 pg/mL) ($p < 0.001$).

Changes in CSF (1→3)-β-D-glucan levels were highly predictive of antifungal therapeutic response, while clearance of *C. albicans* from blood cultures was not predictive of the eradication of organisms from the CNS [17]. The levels of (1→3)-β-D-glucan in CSF significantly decreased in comparison to those in untreated control animals. The levels of CSF (1→3)-β-D-glucan correlated with therapeutic responses to micafungin in a dose-dependent pattern, with a residual fungal burden in the cerebral tissue ($r = 0.842$). Thus, CSF (1→3)-β-D-glucan levels were predictive biomarkers for the detection and the therapeutic monitoring of experimental HCME. Building upon these data, a clinical trial was designed in the attempt to improve the management of HCME in pediatric patients.

Salvatore, Chen, and colleagues measured (1→3)-β-D-glucan levels in serially collected samples of serum and CSF of pediatric patients (aged 0–18 years) with a diagnosis of probable or proven HCME and CNS aspergillosis [19]. Among the nine cases of fungal infections of the central nervous system, seven were caused by HCME. All patients at baseline had detectable (1→3)-β-D-glucan in their CSF. In the six patients who completed the therapy for HCME, the elevated CSF (1→3)-β-D-glucan levels decreased to <31 pg/mL. One patient, who was unable to complete the antifungal therapy, died as the result of an overwhelmingly disseminated candidiasis. Monitoring serial CSF (1→3)-β-D-glucan levels in HCME was critical in determining the length of therapy, which ranged from 3 to 6 months, on the basis of individualized assessments. Subsequent reports have confirmed the utility of measuring CSF (1→3)-β-D-glucan levels for initial diagnosis and therapeutic monitoring of HCME [20–22].

4. Treatment

4.1. Liposomal Amphotericin B in Immunocompromised Children

Liposomal Amphotericin B (L-AMB) is widely used in the treatment of invasive fungal infections in immunocompromised children; however, little is known about its safety and pharmacokinetics in this vulnerable patient population. Seibel and colleagues therefore conducted a study of the safety, tolerability, and pharmacokinetics of L-AMB in 40 immunocompromised children and adolescents in a sequential-dose-escalation, multidose clinical trial [23]. Ten to 13 patients between the ages of 1 and 17 years were enrolled into each of the four dosage cohorts: 2.5, 5.0, 7.5, or 10 mg/kg, to receive empirical antifungal therapy for persistent fever and neutropenia or for the treatment of documented invasive fungal infections.

Serum creatinine increased from a mean of 0.45 ± 0.04 mg/dL to 0.63 ± 0.06 mg/dL across all dosage groups ($p = 0.003$). There was a significant increase in serum creatinine in dosage cohorts of 5.0 and 10 mg/kg/day. A greater frequency of hypokalemia and vomiting was also observed in patients receiving 10 mg/kg. Among the 565 infusions, 63 (11%) infusion-related adverse effects occurred. Five patients experienced acute infusion-related reactions at both the 7.5 and the 10 mg/kg dosage levels.

L-AMB in this patient population exhibited nonlinear pharmacokinetics [24]. The area under the concentration–time curve from 0 to 24 h ($AUC_{0\text{-}24}$) on day 1 increased from 54.7 $\pm$ 32.9 to 430 $\pm$ 566 μg·h/mL in patients receiving 2.5 and 10.0 mg/kg/day. The pharmacokinetic data were best described by a 2-compartment model that incorporated weight and an exponential decay function describing volume of distribution. The population-based model also demonstrated a significant ($p = 0.004$) relationship between the mean $AUC_{0\text{-}24}$ and the probability of nephrotoxicity, with an odds ratio of 2.37 (95% confidence interval, 1.84 to 3.22).

In summary, these data collectively support the use of a range of dosages comparable to those used in adult patients for the treatment of invasive fungal infections, with the understanding that azotemia may occur in direct relation to the $AUC_{0\text{-}24}$.

4.2. *Micafungin in Neonates*

Extensive preclinical studies in the treatment of experimental disseminated candidiasis [25–29] and clinical studies in pediatric patients [30–39] supported the investigation of micafungin in neonates in comparison with that of amphotericin B deoxycholate. Benjamin and colleagues compared the efficacy, safety and pharmacokinetics of intravenous micafungin at 10 mg/kg/d with intravenous amphotericin B deoxycholate at 1 mg/kg/d, in a phase 3, randomized, double-blind, multicenter, parallel-group, noninferiority trial, performed on infants >2–120 days of age with proven invasive candidiasis [40]. A total of 20 infants received micafungin, and 10 received amphotericin B deoxycholate. Although the study was terminated early because of low recruitment, fungal-free survival was observed in 12 out of the 20 [60%; 95% CI: 36–81%] infants treated with micafungin, versus 7 of the 10 (70%; 95% CI: 35–93%) infants treated with amphotericin B deoxycholate. The pharmacokinetic-model-derived mean area under the concentration-time curve (AUC) at steady state for micafungin was 399.3 $\pm$ 163.9 μg·h/mL, with an AUC pharmacodynamic target exposure of micafungin of 170 μg·h/mL. A population-based pharmacodynamic analysis supported a direct relationship between plasma exposure and the successful eradication of candidemia [41].

4.3. *Anidulafungin in Pediatric Patients*

Building upon earlier preclinical and clinical studies of anidulafungin [42,43], a recently published study reports on the safety and efficacy of anidulafungin in pediatric invasive candidiasis [44]. Anidulafungin was administered at a 3 mg/kg loading dose on day 1 and at a 1.5 mg/kg/d maintenance dose thereafter to patients between the ages of 2 and <18 years. Among 49 patients who received $\geq$1 dose of anidulafungin for a median 11 days (range of 1–35 days), all were reported to have a treatment-emergent adverse event (AE), such as, most commonly, diarrhea, vomiting, and fever. Treatment was discontinued due to AEs in four cases which were thought to be related to anidulafungin. Among the 48 patients with an isolate of a *Candida* spp., organisms were identified as *C. albicans* in 37.5%, *C. parapsilosis* in 25.0%, *C. tropicalis* in 14.6%, and *Candida lusitaniae* in 10.4%. One patient did not have an isolate of *Candida* sp. recovered. The global response success rate was 70.8%, while all-cause mortality was 8.2% at the end of intravenous therapy and 14.3% at 6-week follow-up. None of the deaths were considered to be treatment-related. The results of this study support the role of anidulafungin at the studied dosages for the treatment of pediatric invasive candidiasis.

5. Conclusions and Future Directions

During the past several years, important advances have been achieved in key areas of the epidemiology, laboratory diagnosis, and treatment of pediatric invasive candidiasis. There has been a clear downward trend in the incidence of pediatric invasive candidiasis. Nonetheless, pediatric invasive candidiasis remains an important cause of healthcare-associated sepsis and infectious morbidity. The bedside recognition of invasive candidiasis is challenging, and clinical manifestations are usually non-specific. Advances in the laboratory diagnosis of candidemia and deeply invasive candidiasis are helping to improve the recognition of these serious infections. Among these advances is the T2Candida system, which has the ability to detect more cases of candidemia than conventional blood cultures within 3 to 5 h. Another important advance is the detection of CSF (1→3)-β-D-glucan levels, which are highly sensitive in the diagnosis of HCME and can be serially monitored to guide the duration of and evaluate the response to the antifungal therapy.

Recently reported studies of L-AMB, micafungin, and anidulafungin in pediatric patients have been have been important advances in the management of invasive candidiasis in infants can children. A major body of preclinical and clinical studies has established the safety, pharmacokinetic, and efficacy profile of these potent antifungal agents in pediatric patients, including those patients with candidemia and other forms of deeply invasive candidiasis. As resistance to echinocandins and antifungal triazoles develops in *Candida* spp., new antifungal agents will be necessary to treat these emerging medically important pathogens. Among the new antifungal agents in development are the first-in-class molecules SCY-078, which is a triterpene inhibitor of (1→3)-β-D-glucan synthase, and APX-001, which is an inhibitor of fungal glycosyl-phosphatidyl-inositol (GPI) biosynthesis [21]. As these agents are developed, well-defined pediatric studies will need to be designed and implemented for the management of pediatric invasive candidiasis and other mycoses.

Acknowledgments: This paper is based upon a presentation given at the 20th ICHS Symposium on Infections in the Immunocompromised Host, 17–19 June 2018, Athens, Greece.

References

1. Mantadakis, E.; Pana, Z.D.; Zaoutis, T. Candidemia in children: Epidemiology, prevention and management. *Mycoses* **2018**, *61*, 614–622. [CrossRef] [PubMed]
2. Pana, Z.D.; Roilides, E.; Warris, A.; Groll, A.H.; Zaoutis, T. Epidemiology of Invasive Fungal Disease in Children. *J. Pediatr. Infect. Dis.* **2017**, *6*, S3–S11. [CrossRef] [PubMed]
3. Benjamin, D.K., Jr.; Stoll, B.J.; Gantz, M.G.; Walsh, M.C.; Sánchez, P.J.; Das, A.; Shankaran, S.; Higgins, R.D.; Auten, K.J.; Miller, N.A.; et al. Neonatal Candidiasis: Epidemiology, Risk Factors, and Clinical Judgment. *Pediatrics* **2010**, *126*, e865–e873. [CrossRef] [PubMed]
4. Aliaga, S.; Clark, R.H.; Clark, R.H.; Laughon, M.; Walsh, T.J.; Hope, W.; Benjamin, D.K.; Benjamin, D.K., Jr.; Smith, P.B. Decreasing incidence of candidiasis in infants in neonatal intensive care units. *Pediatrics* **2014**, *133*, 236–242. [CrossRef] [PubMed]
5. Invasive Candidiasis Statistics. Available online: https://www.cdc.gov/fungal/diseases/candidiasis/invasive/statistics.html (accessed on 1 December 2018).
6. Benjamin, D.K.; Poole, C.; Steinbach, W.J.; Rowen, J.L.; Walsh, T.J. Neonatal Candidemia and End-Organ Damage: A Critical Appraisal of the Literature Using Meta-analytic Techniques. *Pediatrics* **2003**, *112*, 634–640. [CrossRef] [PubMed]
7. Roilides, E. Invasive candidiasis in neonates and children. *Early Hum. Dev.* **2011**, *87*, S75–S76. [CrossRef] [PubMed]
8. Prasad, P.A.; Fisher, B.T.; Coffin, S.E.; Walsh, T.J.; McGowan, K.L.; Gross, R.; Zaoutis, T.E. Pediatric Risk Factors for Candidemia Secondary to Candida glabrata and Candida krusei Species. *J. Pediatr. Infect. Dis.* **2012**, *2*, 263–266. [CrossRef] [PubMed]
9. Fierro, J.L.; Prasad, P.; Fisher, B.; Gerber, J.; Coffin, S.E.; Walsh, T.J.; Zaoutis, T.E. Ocular manifestations of candidemia in a pediatric population. *Pediatr. Infect. Dis. J.* **2013**, *32*, 84–86. [CrossRef]
10. Gamaletsou, M.N.; Kontoyiannis, D.P.; Sipsas, N.V.; Moriyama, B.; Alexander, E.; Roilides, E.; Brause, B.; Walsh, T.J. Candida Osteomyelitis: Analysis of 207 Pediatric and Adult Cases (1970–2011). *Clin. Infect. Dis.* **2012**, *55*, 1338–1351. [CrossRef] [PubMed]

11. Berenguer, J.; Buck, M.; Witebsky, F.; Stock, F.; Pizzo, P.A.; Walsh, T.J. Lysis—Centrifugation blood cultures in the detection of tissue-proven invasive candidiasis disseminated versus single-organ infection. *Diagn. Microbiol. Infect. Dis.* **1993**, *17*, 103–109. [CrossRef]
12. Huppler, A.R.; Fisher, B.T.; Lehrnbecher, T.; Walsh, T.J.; Steinbach, W.J. Role of Molecular Biomarkers in the Diagnosis of Invasive Fungal Diseases in Children. *J. Pediatr. Infect. Dis.* **2017**, *6*, S32–S44. [CrossRef] [PubMed]
13. McCarthy, M.W.; Walsh, T.J. Molecular diagnosis of invasive mycoses of the central nervous system. *Expert Rev. Mol. Diagn.* **2016**, *17*, 129–139. [CrossRef] [PubMed]
14. Hamula, C.L.; Hughes, K.; Fisher, B.T.; Zaoutis, T.E.; Singh, I.R.; Velegraki, A. T2Candida Provides Rapid and Accurate Species Identification in Pediatric Cases of Candidemia. *Am. J. Clin. Pathol.* **2016**, *145*, 858–861. [CrossRef] [PubMed]
15. Mylonakis, E.; Clancy, C.J.; Ostrosky-Zeichner, L.; Garey, K.W.; Alangaden, G.J.; Vazquez, J.A.; Groeger, J.S.; Judson, M.A.; Vinagre, Y.-M.; Heard, S.O.; et al. T2 Magnetic Resonance Assay for the Rapid Diagnosis of Candidemia in Whole Blood: A Clinical Trial. *Clin. Infect. Dis.* **2015**, *60*, 892–899. [CrossRef]
16. Clancy, C.J.; Pappas, P.G.; Vazquez, J.; Judson, M.A.; Kontoyiannis, D.P.; Thompson, G.R., 3rd; Garey, K.W.; Reboli, A.; Greenberg, R.N.; Apewokin, S.; et al. Detecting Infections Rapidly and Easily for Candidemia Trial, Part 2 (DIRECT2): A Prospective, Multicenter Study of the T2Candida Panel. *Clin. Infect. Dis.* **2018**, *66*, 1678–1686. [CrossRef] [PubMed]
17. McCullers, J.A.; Vargas, S.L.; Flynn, P.M.; Razzouk, B.I.; Shenep, J.L. Candidal Meningitis in Children with Cancer. *Clin. Infect. Dis.* **2000**, *31*, 451–457. [CrossRef]
18. Petraitiene, R.; Petraitis, V.; Hope, W.W.; Mickiene, D.; Kelaher, A.M.; Murray, H.A.; Mya-San, C.; Hughes, J.E.; Cotton, M.P.; Bacher, J.; et al. Cerebrospinal fluid and plasma (1–>3)-beta-D-glucan as surrogate markers for detection and monitoring of therapeutic response in experimental hematogenous Candida meningoencephalitis. *Antimicrob. Agents Chemother.* **2008**, *52*, 4121–4129. [CrossRef]
19. Salvatore, C.M.; Chen, T.K.; Toussi, S.S.; DeLaMora, P.; Petraitiene, R.; Finkelman, M.A.; Walsh, T.J. (1→3)-β-D-glucan in Cerebrospinal Fluid as a Biomarker for Candida and Aspergillus Infections of the Central Nervous System in Pediatric Patients. *J. Pediatr. Infect. Dis. Soc.* **2016**, *5*, 277–286. [CrossRef]
20. Ceccarelli, G.; Ghezzi, M.C.; Raponi, G.; Brunetti, G.; Marsiglia, C.; Fallani, S.; Novelli, A.; Venditti, M. Voriconazole treatment of Candida tropicalis meningitis: Persistence of (1,3)-β-D-glucan in the cerebrospinal fluid is a marker of clinical and microbiological failure: A case report. *Medicine* **2016**, *95*, e4474. [CrossRef]
21. McCarthy, M.W.; Walsh, T.J. Drugs currently under investigation for the treatment of invasive candidiasis. *Expert Opin. Investig. Drugs* **2017**, *26*, 825–831. [CrossRef]
22. Farrugia, M.K.; Fogha, E.P.; Miah, A.R.; Yednock, J.; Palmer, H.C.; Guilfoose, J. Candida meningitis in an immunocompetent patient detected through (1→3)-beta-d-glucan. *Int. J. Infect. Dis.* **2016**, *51*, 25–26. [CrossRef] [PubMed]
23. Seibel, N.L.; Shad, A.T.; Bekersky, I.; Groll, A.H.; Gonzalez, C.; Wood, L.V.; Jarosinski, P.; Buell, D.; Hope, W.W.; Walsh, T.J.; et al. Safety, Tolerability, and Pharmacokinetics of Liposomal Amphotericin B in Immunocompromised Pediatric Patients. *Antimicrob. Agents Chemother.* **2016**, *61*, e01477-16. [CrossRef]
24. Lestner, J.M.; Groll, A.H.; Aljayyoussi, G.; Seibel, N.L.; Shad, A.; Gonzalez, C.; Wood, L.V.; Jarosinski, P.F.; Walsh, T.J.; Hope, W.W. Population Pharmacokinetics of Liposomal Amphotericin B in Immunocompromised Children. *Antimicrob. Agents Chemother.* **2016**, *60*, 7340–7346. [CrossRef] [PubMed]
25. Groll, A.H.; Mickiene, D.; Petraitis, V.; Petraitiene, R.; Ibrahim, K.H.; Piscitelli, S.C.; Bekersky, I.; Walsh, T.J. Compartmental Pharmacokinetics and Tissue Distribution of the Antifungal Echinocandin Lipopeptide Micafungin (FK463) in Rabbits. *Antimicrob. Agents Chemother.* **2001**, *45*, 3322–3327. [CrossRef]
26. Petraitis, V.; Petraitiene, R.; Groll, A.H.; Roussillon, K.; Hemmings, M.; Lyman, C.A.; Sein, T.; Bacher, J.; Bekersky, I.; Walsh, T.J.; et al. Comparative Antifungal Activities and Plasma Pharmacokinetics of Micafungin (FK463) against Disseminated Candidiasis and Invasive Pulmonary Aspergillosis in Persistently Neutropenic Rabbits. *Antimicrob. Agents Chemother.* **2002**, *46*, 1857–1869. [CrossRef] [PubMed]
27. Andes, D.R.; Diekema, D.; Pfaller, M.A.; Marchillo, K.; Bohrmueller, J. In Vivo Pharmacodynamic Target Investigation for Micafungin against Candida albicans and C. glabrata in a Neutropenic Murine Candidiasis Model. *Antimicrob. Agents Chemother.* **2008**, *52*, 3497–3503. [CrossRef] [PubMed]

28. Mickiene, D.; Petraitis, V.; Petraitiene, R.; Bacher, J.; Buell, D.; Heresi, G.; Kelaher, A.M.; Hughes, J.E.; Cotton, M.P.; Hope, W.W.; et al. The Pharmacokinetics and Pharmacodynamics of Micafungin in Experimental Hematogenous Candida Meningoencephalitis: Implications for Echinocandin Therapy in Neonates. *J. Infect. Dis.* **2008**, *197*, 163–171.
29. Simitsopoulou, M.; Chlichlia, K.; Kyrpitzi, D.; Walsh, T.J.; Roilides, E. Pharmacodynamic and Immunomodulatory Effects of Micafungin on Host Responses against Biofilms of Candida parapsilosis in Comparison to Those of Candida albicans. *Antimicrob. Agents Chemother.* **2018**, *62*. [CrossRef]
30. Seibel, N.L.; Schwartz, C.; Arrieta, A.; Flynn, P.; Shad, A.; Albano, E.; Keirns, J.; Lau, W.M.; Facklam, D.P.; Buell, D.N.; et al. Safety, Tolerability, and Pharmacokinetics of Micafungin (FK463) in Febrile Neutropenic Pediatric Patients. *Antimicrob. Agents Chemother.* **2005**, *49*, 3317–3324. [CrossRef]
31. Santos, R.P.; Sánchez, P.J.; Mejias, A.; Benjamin, D.K., Jr.; Walsh, T.J.; Patel, S.; Jafri, H.S. Successful medical treatment of cutaneous aspergillosis in a premature infant using liposomal amphotericin B, voriconazole and micafungin. *Pediatr. Infect. Dis. J.* **2007**, *26*, 364–366. [CrossRef]
32. Hope, W.; Seibel, N.L.; Schwartz, C.L.; Arrieta, A.; Flynn, P.; Shad, A.; Albano, E.; Keirns, J.J.; Buell, D.N.; Gumbo, T.; et al. Population Pharmacokinetics of Micafungin in Pediatric Patients and Implications for Antifungal Dosing. *Antimicrob. Agents Chemother.* **2007**, *51*, 3714–3719. [CrossRef] [PubMed]
33. Queiroz-Telles, F.; Berezin, E.; Leverger, G.; Freire, A.; van der Vyver, A.; Chotpitayasunondh, T.; Konja, J.; Diekmann-Berndt, H.; Koblinger, S.; Groll, A.H.; et al. Micafungin versus liposomal amphotericin B for pediatric patients with invasive candidiasis: Substudy of a randomized double-blind trial. *Pediatr. Infect. Dis. J.* **2008**, *27*, 820–826. [CrossRef] [PubMed]
34. Smith, P.B.; Walsh, T.J.; Hope, W.; Arrieta, A.; Takada, A.; Kovanda, L.L.; Kearns, G.L.; Kaufman, D.; Sawamoto, T.; Buell, D.N.; et al. Pharmacokinetics of an Elevated Dosage of Micafungin in Premature Neonates. *Pediatr. Infect. Dis. J.* **2009**, *28*, 412–415. [CrossRef] [PubMed]
35. Benjamin, D.K.; Arrieta, A.; Castro, L.; Sánchez, P.J.; Kaufman, D.; Arnold, L.J.; Kovanda, L.L.; Sawamoto, T.; Buell, D.N.; Hope, W.; et al. Safety and Pharmacokinetics of Repeat-Dose Micafungin in Young Infants. *Clin. Pharmacol. Ther.* **2009**, *87*, 93–99. [CrossRef] [PubMed]
36. Walsh, T.J.; Goutelle, S.; Jelliffe, R.W.; Golden, J.A.; Little, E.A.; DeVoe, C.; Mickiene, D.; Hayes, M.; Conte, J.E., Jr. Intrapulmonary Pharmacokinetics and Pharmacodynamics of Micafungin in Adult Lung Transplant Patients. *Antimicrob. Agents Chemother.* **2010**, *54*, 3451–3459. [CrossRef] [PubMed]
37. Hope, W.; Smith, P.B.; Arrieta, A.; Buell, D.N.; Roy, M.; Kaibara, A.; Walsh, T.J.; Cohen-Wolkowiez, M.; Benjamin, D.K., Jr. Population Pharmacokinetics of Micafungin in Neonates and Young Infants. *Antimicrob. Agents Chemother.* **2010**, *54*, 2633–2637. [CrossRef]
38. Arrieta, A.C.; Maddison, P.; Groll, A.H. Safety of Micafungin in Pediatric Clinical Trials. *Pediatr. Infect. Dis. J.* **2011**, *30*, e97–e102. [CrossRef]
39. Bochennek, K.; Balan, A.; Müller-Scholden, L.; Becker, M.; Farowski, F.; Müller, C.; Groll, A.H.; Lehrnbecher, T. Micafungin twice weekly as antifungal prophylaxis in paediatric patients at high risk for invasive fungal disease. *J. Antimicrob. Chemother.* **2015**, *70*, 1527–1530. [CrossRef]
40. Benjamin, D.K., Jr.; Kaufman, D.A.; Hope, W.W.; Smith, P.B.; Arrieta, A.; Manzoni, P.; Kovanda, L.L.; Lademacher, C.; Isaacson, B.; Jednachowski, D.; et al. A Phase 3 Study of Micafungin Versus Amphotericin B Deoxycholate in Infants with Invasive Candidiasis. *Pediatr. Infect. Dis. J.* **2018**, *37*, 992–998. [CrossRef]
41. Kovanda, L.L.; Walsh, T.J.; Benjamin, D.; Arrieta, A.; Kauffman, D.; Smith, P.B.; Manzoni, P.; Desai, A.V.; Kaibara, A.; Bonate, P.; et al. Exposure-response analysis of micafungin in neonatal candidiasis: Pooled analysis of two clinical trials. *Pediatr. Infect. Dis. J.* **2008**, *37*, 580–585. [CrossRef]
42. Groll, A.H.; Mickiene, D.; Petraitiene, R.; Petraitis, V.; Lyman, C.A.; Bacher, J.S.; Piscitelli, S.C.; Walsh, T.J. Pharmacokinetic and Pharmacodynamic Modeling of Anidulafungin (LY303366): Reappraisal of Its Efficacy in Neutropenic Animal Models of Opportunistic Mycoses Using Optimal Plasma Sampling. *Antimicrob. Agents Chemother.* **2001**, *45*, 2845–2855. [CrossRef] [PubMed]
43. Benjamin, D.K.; Driscoll, T.; Seibel, N.L.; González, C.E.; Roden, M.M.; Kilaru, R.; Clark, K.; Dowell, J.A.; Schranz, J.; Walsh, T.J.; et al. Safety and Pharmacokinetics of Intravenous Anidulafungin in Children with Neutropenia at High Risk for Invasive Fungal Infections. *Antimicrob. Agents Chemother.* **2006**, *50*, 632–638. [CrossRef] [PubMed]

44. Roilides, E.; Carlesse, F.; Leister-Tebbe, H.; Conte, U.; Yan, J.L.; Liu, P.; Tawadrous, M.; Aram, J.A.; Queiroz-Telles, F.; Anidulafungin A8851008 Pediatric Study Group. A Prospective, Open-label Study to Assess the Safety, Tolerability, and Efficacy of Anidulafungin in the Treatment of Invasive Candidiasis in Children 2 to <18 Years of Age. *Pediatr. Infect. Dis. J.* **2018**. [CrossRef]

9

Host-Pathogen Interactions Mediated by MDR Transporters in Fungi: As Pleiotropic as it Gets!

Mafalda Cavalheiro [1,2], Pedro Pais [1,2], Mónica Galocha [1,2] and Miguel C. Teixeira [1,2,*]

[1] Department of Bioengineering, Instituto Superior Técnico, Universidade de Lisboa, 1049-001 Lisbon, Portugal; mafalda.cavalheiro@tecnico.ulisboa.pt (M.C.); pedrohpais@tecnico.ulisboa.pt (P.P.); monicagalocha@tecnico.ulisboa.pt (M.G.)

[2] Biological Sciences Research Group, iBB—Institute for Bioengineering and Biosciences, Instituto Superior Técnico, Universidade de Lisboa, 1049-001 Lisboa, Portugal

* Correspondence: mnpct@tecnico.ulisboa.pt

Abstract: Fungal infections caused by *Candida*, *Aspergillus*, and *Cryptococcus* species are an increasing problem worldwide, associated with very high mortality rates. The successful prevalence of these human pathogens is due to their ability to thrive in stressful host niche colonization sites, to tolerate host immune system-induced stress, and to resist antifungal drugs. This review focuses on the key role played by multidrug resistance (MDR) transporters, belonging to the ATP-binding cassette (ABC), and the major facilitator superfamilies (MFS), in mediating fungal resistance to pathogenesis-related stresses. These clearly include the extrusion of antifungal drugs, with *C. albicans CDR1* and *MDR1* genes, and corresponding homologs in other fungal pathogens, playing a key role in this phenomenon. More recently, however, clues on the transcriptional regulation and physiological roles of MDR transporters, including the transport of lipids, ions, and small metabolites, have emerged, linking these transporters to important pathogenesis features, such as resistance to host niche environments, biofilm formation, immune system evasion, and virulence. The wider view of the activity of MDR transporters provided in this review highlights their relevance beyond drug resistance and the need to develop therapeutic strategies that successfully face the challenges posed by the pleiotropic nature of these transporters.

Keywords: fungal pathogens; multidrug transporters; host-pathogen interaction; virulence

---

1. Introduction

Species belonging to the *Aspergillus*, *Cryptococcus*, and *Candida* genera constitute the most relevant human fungal pathogens. Infections caused by these pathogens are especially severe in immunocompromised patients, particularly HIV-infected patients, cancer patients, and transplant recipients [1–3]. *Candida albicans* and *Candida glabrata* are the most prevalent of the pathogenic *Candida* species, being responsible for more than 400,000 life-threatening infections worldwide every year [4], as well as persistent mucosal infections [5,6]. *Aspergillus fumigatus* is the most frequent pathogenic species of the *Aspergillus* genus found to cause life-threatening pulmonary disease [7]. Central nervous system manifestations of meningitis or meningoencephalitis are recurrent manifestations associated with *Cryptococcus neoformans* infections [8].

One very resourceful feature of pathogenic fungi is the expression of multidrug resistance (MDR) transporters, which allow the development of antifungal drug resistance, being responsible for many cases of therapeutic failure [9,10]. MDR transporters belong mainly to two superfamilies, the ATP-binding cassette (ABC) and the major facilitator superfamilies (MFS). The ABC transporters have two main domains, each including a transmembrane domain (TMD) with six trans-membrane segments and a nucleotide-binding domain (NBD). This structure usually allows the transport of different molecules against an electrochemical gradient at the direct expense of ATP hydrolysis [11–13]. On the other hand, the transport performed by MFS transporters is driven by a proton-motive force. The MFS-MDR transporters are clustered into two families in fungi, the drug:H^+ antiporter 1 (DHA1), including 12 transmembrane segment proteins, and the drug:H^+ antiporter 2 (DHA2), including 14 transmembrane segment proteins [14]. Numerous molecules are proposed to be transported by MDR transporters of both superfamilies, including steroids, lipids, anti-cancer molecules, antifungals, herbicides, antibiotics, fluorescent dyes, carbohydrates, metabolites, neurotransmitters, nucleosides, amino acids, peptides, organic and inorganic anions, cations, and various Kreb's cycle intermediates [15,16], strongly suggesting either a promiscuous nature for MDR transporters or that they may indirectly affect the accumulation of these very diverse compounds, as a consequence of the transport of their physiological substrates.

The best-studied families of fungal drug efflux pumps are those from the model yeast *Saccharomyces cerevisiae* [17], in part, because it was the first eukaryote to have its genome sequenced [18]. In this model eukaryote, the ABC transporters have been classified into three main subfamilies, namely, the pleiotropic drug resistance (PDR), MDR, and multidrug resistance-associated protein (MRP), composing a total of 21 ABC drug resistance-related transporters [17,19]. Additionally, a total of 22 MFS drug transporters were reported in the genome of *S. cerevisiae* [20].

Genome sequencing has revealed that there is a wide repertoire of predicted ABC drug efflux pumps among pathogenic fungal species. However, only a few of these proteins have been functionally characterised, including those reported to be involved in multidrug resistance in human pathogens, such as *Candida albicans* [21–23], *Candida glabrata* [24–27], *A. fumigatus* [28,29], and *C. neoformans* [30,31]. Gaur et al. [32] constructed a complete inventory of ABC proteins in the genome of *C. albicans*, based on sequence similarities with ABC systems in other living organisms, and they found that *C. albicans* possesses 28 putative ABC proteins. The genome of the second most prevalent *Candida* species, *C. glabrata*, is predicted to have approximately two-thirds the number of ABC transporters predicted for *C. albicans* (18) [33]. Otherwise, much larger numbers of ABC proteins are predicted in the genomes of *A. fumigatus* and *C. neoformans*. The *A. fumigatus* genome is predicted to encode 49 ABC transporters, 35 of which are predicted to be multidrug efflux pumps [7,34]. *C. neoformans* is predicted to encode 54 ABC transporters [35].

The MFS transporters constitute the largest group of secondary active transporters, functioning as uniporters, symporters, or antiporters [16]. A subset of these transporters is involved in drug efflux [36]. Costa et al. [20] listed the DHA-MFS transporters found to occur, based on phylogenetic analysis with the model yeast *S. cerevisiae*, in the pathogenic yeasts of the *Candida* genus and also in *C. neoformans*, and *A. fumigatus*. Within the DHA1-MFS family, it was found 18, 10, 9, and 54 predicted transporters in the genome of *C. albicans*, *C. glabrata*, *C. neoformans*, and *A. fumigatus*, respectively. Regarding the DHA2-MFS family, 8, 5, 7, and 32 were found as predicted transporters in the genome of *C. albicans*, *C. glabrata*, *C. neoformans*, and *A. fumigatus*, respectively.

Although the main studied function of MDR transporters in fungi is related to the efflux of antifungal drugs, whose importance in azole resistance is reviewed herein, these transporters have different physiological roles that are also determinant for the survival of fungal pathogens in the human host. In this review, a collection of the identified physiological functions of the MDR transporters is compiled, highlighting how certain roles are necessary for the adaptation of fungi to the host niches, as well as in the fight against stresses imposed by the immune response of the host. Clues on the function of MDR transporters are also extracted from the gathered information on their transcription regulators.

2. MDR Transporters in Fungal Pathogens: Mediators of Azole Drug Resistance

Efflux-mediated drug resistance appears to be the most widespread mechanism of azole drug resistance among pathogenic fungal species [37–39]. The ABC drug efflux pumps have, in general, been linked to greater clinical significance [40]. However, and unlike what has been observed for ABC drug efflux pumps, which are widespread from bacteria to man, the MFS-MDR family appears to be strictly conserved within bacteria and fungi, turning these proteins into interesting candidates for targets for the development of new antifungal drugs [20].

The ABC transporters implicated in azole drug resistance in *C. albicans* are described as *Candida* Drug Resistance *(CDR)* genes , with *CaCDR1* encoding the best characterised multidrug transporter [41]. Together with *CaCDR1, CaCDR2* also contributes to azole resistance mediated by increased drug efflux [23,42]. In the non-*albicans Candida* species, the *CDR* genes have also been shown to play a role in azole resistance. In *Candida dubliniensis, CdCDR1* is overexpressed in the fluconazole-resistant strains [43]. In addition, *CDR1* is also induced in azole resistant *Candida parapsilosis* and *Candida tropicalis* clinical isolates [44–46]. In turn, the expression of the ABC transporters CgCdr1 and CgCdr2 in *C. glabrata* is related with the frequent azole resistance observed in this species [47]. Additionally, the ABC transporters CgSnq2 and CgYor1 have also been implicated in azole stress response in *C. glabrata* [26,48]. *Candida krusei,* which displays intrinsic azole resistance, harbors two ABC drug efflux pumps (CkAbc1 and CkAbc2) that are upregulated during azole stress [49]. *Candida krusei* CkAbc1 is involved in intrinsic fluconazole resistance [50] and confers fluconazole resistance through drug efflux upon overexpression in *S. cerevisiae* [51]. *CkABC2* expression was correlated with itraconazole resistance [52].

In *A. fumigatus,* the mechanisms of antifungal resistance have deserved more intensive investigations in the past ten years. Alteration of the azole target *cyp51A* is a major mechanism in clinical and environmental isolates. However, there are now also several non-*cyp51A*-mediated azole-resistant isolates in which the underlying mechanisms remain partially unsolved [53]. The reduced intracellular accumulation of drugs has also been correlated with the overexpression of MDR efflux transporter genes in this pathogen [38]. In contrast to the extensive number of genes predicted to encode transporters in *A. fumigatus* [54], there are very few studies characterizing these transporters and their relationship with multidrug resistance. However, decreased intracellular accumulation of itraconazole was verified in *A. fumigatus,* hinting for a possible participation of efflux pumps in azole resistance in this fungus. Slaven et al. [29] and Nascimento et al. [55] have characterised AfuAtrF and AfuMdr4, respectively, as ABC transporters, and correlated them with itraconazole resistance. Additionally, genes encoding the set of transporters AfuAbcA-E, AtrF, and AtrI are induced during voriconazole stress [53,56].

In *C. neoformans*, the reduced intracellular accumulation of drugs has been correlated with the overexpression of MDR efflux transporter genes [39]. The genome of this pathogen is predicted to encode nearly 86 DHA-MFS transporters and 54 ABC transporters. Nevertheless, only three efflux pumps have been related with drug extrusion, CnAfr1, CnAfr2, and CnMdr1 [30,57,58]. A recent study by Chang et al. [57] demonstrated that CnAfr1 is a crucial for azole efflux and is important for handling other xenobiotics, including cycloheximide, nocodazole, and trichostatin A. The overexpression of the *C. neoformans* ABC transporter CnAfr1 is known to underlie clinical fluconazole resistance [31], while CnMdr1 confers itraconazole resistance upon overexpression in *S. cerevisiae* [51]. However, these three efflux pumps appeared to play no clear role in susceptibility towards amphotericin B and 5-fluorocytosine.

Although transporter-mediated azole resistance has been initially associated with ABC drug efflux pumps, further insights have shown that MFS-MDR transporters also play a relevant role in this phenomenon. In fact, several transporters from the MFS-MDR family are also relevant players in clinical azole resistance phenotypes, as is the case with the *C. albicans* CaMdr1. Considered a major mediator of azole resistance, it is overexpressed in some resistant clinical isolates, underlying fluconazole resistance [59]. A similar case was also identified in *Candida dubliniensis*, with increased *CdMDR1* transcript levels associated with clinical resistance phenotypes to fluconazole, but not to ketoconazole [43,60]. Moreover, *C. parapsilosis* azole resistant clinical isolates overexpress CpMdr1 [44,45], and such a response is also observed during the in vitro induction of azole resistance [61]. Resistant clinical isolates of *C. tropicalis* were found to overexpress the CtMdr1 transporter [46,62]. The *C. albicans* MFS transporter CaFlu1 confers fluconazole resistance in *S. cerevisiae*, but it plays a secondary role in *C. albicans* [63,64].

A relevant role of MFS efflux pumps in azole response is also observed in *C. glabrata*, translated by the increased expression of CgAqr1, CgQdr2, CgTpo1_1, and CgTpo3, found to mediate clotrimazole resistance in clinical isolates [10]. These transporters were previously found to mediate azole resistance in laboratory strains as well [24,25,27,65]. Interestingly, the level of correlation between the increased expression of these transporters and the azole drug resistance was similar to that observed for the *CgCDR2* gene, thus highlighting the importance of MFS-MDR transporters in the clinical setting [10]. More recently, the MFS-MDR transporters CgTpo1_2, CgFlr1, and CgFlr2, were also found to confer azole resistance, by mediating the decreased intracellular accumulation of these drugs [65,66]. In *A. fumigatus*, the MFS transporters can potentially have a relevant role in azole resistance, since AfuMdr3 displays an increased expression in itraconazole-resistant mutants [55]. In addition, three transporters (AfuMfsA–C) are highly expressed during voriconazole stress [56].

Within the MFS-MDR transporters, only eight (CaMdr1, CaFlu1, CaNag3, CaNag4, CaNag6, CaQdr1, CaQdr2, and CaQdr3), seven (CgAqr1, CgFlr1, CgFlr2, CgTpo1_1, CgTpo1_2, CgTpo3, CgQdr2), three (CNA07070, CNC03290, and CND00440/aflT), and six (gliA, mfs56, Mdr3, and MfsA–C), were already characterised in *C. albicans*, *C. glabrata*, *C. neoformans*, and *A. fumigatus*, respectively [20].

Not only is there a wide variety of MDR transporters involved in azole resistance in several fungal pathogens, but the regulation of their expression is also diverse. The most prominent mechanism of azole resistance acquisition involves increased drug efflux pumps gene expression, which is mediated by master regulators of azole resistance. They include Tac1 and Mrr1 in *C. albicans* and related species; and CgPdr1 in *C. glabrata*. These transcription factors are subjected to gain-of-function (GOF) mutations in their protein sequence, which result in hyperactive forms, responsible for constitutive increased transcription of their target genes [44,61,67–72]. Additionally, each transcription factor regulates its own expression, increasing their own transcript levels in response to azole stress [67,73–75]. ABC transporters in particular have been first described as targets of CaTac1 and CgPdr1 [26,48,76–78], but several MFS transporters are also activated by CaMrr1 and CgPdr1 [65,66,71,72], thus reinforcing the role of multiple transporters in azole resistance pathways.

Other than mutations in transcriptional regulators, another regulatory mechanism mediating azole resistance is chromosomal abnormalities. These can include loss of heterozygosity (LOH), chromosomal aneuploidies, or increased gene copy number. Development of azole resistance by LOH events is known to occur in *C. albicans*, namely in the genomic regions containing *CaTAC1* or *CaMRR1*. Mutations in *MRR1* followed by the loss of heterozygosity, contribute to the overexpression of this gene [72]. This phenomenon also occurs to give rise to *CaTAC1* homozygous mutations because of the loss of heterozygosity in chromosome 5 [70]. Chromosomal rearrangements also contribute to the amplification of the *CaTAC1* gene [79]. In *C. glabrata*, the existence of differential chromosome configurations and segmental aneuploidies was observed in azole-resistant strains [80]. Alterations in chromosome copy number is related with *C. neoformans* resistance to azoles. In particular, CnAfr1 overexpression due to chromosome 1 duplication results in resistant populations in response to selection [81].

Although the transcriptional regulation of MDR transporters in *A. fumigatus* and *C. neoformans* have not yet been deeply studied, Hagiwara and colleagues [82] reported a novel Zn_2–Cys_6 transcription factor, AfuAtrR, as playing a key role in an azole resistance mechanism of *A. fumigatus*, by regulating the drug target AfuCyp51A (14-α sterol demethylase) and the putative drug efflux pump AfuCdr1B (AfuAbcC) expression. Additionally, through the screening of a library of transcription factor mutants, different transcription factors regulating the expression of efflux pumps genes in response to fluconazole exposure were identified in *C. neoformans*. These include *CnCRZ1* and *CnYAP1*, which had been previously characterised as transcription factors functioning in response to environmental stress, including thermal, hypoxic, and fluconazole, as well as oxidative stress in *C. neoformans* [83,84]. Chang and co-workers [57] determined that CnAfr1 expression was positively regulated by CnCrz1 and CnYap1 in response to fluconazole.

3. MDR Transporters in Fungal Pathogens: Mediating the Transport of Physiological Substrates as a Way to Adapt to Host Niches

Fungal pathogens have different strategies to colonize, survive, and infect the human host. Each species has preferential niches, developing specific mechanisms that allow adaptation to each microenvironment and evasion from the immune system. For instance, *C. albicans* exhibits different morphologies to better adapt to each niche, for example switching from the hyphal morphology used to penetrate host epithelial cells to the yeast shape to circulate in the bloodstream [85]. The preferential niches for *C. albicans* and other *Candida* species include the oral cavity, the skin, the urogenital, and gastrointestinal tracts, whose infection might lead to disseminated disease [85,86]. In the case of the *Cryptococcus* species, the preferable niches of the human host include the pulmonary tissue and the central nervous system. The establishment of a *Cryptococcus* invasive disease often starts with infection of the lung tissue, followed by invasion of the bloodstream, and subsequent dissemination of *Cryptococcus* cells to the central nervous system [87,88]. Likewise, *A. fumigatus* infects primarily the lungs, disseminating from there to any possible organ [89].

In each specific niche, different stresses like heat shock, osmotic, oxidative and nitrosative stresses, pH variations, and hypoxia might be encountered, forcing the development of stress resistance mechanisms by fungal pathogens [90]. Given the different stresses and different nutrient availability, fungal pathogens must have increased flexibility to adapt and respond to the environment. This wide capacity of metabolic adaptation and resistance to stress also promotes virulence in fungal pathogens, as it lessens their vulnerability to the surrounding environment [86].

In the oral cavity, different factors protect the host from the presence of fungal pathogens. First of all, different cell types are ready to identify them, including polymorphonuclear leukocytes, monocytes/macrophages, non-major histocompatibility complex (MHC)-restricted $CD8^+$ T cells, and oral epithelial cells [91]. Upon the presence of *Candida* cells, the epithelial cells from the oral mucosa induce expression of a nitric oxide synthase, which leads to increased levels of nitric oxide believed to have a candidacidal activity, helping in the resistance to mucosal candidiasis [91]. These cells are also able to secrete different antimicrobial peptides, including members of the β-defensin family [92]. Additionally, the saliva has powerful antimicrobial peptides, such as histatins. These are known to promote cell cycle disturbance, increased intracellular reactive oxygen species (ROS), and loss of cell volume in *C. albicans*, ultimately leading to the apoptosis of yeast cells. Histatin-1, -3, and -5 are produced by acinar cells present in human salivary glands [93].

The lungs constitute the first site for *Cryptococcus* infection. This niche also has its strategies of protection against invasion. As a first defense mechanism of the innate immune system is the presence of bronchial and alveolar Type I and Type II epithelial cells that, besides forming a physical barrier, also release several cytokines and chemokines to activate an immunologic response [94]. Also important for this response is the presence in the lung tissue of inflammatory monocytes, alveolar macrophages, dendritic cells, and neutrophils [95,96]. M1 macrophages produce ROS and reactive nitrogen species (RNS), including nitric oxide, known to have anti-cryptococcal properties [96]. *Aspergillus fumigatus* also enters the host by inhalation, facing the action of alveolar macrophages, neutrophils, and dendritic cells [97,98].

In turn, the vaginal mucosa is a low pH environment with the presence of weak acids, like acetic and lactic acids [99,100], protected by *Candida*-specific cell-mediated immunity. This immunity is mediated by T helper (Th) 1-type responses [101]. Additionally, the established microbiome present in this niche is also responsible for its protection. A good example is the role of *Lactobacillus crispatus* in this context, found to mediate the immune response of vaginal epithelial cells deployed in the presence of *C. albicans* [102].

Although generally associated to multidrug resistance, some MDR transporters have been found to contribute to the adaptation of fungal pathogens to human host niches. This role of MDR transporters seems to be linked to a general function of cellular detoxification, given their ability to catalyse the efflux of antifungal drugs, but also other toxic metabolites present mainly in the stationary phase of cellular growth [103]. Interestingly, the ability to control the concentration of some of these physiological substrates is likely to confer a selective advantage when growing, both as commensals and pathogens in human host niches.

For example, the *C. albicans* ABC transporter Cdr1 was found to transport steroids. Accumulation assays with radiolabelled β-estradiol and corticosterone have demonstrated the ability of CaCdr1, expressed in the AD1234568 (AD)-*CDR1 S. cerevisiae* strain, to enhance the efflux of these human steroids, that appear to compete with drugs such as cycloheximide, O-phenanthroline, chloramphenicol, fluconazole, or rhodamine 123 as Cdr1 substrates [104]. However, the transport of [^{3}H]-β-estradiol was not affected by the truncation of domain 12 of CaCdr1, a mutation that affects drug transport, suggesting that Cdr1 displays different binding sites for these different substrates [105]. Interestingly, increased incidence of vulvovaginal candidiasis has been linked to the presence of elevated estrogen levels during pregnancy or to the presence of exogenous estrogens from oral contraceptives [106–109]. The effect of β-estradiol or ethynyl estradiol, but not α-estradiol or estriol, on the formation of germ tubes has been reported, revealing the specificity of such an induction [110,111]. *Candida albicans* strain SC5314 and the vaginal isolate GC15 in Roswell Park Memorial Institute (RPMI)-free supplemented with supraphysiological (10^{-5} M) or physiological (10^{-10} M) concentrations of 17-β-estradiol and estradiol, respectively, during different time points, exhibit the upregulation of *CaCDR1* and *CaCDR2*. When both genes were disrupted, the *C. albicans* cells exposed to 17-β-estradiol had a decreased germ tube formation [111]. These evidences point out the importance that MDR efflux pump-mediated resistance to chemical compounds present in human body niches have in the success of fungal infections.

In *S. cerevisiae*, sterol uptake requires the involvement of the ABC transporters Pdr11 and Aus1. These are necessary for the nonvesicular movement, from the plasma membrane to the endoplasmatic reticulum, a movement needed for the sterol ester synthesis required for sterol uptake [112]. The *S. cerevisiae* Upc2 transcription factor is known to induce the *AUS1* and *PDR11* expression under anaerobiosis conditions, when the sterol uptake is essential. The absence of these two genes leads to defects in sterol uptake [113]. Although, in *S. cerevisiae*, no connection to MDR has been observed for these transporters; in *Cryptococcus gattii*, Pdr11 was found to be necessary for fluconazole resistance in the VGII clinical strain [114]; and *C. glabrata* Aus1 has been linked to sterol transport associated with the presence of azole drugs, being upregulated in anaerobic conditions [115]. In fact, sterol uptake was found to be used by *C. glabrata* strains defective in ergosterol [116] and in *C. glabrata* clinical isolates [117]. In fact, upon the use of azoles, which affect the production of ergosterol, the sterol uptake response is activated as a resistance mechanism that allows *C. glabrata* cells to survive ergosterol defects with host sterols, like cholesterol [118]. Sterol uptake might also be necessary for *C. glabrata* virulence, as Aus1 is necessary in a mice model of disseminated infection, being significantly upregulated in such conditions [115]. Therefore, sterol uptake is an important strategy developed by *C. glabrata* to survive in the human host, ensuring its virulence and antifungal resistance in mucosal niches.

Major facilitator superfamilies multidrug transporters have also been found to contribute to lipid homeostasis in *C. albicans* and *C. glabrata*. The MFS-MDR transporters Qdr1, Qdr2, and Qdr3 of *C. albicans* were found to be localized in the plasma membrane, with preferential localization of Qdr1 and Qdr2 in lipid rafts. These transporters do not participate in the resistance to any type of known antifungals [119], although their homologs in *C. glabrata* and in *S. cerevisiae* are recognized drug transporters [25,120–122]. Nevertheless, they seem to have other important functions for the survival of *C. albicans*. When absent, *CaQDR1*, *CaQDR2*, or *CaQDR3* lead to the accumulation of phosphatidylinositol and phosphatidylserine, as well as of sphingolipids, thus indicating a role of these transporters in lipid homeostasis [119]. On the other hand, the *C. glabrata* Tpo1_2 MFS-MDR transporter has also been linked to fatty acid and sterol homeostasis, especially during biofilm formation. The absence of *CgTPO1_2* upon biofilm formation leads to a decrease of very long fatty acids. Moreover, ergosterol content in the Δ*cgtpo1_2* deletion mutant was found to be 30% higher than in its parental strain [123]. This physiological function of lipid transportation in *C. glabrata* seems to be important for to the adaptation to low pH environments with organic acids, as alterations in the membrane lipid composition have been described as a mechanism to surpass the stress on such environment [124].

The CgTpo1_2 homolog, CgTpo1_1, is also an MFS drug transporter with an interesting proposed role in the survival of *C. glabrata* in the oral cavity. One of the mechanisms used by the host to resist candidiasis is the release of the antimicrobial peptide histatin-5 in the saliva [93], as described above. Interestingly, the CgTpo1_1 transporter was found to be necessary for the resistance of *C. glabrata* to this antimicrobial peptide [123]. Another similar player in histatin-5 resistance is the *C. albicans* Flu1 MFS transporter involved in the resistance towards fluconazole, ketoconazole, and itraconazole [63]. In fact, the absence of *CaFLU1* significantly defects cellular growth and biofilm formation upon the exposure to this antimicrobial peptide [125]. Both studies give evidence of the role of MDR transporters' action against antimicrobial peptides, a usually effective weapon of the human immune system against microbial infections.

The roles of the Ste6 ABC transporter of *S. cerevisiae* are also different and interesting. This transporter was found to be responsible for the secretion of a lipopeptide mating pheromone, designated a-factor, but also for the resistance of this species to valinomycin, an antibiotic peptide [126]. Interestingly, *C. albicans* homolog of Ste6, designated Hst6, was found to be able to complement the role of *S. cerevisiae* Ste6 in a Δ*scste6* deletion mutant [127]. Nevertheless, its specific function in *C. albicans* remains to be discovered, as this species is not known to secrete mating pheromones. On the other hand, the Ste6 homolog in *C. neoformans* has been shown to be involved in the mating process of this pathogen [128]. In turn, *A. fumigatus* Afu3g03430, which is also similar to *S. cerevisiae* Ste6, has been indicated as being involved in iron uptake [129–131]. Iron uptake is an important function for the survival of any fungal pathogen, as this cofactor is necessary for several enzymatic reactions and is withheld in the human host as a protective mechanism against microbial infections [132].

Another example of the importance of MDR transporters in the adaptation to human niches is their role in polyamine resistance. Polyamines like spermine, spermidine, and putrescine are essential organic polycations, which are usually involved in the regulation of nucleic acid and protein synthesis, as well as cell growth [14]. The plasma membrane MFS-MDR transporters, Tpo1–4 and Qdr3, were the first identified as important players in the resistance to polyamines in *S. cerevisiae* [133–135]. In *C. glabrata*, MFS-MDR transporters have also been found to contribute to the resistance to polyamines, which may become toxic above certain concentrations, such as those found in the human urogenital tract [136]. The prevalence of *Candida* species in this niche is likely facilitated by two homologs of ScTpo1 in *C. glabrata*, CgTpo1_1 and CgTpo1_2, which have been identified as determinants in spermine resistance [65]. In turn, the CgTpo3 transporter, known to be involved in *C. glabrata* azole resistance, presents the same physiological role as its *S. cerevisiae* homolog, Tpo3, in polyamine resistance [24].

Since the vaginal tract is characterised by an acidic pH of about 4, as well as the presence of weak acids, like acetic and lactic acids [99,100], the ability to tolerate the stress induced by weak acids is crucial for *Candida* colonization and successful infection. Interestingly, *S. cerevisiae* MFS-MDR transporters, like Aqr1 and Qdr1, are important determinants in short-chain monocarboxylic acid resistance [120,137]. *S. cerevisiae* Aqr1 has also been implicated in the excretion of homoserine, threonine, alanine, glutamate, and aspartate, probably through vesicles, releasing the amino acids to the extracellular environment through exocytosis [138]. The homolog of *S. cerevisiae* Aqr1 in *C. glabrata*, CgAqr1, has been linked to flucytosine and clotrimazole resistance, as well as resistance against acetic acid [27]. Such a role in the resistance to acetic acid is also performed by the MFS-MDR CgDtr1 and CgTpo3 transporters [139,140], being the later controlled by the CgHaa1 transcription factor, known to regulate the response of *C. glabrata* to acetic acid [140]. These different roles of MFS transporters [14,20] point out their importance for the survival of such pathogens in acidic human microenvironments.

4. MDR Transporters in Fungal Pathogens: Playing a Role in Virulence, Biofilm Formation, and Phagocytosis Evasion

To persist in the human host, fungal pathogens need to survive in the first site of infection, and disseminate to other niches of the host. To achieve this goal, several barriers imposed by the niches need to be surpassed, as well as the ones imposed by the immune response (Figure 1). To face and resist such offenses, fungal pathogens develop strategies of survival, including biofilm formation, macrophage evasion mechanisms, and virulence factors, where the role of given MDR transporters becomes important.

For example, similarly to the *S. cerevisiae* Pdr5 and Yor1 ABC transporters [17], *C. albicans* CaCdr1, CaCdr2, and CaCdr3 have been shown to play a role in phospholipid translocation when expressed in *S. cerevisiae*. CaCdr1 and CaCdr2 conduct an in-to-out movement of phospholipids through the plasma membrane bilayer in an energy-dependent manner, while CaCdr3, which is not involved in antifungal drug resistance, produces the opposite movement, from the outer to the inner leaflet of the plasma membrane [141]. The transport of phospholipids by Cdr1 may be extremely important for *C. albicans* evasion to the host immune system, as some phospholipids have been identified as lipid antigens and precursors of lysophospholipids, also known to be lipid antigens recognized by human natural killer T lymphocytes [142,143]. For instance, to avoid identification by the host immune response, *C. albicans* relies on CaQdr2 and CaQdr3 transporters, given that they are necessary for the maintenance of phosphatidylinositol, which is a lipid antigen recognized by the CD1 antigen-presenting cells from the host [144]. Interestingly, the absence of *CaQDR2* and *CaQDR3* genes have shown to attenuated *C. albicans* virulence in a murine model of hematogenously disseminated candidiasis [119].

When fungal evasion is not effective, pathogens are phagocyted and a new environment is set upon them, to which they have to adapt to survive. Different host cells are able to perform phagocytosis, including monocytes/macrophages, neutrophils, and dendritic cells [145,146]. All these lead to the formation of phagolysosomes that attempt to kill pathogens by producing ROS and RNS, activating the action of proteases and decreasing the pH, resorting to K^+ fluxes [146]. *Candida* species display an activation of oxidative stress response in this environment, as well as other survival mechanisms [147]. In particular, *C. glabrata* cells are known to be able to resist and proliferate inside mammalian macrophages for a very long time [148]. Together with other more specific mechanisms, *C. glabrata* is known to count with two transporters from the MFS-MDR family, CgAqr1 and CgDtr1, which are responsible for the resistance to weak acids and oxidative stress [27,139]. CgAqr1 was found to confer resistance to acetic acid [27], like its homolog in *S. cerevisiae* [137], and CgDtr1 was identified as an acetic acid exporter, allowing the resistance to this acid and oxidative stress [139]. It is likely that the role of CgDtr1 in weak acid and oxidative stress resistance underlies its contribution to the survival of *C. glabrata* in the macrophages and, indirectly, to increase virulence. Indeed, the *CgDTR1* expression is upregulated in cells phagocytozed by *Galleria mellonella,* hemocytes and the overexpression of this gene leads to an increase in the survival of *C. glabrata* cells in *G. mellonella* hemocytes. Furthermore, CgDtr1 was found to be necessary for the full virulence of *C. glabrata* in the infection model *G. mellonella* [139].

Cryptococcus neoformans survival in phagocytic cells also depends on its reaction to the new environment with low pH, ROS, and nitric oxide [96]. Upon *C. neoformans* phagocytosis by macrophages in vitro, the overexpression of the *CnAFR1* gene takes place [39]. The Afr1 ABC transporter is known for the in vitro and in vivo resistance to fluconazole [31,39,58], but has also been linked to the virulence of *C. neoformans*, in intravenous and in inhalation mouse models [39]. Although not helping to avoid phagocytosis, CnAfr1 delays the maturation of the phagolysosome, which exhibits less acid vacuoles. CnAfr1 seems to interfere with the pathway of phagolysosome maturation, as the early endosome marker Rab5 and late marker Rab7 are less detected upon the overexpression of the *CnAFR1* gene [149]. Moreover, Goulart and colleagues have reported the upregulation of other ABC transporters in *C. neoformans* cells phagocyted by peritoneal macrophages [150], highlighting the importance these transporters within the study of the *Cryptococcus* species survival in the host.

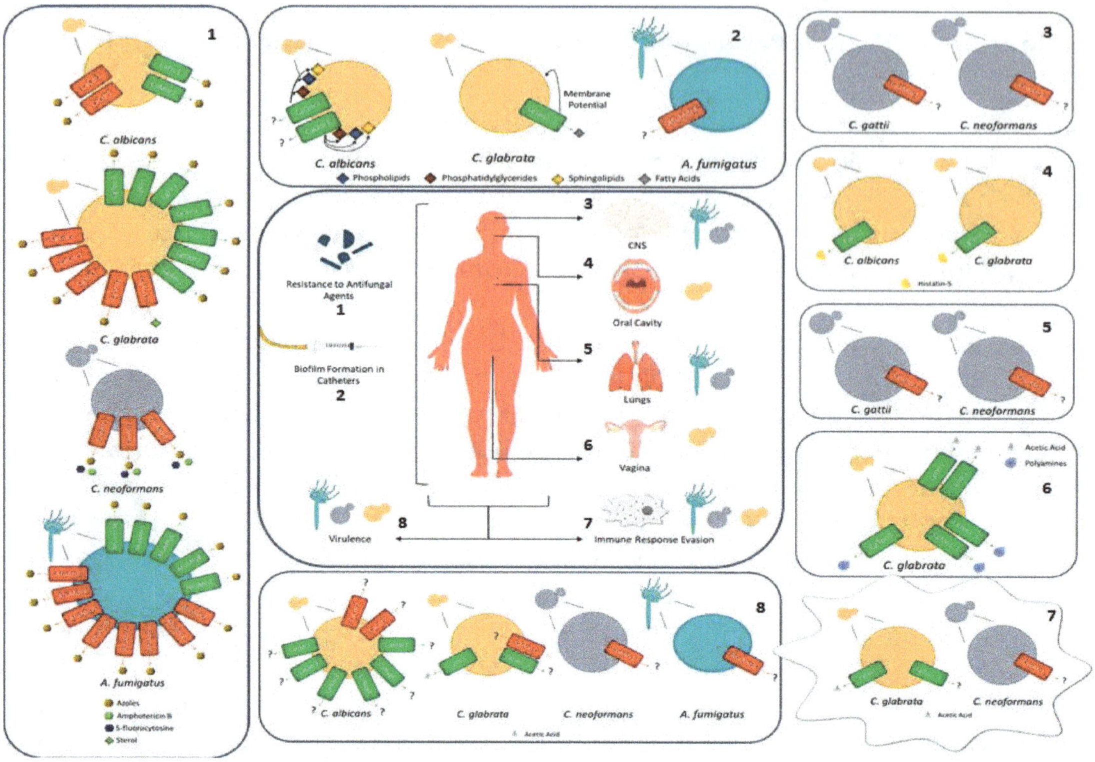

Figure 1. The role of multidrug resistance (MDR) transporters in the survival of *Candida*, *Cryptococcus*, and *Aspergillus* species upon infection in the human host. (1) MDR transporters involved in multiple azole resistance; (2) MDR transporters necessary for biofilm formation; (3) MDR transporters involved in *Cryptococcus* species virulence in the central nervous system (CNS); (4) MDR transporters involved in the efflux of histatin-5 in the oral cavity; (5) MDR transporters involved in *Cryptococcus* species virulence in the lungs; (6) *Candida glabrata* MDR transporters involved in polyamine or acetic acid export for the survival in the vaginal tract; (7) MDR transporters involved in the fight against the immune response of the host; and (8) MDR transporters known to be essential for normal virulence of fungal pathogens. The central picture summarizes the niches of infection in which the referred fungal pathogens are found. ATP-binding cassette (ABC) transporters are highlighted in red and major facilitator superfamilies (MFS) transporters are highlighted in green.

Cryptococcus gattii seems to count with drug transporters for its full virulence in the brain and the pulmonary tissue, like the MFS Mdr1 and the ABC Pdr11 transporters, determinants of *C. gattii* MDR [58,114]. The *MDR1* gene was found to be upregulated in cells recovered from the brain and lungs of infected mice, while *PDR11* was overexpressed in cells recovered from the lungs of infected mice [151]. Both Mdr1 and Pdr11 were proposed to play an additional role *C. gattii* virulence and adaptation to the host environment, although the exact mechanism underlying this observation is unclear.

Likewise, *A. fumigatus* infects primarily the lungs disseminating to any possible organ [89]. Such infections are believed to make use of the 49 ABC-like genes and 278 MFS-like genes present in this species [54], which, given their elevated number, indicate a major role in *A. fumigatus*. From all these, some have been identified as antifungal resistant players [28,29,55,56], but having additional roles in expelling toxic molecules [54]. abcA and abcB are two *A. fumigatus* transporters, with a high similarity to the *S. cerevisiae* Pdr5 drug efflux pump. abcB is necessary for full virulence of *A. fumigatus* in the *G. mellonella* model of infection and the overexpression of the *abcA* gene leads to an augmentation of virulence in the presence of voriconazole, in the same infection model [152].

The *C. albicans* Mdr1 MFS transporter is well known for its role in MDR [9,153,154]. Nevertheless, this transporter has been identified as necessary for full virulence in *C. albicans* in immunocompetent and immunocompromised mice models [155], although its specific functions in virulence have not yet been assessed. Moreover, the CaNag3, CaNag4, and CaNag6 MFS transporters are necessary for the full virulence of *C. albicans* in a mouse model [156].

Several MDR transporters have also been shown to have roles in biofilm formation, an important feature that allows the persistence of fungal pathogens in the host [157]. One specific case is the activity displayed by CaQdr2 and CaQdr3 in the architecture of *C. albicans* biofilm, which, although not contributing for the total biomass produced, help to shape the structure of the biofilm [119]. In *C. glabrata*, the CgTpo1_2 has been highlighted as an important player in biofilm formation, being necessary for the normal expression of *CgALS1*, *CgEAP1*, and *CgEPA1* genes encoding adhesins. Its role in biofilm formation seems to be linked to its importance in fatty acids homeostasis, as it affects the incorporation of very long chain fatty acids, which are usually found in *C. glabrata* biofilms [123]. In turn, *A. fumigatus* Mdr4 transporter has been identified as upregulated upon voriconazole exposure and biofilm formation conditions [129,158], indicating a possible role in the development of biofilm. Interestingly, GOF mutations in the multidrug resistance transcription factor Pdr1 were also found to be required for increased virulence and biofilm formation, by controlling the expression of the adhesion encoding gene *EPA1* [159,160].

5. Hints on the Function of MDR Transporters Based on Transcription Regulation

Recently, clues on the physiological roles of MDR transporters, including the transport of lipids, ions, and small metabolites, have emerged from transcriptional regulation data, linking these transporters to important pathogenesis features such as resistance to host niche environments, biofilm formation, immune system evasion, and virulence. In this section, all available information on the transcriptional regulation of ABC/MFS-MDR transporter genes in the human pathogens *C. albicans* and *C. glabrata* is reviewed. Although a similar analysis would be very interesting for *A. fumigatus* and *C. neoformans*, the available information is very limited and scattered. On the contrary, information on *C. albicans* and *C. glabrata* has been recently gathered in the PathoYeastract database (www.pathoyeastract.org) [161], enabling the analysis of MDR transporter regulation, not only in the multidrug resistance context, but also within the perspective of their physiological roles and their implication in other pathogenesis-related phenotypes.

Besides the expected role of the MDR transcription factors, transcription factors controlling stress response, cell cycle, cell wall dynamics, biofilm formation, lipid and carbohydrate metabolism, and nutrient availability have been found to regulate the expression of the MDR transporter encoding genes in *C. albicans*. In fact, the number of regulatory associations with MDR transporter genes involving transcription factors virtually not related to MDR is much higher than that involving recognized MDR transcription factors. Surprisingly, with regards to multidrug resistance, only 36% (12 out of 33) of the MDR-related transporters in *C. albicans* are reported to be regulated by at least one MDR-related transcription factor, more specifically, 57% (8 out of 14) of the ABC transporters and nearly 21% (4 out of 19) of the MFS-MDR transporters (Figure 2A). Expectably, the transcription factor CaMrr1, a multidrug resistance regulator in *C. albicans*, was found to regulate 11 out of the 12 MDR transporters reported to be regulated by at least one MDR-related transcription factor, including the MFS-MDR transporter, CaMdr1, a key player in the acquisition of azole resistance in clinical isolates [71]. Transporters that have been clearly linked to resistance of a wider range of drugs are indeed those that are regulated by a higher number of MDR transcription factors. This is the case for *CaCDR1* and *CaCDR2*, which are the main ABC transporter genes responsible for azole drug resistance in *C. albicans*. *CaCDR1* is regulated by CaFcr1, CaMrr1, CaMrr2, and CaTac1, whereas *CaCDR2* is reported to be regulated by CaMrr1 and CaTac1. In particular, the *CaCDR1* regulation appears to be highly complex, being controlled by at least 19 transcription factors not only related to MDR, but also with biofilm formation, stress response, cell-wall dynamics, carbohydrate metabolism, cell-cycle, and lipid metabolism. Besides CaMrr1, *C. albicans* carries yet another major regulator of multidrug resistance transporters, CaTac1, which is described as the major factor needed for the regulation of

CaCDR1 and *CaCDR2* [76]. Nevertheless, contrasting with CaMrr1, CaTac1 appears to regulate no other MDR transporter genes besides *CaCDR1* and *CaCDR2* (Figure 2A).

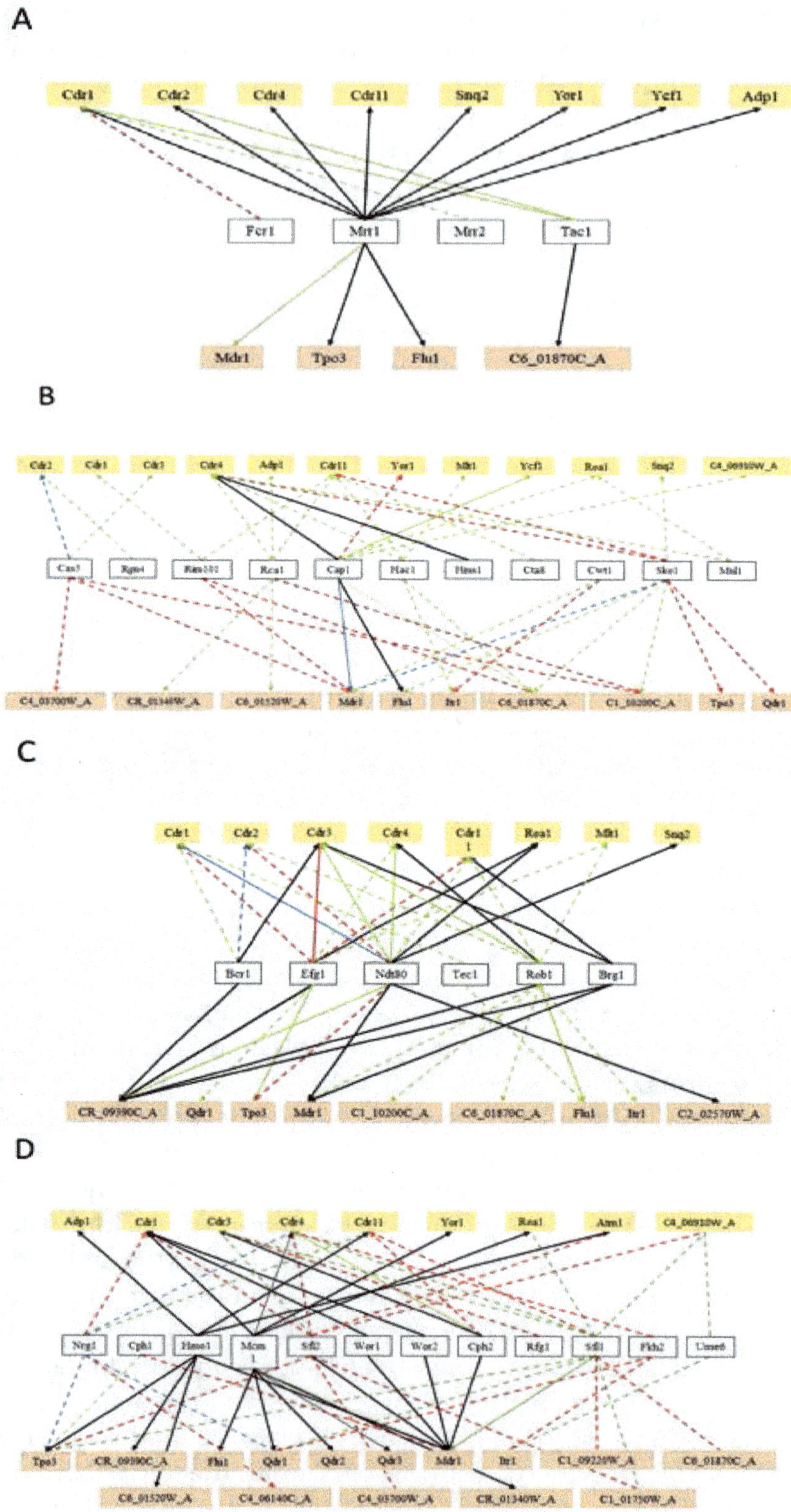

Figure 2. *Cont.*

E

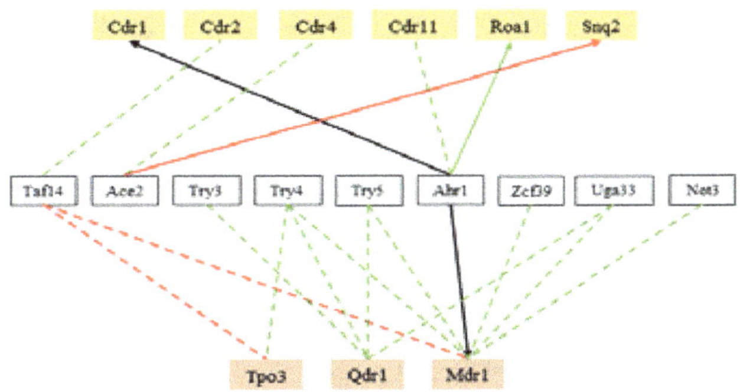

F

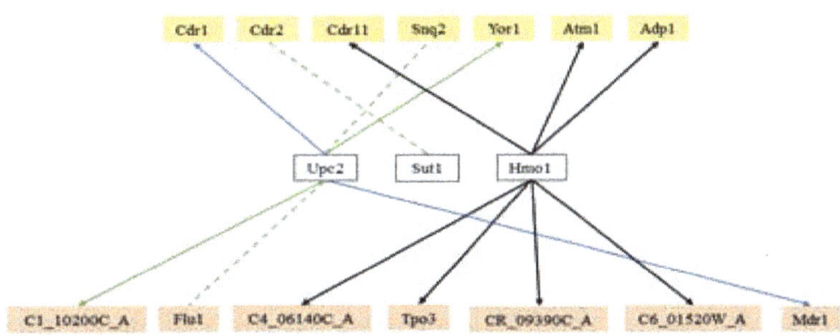

Figure 2. Transcriptional regulatory networks that control the expression of MDR transporter genes in *C. albicans*, considering the subgroups of transcription factors known to be involved in multidrug resistance (**A**); in stress response (**B**); biofilm formation (**C**); cell-cycle/morphology (**D**); cell-wall dynamics (**E**); and lipid (**F**). The displayed regulatory associations are according to the data present in the Pathoyeastract database (http://pathoyeastract.org/) [161]. The ABC transporters are highlighted by the yellow colour and the MFS transporters are highlighted by the orange colour. Arrows indicate the experimental basis of the documented regulatory associations, either expression evidence (dashed line) or DNA-binding evidence (filled line). Green, red, blue, or black arrows indicate a positive, negative, positive and negative, or unspecified association, respectively.

It is surprising the number of stress-related transcription factors reported to regulate MDR transporters in *C. albicans*. Nearly 67% (22 out of 33) of the *C. albicans* MDR transporters have been found to be regulated by at least one stress-related transcription factor, with the transcription factors CaCap1 and CaSko1 regulating the highest number of transporters (eight and nine, respectively) (Figure 2B). These two transcription factors are known to be required for oxidative stress tolerance in *C. albicans* [162,163], which is a vital process for this pathogen to survive in healthy hosts, especially during phagocytosis. Additionally, the transcription factor CaRim101 was found to regulate the expression of a considerable number of MDR transporter genes (7). This regulator plays a crucial role in pH-response [164], and the Rim101 pathway is required for host-pathogen interactions, as it regulates the expression of genes that stimulate host cell damage [165]. Among other stress-related transcription factors that were found to control MDR transporter genes are CaCta8, an essential transcription factor that mediates heat shock response [166]; CaRpn4 and CaHac1, key regulators of unfolded protein response (UPR), which is a crucial phenomenon for cellular protein homeostasis maintenance, which is often lost when cells are under stress such as that induced by antifungals [167]; and Cas5, a zinc finger transcription factor that controls the response to cell wall stress, including those induced by echinocandins [168], but also the response to membrane stress exerted by the azole antifungal drugs [169].

Transcription factors related to biofilm formation were also found to regulate a significant number of MDR transporters in *C. albicans* (nearly 52%, 17 out of 33) (Figure 2C). Nobile et al. [170] described and analysed the transcriptional network controlling the biofilm formation in *C. albicans*, whose biofilms are a major source of medical device-associated infections. They demonstrated that CaBcr1, CaTec1, CaEfg1, CaNdt80, CaRob1, and CaBrg1 are the major players in the transcriptional network controlling the biofilm development in this human pathogen, including many MDR transporters. In fact, genes encoding for drug efflux pumps had been previously been reported in biofilms to be differentially regulated during development, as well as upon exposure to antimicrobial agents, including *CaCDR1*, *CaCDR2*, *CaMDR1*, *CaNAG3*, and *CaNAG4* [171–173]. CaRob1 and CaNdt80 were found to regulate the highest number of MDR transporters (nearly 65%, 11 out of 17 each), whereas CaTec1 was found to regulate a smaller portion of those (approximately 12%, 2 out of 17). These associations corroborate the observation that efflux pump-mediated multidrug resistance is an important trait of biofilm cells [174].

In *C. albicans*, the ability to undergo morphological switching from yeast cells to hyphae, in response to various environmental signals, is an important virulence factor that contributes to biofilm formation, invasion and dissemination of *Candida* in host tissues, and resistance to macrophage and neutrophil engulfment [171,175,176]. Interestingly, cell-cycle/morphology related transcription factors were found to regulate the highest portion of MDR transporters, 72% (24 out of 33), including the *CDR* genes and *MDR1* (Figure 2D). In fact, despite the fact that cell-cycle related transcriptional regulators have never been demonstrated to be crucial for efflux pump expression, a positive correlation between the level of antifungal drug resistance and the ability to form hyphae in the presence of azole drugs has been identified [176]. For instance, Mcm1, which is an essential transcription factor in *C. albicans* crucial for morphogenesis [177], was found to regulate the expression of several MDR transporters (10 out of 24), including *CaCDR1* and *CaMDR1*. CaMcm1 was previously demonstrated to be dispensable for *CaMDR1* upregulation in response to H_2O_2 , but was required for full *CaMDR1* induction by benomyl [177]. The transcription factors CaSfl1 and CaSfl2, two homologous heat shock factor-type transcriptional regulators that antagonistically control morphogenesis in *C. albicans*, while being required for full pathogenesis and virulence [178], were also found to regulate a number of MDR transporters (11 and 9, respectively). Finally, CaWor1 and CaWor2 are transcriptional regulators of *C. albicans* opaque cell formation, and were also found to regulate MDR transporters.

Also, cell-wall dynamics related transcription factors regulate MDR transporters in *C. albicans* (9), including the *CDR* gene family and *CaMDR1* (Figure 2E). The Try transcription factors and Taf14, Ahr1, Uga33, and Zcf39 are all reported regulators of *C. albicans* yeast form adherence, and they were found to regulate at least one MDR transporter.

Additionally, CaUpc2, the master regulator of the ergosterol biosynthesis (*ERG*) genes [179], and CaHmo1, which was also shown to bind promoters of ergosterol metabolism genes [180], regulate the expression of 13 MDR transporters (Figure 2F). The regulation of ABC drug efflux pumps by the lipid metabolism related transcription factor, is likely to be due to the activity of some of these MDR transporters in phospholipid translocation or ergosterol transport. It is not likely that all drug pumps involved in multidrug resistance are phospholipid translocators. For instance, *CaMDR1* shows no detectable phospholipid exchange activity [181]. However, the observation that these transcription factors also control the expression of MDR-MFS transporters, suggest that they may also play a role in this lipid metabolism. This hypothesis is consistent with the observation that the deletion of MFS-MDR genes *CaQDR1*, *CaQDR2*, and *CaQDR3* [119], or *CgTPO1_2* [123], does affect lipid composition.

In the case of *C. glabrata*, only a few regulators of MDR transporter genes have yet been unveiled, reflecting the fact that the study of transcriptional regulation in this yeast is still in its infancy, especially in biological processes beyond drug resistance. The transcription factor CgPdr1 is described as the master regulator of multidrug resistance in this organism, regulating the expression of several MDR transporter genes [48]. CgPdr1 is thought to form a heterodimer with CgStb5, as it happens in the closely related *S. cerevisiae*. The overexpression of *CgSTB5* in *C. glabrata* represses azole resistance, while its deletion produces a shy intensification in resistance. Expression analysis assays established that CgStb5p shares many transcriptional targets with CgPdr1, but, unlike the second, it is a negative regulator of pleiotropic drug resistance [68,182]. These two MDR-related transcription factors were found to regulate a total of 12 MDR transporters (seven ABC and five MFS) (Figure 3A).

Besides the expected role of MDR transcription factors, stress response transcription factors have been found to regulate the MDR transporter encoding genes in *C. glabrata*. Five stress-responsive transcription factors are reported to regulate the expression of at least one MDR transporter gene (Figure 3B). CgYap1 is the major regulator of oxidative stress response genes in *C. glabrata* [183], and it was also demonstrated to induce the expression of multidrug transporters [184]. As antifungals induce the endogenous production of ROS, thus inducing oxidative stress response mediated by CgYap1, it is likely that CgYap1 targets the MDR transporters that play a role in the extrusion of oxidative stress generating molecules from the cells. Otherwise, CgYap7 is a transcriptional repressor of nitric oxide oxidase and also regulates the iron–sulfur cluster biogenesis [185]. The remaining transcription factors present in this group were not yet characterised. However, they are thought to be involved in salt tolerance (CgHal9 and CgYap6) and weak acid response (CgWar1), based on the function of their *S. cerevisiae* homologs. It is interesting to note that the ABC transporter encoding ORF *CAGL0M07293g*, although uncharacterised, is reported to be regulated by CgYap7, CgYap6, CgHal9, and CgWar1 transcription factors. This is in accordance with its predicted function as a weak-acid-inducible multidrug transporter required for weak organic acid resistance, based on the function of its closest *S. cerevisiae* homolog ScPdr12.

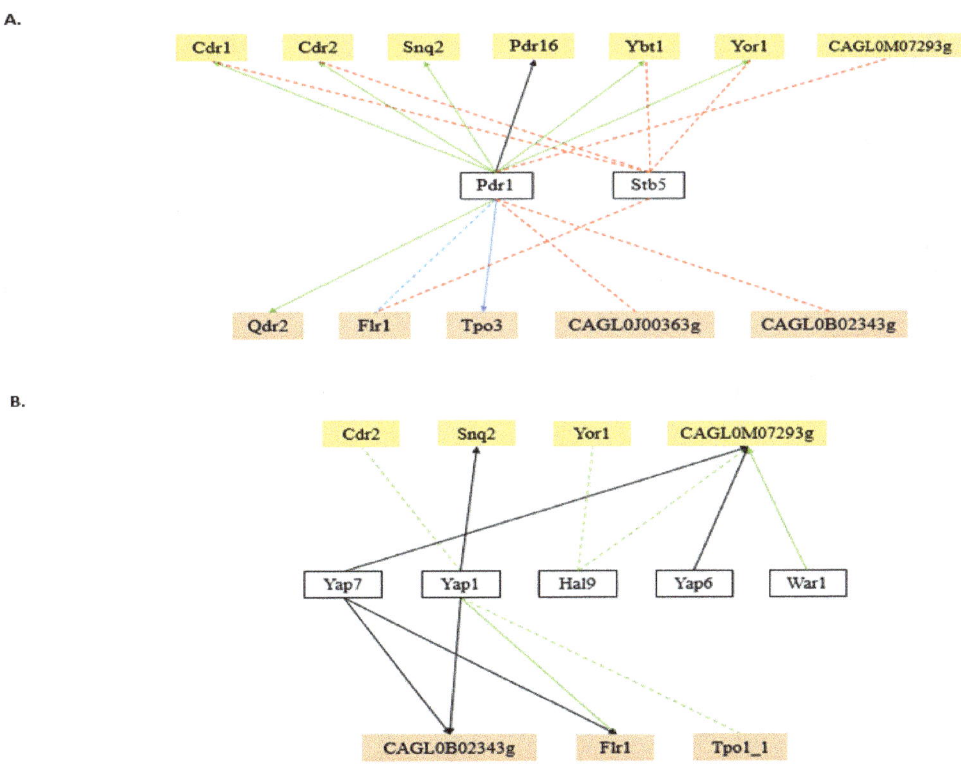

Figure 3. Transcriptional regulatory networks that control the expression of MDR transporter genes in *C. glabrata*, considering the subgroups of transcription factors known to be involved in multidrug resistance (**A**) and in stress response (**B**). The displayed regulatory associations are according to the data present in the Pathoyeastract database (http://pathoyeastract.org/) [161]. ABC transporters are highlighted by the yellow colour and MFS transporters are highlighted by the orange colour. Arrows indicate the experimental basis of the documented regulatory associations, either expression evidence (dashed line) or DNA-binding evidence (filled line). Green, red, blue, or black arrows indicate a positive, negative, positive and negative, or unspecified association, respectively.

6. Conclusions and Perspectives.

MDR transporters are undoubtedly necessary players for the successful survival of fungal pathogens in the human host (Tables 2 and 2). As reviewed herein, their prominent role in MDR has a real impact in the clinical acquisition of drug resistance, allowing these pathogens to persist even upon treatment with different antifungal agents. Indeed, within the characterised MDR transporters, 88.5% and 71.4% of the ABC and MFS, respectively, have been shown to contribute to drug resistance, suggesting that this is their most relevant feature.

This review, however, highlights the observation that both ABC and MFS-MDR transporters contribute to the ability of fungal pathogens to colonize the host and evade host induced defenses, by executing other functions not directly connected with MDR. The study of the transcriptional networks controlling the expression of drug transporters in *C. albicans* and *C. glabrata* points towards possible links between MDR transporters and several cellular processes, including stress response, morphological switching, cell wall, and lipid homeostasis. Indeed, mounting evidence suggests that the function of MDR transporters goes well beyond their traditional role in drug resistance. Clues on what may be the physiological role of these transporters, suggest that their natural activity is not linked to the transport of chemical compounds that are not found in nature, but rather the transport of metabolites that can be found in the natural ecosystems where pathogenic fungi thrive. Among the characterised ABC and MFS transporters, 19.2% and 42.8%, respectively have been associated to the transport of such biomolecules. Significantly, MDR transporter roles associated to phospholipid and ergosterol incorporation, as well as in the excretion of metabolites that reach toxic concentrations in host niches, such as polyamines and weak acids, establish a strong link between the MDR transporters and the survival of fungal pathogens in several human microenvironments. Additionally, a few MDR transporters have been linked to the resistance to stress imposed by the host immune system, including phagocytosis and antimicrobial peptides, such as histatin-5. Not surprisingly, a high proportion of the characterised ABC (43.5%) and MFS (39.3%)-MDR transporters were found to be required for full virulence in infection models, several of which, however, for unknown reasons. It will be interesting to ascertain the precise function of these transporters in the context of virulence.

Despite their crucial role in several aspects of pathogenesis, there is still a striking lack of knowledge about the function of the majority of the MDR transporters. Indeed, among the 241 predicted ABC drug transporters in the fungal pathogens approached in this review, only 10.8%, that is 26, have been characterised. In the case of the predicted MFS-MDR transporters, only 5.8% (28 out of 479), have been functionally analysed. This observation highlights the pressing need to invest in the study of these two families of drug transporters, with special emphasis on less studied organisms, which in this context includes *A. fumigatus*, for which only 2.1% of the MFS-MDR transporters have been characterised, or *C. tropicalis*, for which only 4.5% of the ABC drug efflux pumps have been studied.

Overall, this review gathers evidence of the multitasking capacity of MDR transporters in fungal pathogens, while highlighting their key role in the successful colonization, persistence, and virulence in the human host. The truly pleiotropic activity of the ABC and MFS-MDR transporters underlines their importance in fungal pathogenesis, and highlights them as very promising drug targets for the development of new antifungals.

Table 1. ATP-binding cassette (ABC) transporters of *Candida, Aspergillus,* and *Cryptococcus* species focusing their roles in multidrug resistance (MDR) and physiological functions, as well as their pathogenicity and virulence features.

	Species	Total #	Characterised #	Characterised ORFs	Role in MDR	Physiological Role	Pathogenicity and Virulence Features
ABC Proteins	*Candida albicans*	28	4	*orf19.6000/CDR1*	Multidrug transporter of ABC superfamily	Transport of phospholipids (in-to-out direction), steroids	Induced by β-estradiol, progesterone, corticosteroid, or cholesterol; Spider biofilm induced
				orf19.5958/CDR2	Multidrug transporter of ABC superfamily, overexpressed in azole-resistant isolates	Transports phospholipids (in-to-out direction)	Repressed in young biofilms
				orf19.1313/CDR3	-	Transporter of the Pdr/Cdr family of the ATP-binding cassette superfamily; transports phospholipids (out-to-in direction); expressed in opaque-phase cells	Induced by macrophage interaction; Spider biofilm induced
				orf19.5079/CDR4	-	-	Rat catheter and flow model biofilm induced
	Candida glabrata	18	5	*CAGL0M01760g/CDR1*	Multidrug transporter of ABC superfamily, involved in resistance to azoles, expression regulated by Pdr1p, increased abundance in azole resistant strains	Expression increased by loss of the mitochondrial genome	-
				CAGL0F02717g/CDR2 (PDH1)	Multidrug transporter, predicted plasma membrane ATP-binding cassette (ABC) transporter; regulated by Pdr1p; involved in fluconazole resistance	-	-
				CAGL0I04862g /SNQ2	Predicted plasma membrane ATP-binding cassette (ABC) transporter, putative transporter involved in multidrug resistance; involved in Pdr1p-mediated azole resistance	-	-
				CAGL0G00242g/YOR1	Putative ABC transporter involved in multidrug efflux; gene is upregulated in azole-resistant strain	-	-
				CAGL0F01419g/AUS1	-	ATP-binding cassette transporter involved in sterol uptake	Necessary for *C. glabrata* virulence in a mice model of disseminated infection
	Candida tropicalis	22	1	*CDR1*	Induced in clinical azole resistant isolates	-	-
	Candida parapsilosis	19	1	*CPAR2_405290/CDR1*	Induced in clinical azole resistant isolates	-	-
	Candida dubliniensis	19	1	*Cd36_85210/CDR1*	Predicted multidrug transporter of ABC superfamily, involved in multidrug resistance, overexpressed in fluconazole-resistant derivatives obtained in vitro	-	-
	Candida krusei	9	2	*ABC1*	Upregulated during azole stress, involved in innate fluconazole resistance, confers	-	-

Table 1. *Cont.*

					fluconazole resistance through drug efflux upon hyperexpression in *S. cerevisiae*		
				ABC2	Upregulated during azole stress, expression correlated with itraconazole resistance	-	-
	Aspergillus fumigatus	49	7	*Afu6g04360/ATRF*	Putative ABC transporter; drug efflux pump; involved in itraconazole resistance	-	-
				Afu1g12690/MDR4	ABC multidrug transporter; induced by voriconazole exposure in vitro and in mice; involved in itraconazole resistance	-	Biofilm growth regulated protein
				Afu1g17440/ABCA	ABC drug exporter; induced during voriconazole stress	-	Overexpression leads to an augmentation of virulence in the presence of voriconazole in the *G. mellonella* model of infection
				Afu1g10390/ABCB	Putative ABC multidrug transporter; transcript induced by voriconazole	-	Necessary for full virulence of *A. fumigatus* in the *G. mellonella* model of infection
				Afu1g14330/ABCC	Putative ABC transporter; induced during voriconazole stress; mutation causes increased itraconazole, voriconazole and posaconazole sensitivity	-	-
				Afu6g03470/ABCD	Putative *MDR1* family ABC transporter; induced during voriconazole stress	-	Biofilm growth regulated protein
				Afu7g00480/ABCE	Putative ABC transporter; induced during voriconazole stress	-	Biofilm growth regulated protein
				Afu3g07300/ATRI	Putative ABC transporter; induced during voriconazole stress mutation causes increased itraconazole and voriconazole sensitivity	-	-
	Cryptococcus neoformans	54	3	*AFR1*	Pump required for azole efflux and other xenobiotics, including cycloheximide, nocodazole, and trichostatin A; involved in clinical fluconazole resistance; role in susceptibility towards amphotericin B and 5-fluorocytosine: expression was positively regulated by CnCrz1 and CnYap1 in response to fluconazole	-	Necessary for full virulence of *C. neoformans* in intravenous and in inhalation mouse models; overexpression upon *C. neoformans* phagocytosis; and involved in the resistance against microglia
				AFR2	Role in susceptibility towards amphotericin B and 5-fluorocytosine	-	-
				MDR1	Confers itraconazole resistance upon hyperexpression in *S. cerevisiae;* role in susceptibility towards amphotericin B and 5-fluorocytosine	-	-
	Cryptococcus gattii	23	2	*MDR1*	Confers fluconazole resistance in *S. cerevisiae*	-	Overexpressed in cells recovered from the brain of infected mice
				PDR11	Necessary for fluconazole resistance in the VGII clinical strain	-	Overexpressed in cells recovered from the lungs of infected mice

Table 2. MFS transporters of *Candida*, *Aspergillus*, and *Cryptococcus* species, focusing their roles in MDR and physiological functions, as well as their pathogenicity and virulence features.

	Species	Total #	Characterised #	Characterised ORFs	Role in MDR	Physiological Role	Pathogenicity and Virulence Features
MFS Proteins	*Candida albicans*	26	8	*orf19.5604/MDR1*	Major mediator of azole resistance; methotrexate is preferred substrate; overexpression in drug-resistant clinical isolates confers fluconazole resistance; repressed in young biofilm	-	Necessary for full virulence in *C. albicans* in immunocompetent and immunocompromised mice models
				orf19.6577/FLU1	Involved in the resistance towards fluconazole, ketoconazole, and itraconazole; confers fluconazole resistance in *S. cerevisiae*	Involved in histatin-5 efflux	-
				orf19.2160/NAG4	Required for wild-type cycloheximide resistance	-	Required for wild-type mouse virulence
				orf19.2158/NAG3	Required for wild-type cycloheximide resistance	-	Required for wild-type mouse virulence; Spider biofilm repressed
				orf19.2151/NAG6	Required for wild-type cycloheximide resistance	-	Required for wild-type mouse virulence
				orf19.508/QDR1	-	Involved in lipid homeostasis	Involved in biofilm architecture and thickness and virulence
				orf19.6992/QDR2	-	Involved in lipid homeostasis	Involved in biofilm architecture and thickness and virulence in a murine model of hematogenously disseminated candidiasis
				orf19.136/QDR3	-	Involved in lipid homeostasis	Involved in biofilm architecture and thickness and virulence in a murine model of hematogenously disseminated candidiasis
	Candida glabrata	15	8	*CAGL0J09944g/AQR1*	Involved in resistance to flucytosine and imidazoles	Involved in resistance to acetic acid	-
				CAGL0G03927g/TPO1_1	Putative drug:H^+ antiporter, involved in efflux of clotrimazole; required for resistance to clotrimazole and other drugs	Involved in the resistance to histatin-5; involved in spermine resistance	Involved in virulence
				CAGL0E03674g/TPO1_2	Putative drug:H^+ antiporter, involved in efflux of clotrimazole; required for resistance to clotrimazole and other drugs	Involved in fatty acid and sterol homeostasis upon biofilm formation; involved in spermine resistance	Involved in virulence in the *G. mellonella* model and biofilm formation
				CAGL0I10384g/TPO3	Confers imidazole and triazole drug resistance; activated by CgPdr1	Involved in polyamine homeostasis	-
				CAGL0G08624g/QDR2	Confers imidazole drug resistance, involved in clotrimazole efflux; activated by CgPdr1; upregulated in azole-resistant strain	-	-
				CAGL0H06017g/FLR1	Confers resistance to benomyl; gene is downregulated in azole-resistant strain	-	-
				CAGL0H06039g/FLR2	Multidrug transporter of the major facilitator superfamily involved in 5-flucytosine resistance	-	-
				CAGL0M06281g/DTR1	-	Acetate exporter in the plasma membrane	Required for virulence in *G. mellonella* model
	Candida tropicalis	26	1	*MDR1*	Overexpression in resistant clinical isolates and upon biofilm formation	-	-

Table 2. *Cont.*

	Candida parapsilosis	34	1	*CPAR2_301760/MDR1*	Member of the MDR family of major facilitator transporter superfamily; putative drug transporter; expression increased in fluconazole and voriconazole resistant strains	-	-
	Candida dubliniensis	14	1	*Cd36_63890/MDR1*	Predicted multidrug transporter of ABC superfamily, involved in multidrug resistance	-	-
	Aspergillus fumigatus	278	6	*Afu6g09710/GLIA*	-	Predicted major facilitator type glioxin transporter, encoded in the putative gliotoxin biosynthetic gene cluster	
				Afu1g05010/MFS56	Putative MFS transporter; mutation causes increased azole sensitivity	-	-
				Afu3g03500/MDR3	Putative multidrug resistance protein; transcript upregulated in response to amphotericin B; displays itraconazole-increased expression in resistant mutants	-	-
				Afu8g05710/MFSA	Highly expressed during voriconazole stress	Putative major facilitator superfamily (MFS) sugar transporter	Calcium induced; transcript upregulated in conidia exposed to neutrophils
				Afu1g15490/MFSB	Putative major facilitator superfamily (MFS) transporter; highly expressed during voriconazole stress	-	-
				Afu1g03200/MFSC	Putative major facilitator superfamily (MFS) transporter; highly expressed during voriconazole stress	-	-
	Cryptococcus neoformans	86	3	*CNA07070*	-	Dityrosine transporter	-
				CNC03290	-	-	-
				CND00440/AFLT	-	-	-

References

1. Sims, C.R.; Ostrosky-Zeichner, L.; Rex, J.H. Invasive candidiasis in immunocompromised hospitalized patients. *Arch. Med. Res.* **2005**, *36*, 660–671. [CrossRef] [PubMed]
2. Chauhan, N.; Latge, J.-P.; Calderone, R. Signalling and oxidant adaptation in *Candida albicans* and *Aspergillus fumigatus*. *Nat. Rev. Microbiol.* **2006**, *4*, 435–444. [CrossRef] [PubMed]
3. Schmalzle, S.A.; Buchwald, U.K.; Gilliam, B.L.; Riedel, D.J. *Cryptococcus neoformans* infection in malignancy. *Mycoses Diagn. Ther. Prophyl. Fungal Dis.* **2016**, *59*, 542–552. [CrossRef]
4. Wisplinghoff, H.; Bischoff, T.; Tallent, S.M.; Seifert, H.; Wenzel, R.P.; Edmond, M.B. Nosocomial bloodstream infections in US hospitals: Analysis of 24,179 cases from a prospective nationwide surveillance study. *Clin. Infect. Dis.* **2004**, *39*, 309–317. [CrossRef] [PubMed]
5. Fidel, P.L.; Vazquez, J.A.; Sobel, J.D. *Candida glabrata*: Review of epidemiology, pathogenesis, and clinical disease with comparison to *C albicans*. *Clin. Microbiol. Rev.* **1999**, *12*, 80–96. [PubMed]
6. Mccullough, M.J.; Ross, B.C.; Reade, P.C. *Candida albicans*: A review of its history, taxonomy, epidemiology, virulence attributes, and methods of strain differentiation. *Oral Maxillofac. Surg.* **1996**, *25*, 136–144. [CrossRef]
7. Da Silva Ferreira, M.E.S.; Colombo, A.L.; Paulsen, I.; Ren, Q.; Wortman, J.; Huang, J.; Goldman, M.H.S.; Goldman, G.H. The ergosterol biosynthesis pathway, transporter genes, and azole resistance in *Aspergillus fumigatus*. *Med. Mycol.* **2005**, *43*, S313–S319. [CrossRef]
8. Dou, H.-T.; Xu, Y.-C.; Wang, H.-Z.; Li, T.-S. Molecular epidemiology of *Cryptococcus neoformans* and *Cryptococcus gattii* in China between 2007 and 2013 using multilocus sequence typing and the DiversiLab system. *Eur. J. Clin. Microbiol. Infect. Dis.* **2015**, *34*, 753–762. [CrossRef] [PubMed]
9. Sanglard, D.; Kuchler, K.; Ischer, F.; Pagani, J.L.; Monod, M.; Bille, J. Mechanisms of resistance to azole antifungal agents in *Candida albicans* isolates from AIDS patients involve specific multidrug transporters. *Antimicrob. Agents Chemother.* **1995**, *39*, 2378–2386. [CrossRef] [PubMed]
10. Costa, C.; Ribeiro, J.; Miranda, I.M.; Silva-dias, A.I.; Cavalheiro, M.; Costa-de-oliveira, S.; Rodrigues, A.G.; Teixeira, M.C. Clotrimazole drug resistance in *Candida glabrata* clinical isolates correlates with increased expression of the drug: H^+ antiporters CgAqr1, CgTpo1_1, CgTpo3 and CgQdr2. *Front. Microbiol.* **2016**. [CrossRef] [PubMed]
11. Prasad, R.; Khandelwal, N.K.; Banerjee, A. Yeast ABC transporters in lipid trafficking. *Fungal Genet. Biol.* **2016**, *93*, 25–34. [CrossRef] [PubMed]
12. Cannon, R.D.; Holmes, A.R. Learning the ABC of oral fungal drug resistance. *Mol. Oral Microbiol.* **2015**, *30*, 425–437. [CrossRef] [PubMed]
13. Del Sorbo, G.; Schoonbeek, H.J.; De Waard, M.A. Fungal transporters involved in efflux of natural toxic compounds and fungicides. *Fungal Genet. Biol.* **2000**, *30*, 1–15. [CrossRef] [PubMed]
14. Sá-Correia, I.; dos Santos, S.C.; Teixeira, M.C.; Cabrito, T.R.; Mira, N.P. Drug: H^+ antiporters in chemical stress response in yeast. *Trends Microbiol.* **2008**, *17*, 22–31. [CrossRef] [PubMed]
15. Prasad, R.; Banerjee, A.; Khandelwal, N.K.; Dhamgaye, S. The ABCs of *Candida albicans* multidrug transporter Cdr1. *Eukaryot. Cell* **2015**, *14*, 1154–1164. [CrossRef] [PubMed]
16. Pao, S.S.; Paulsen, I.T.; Saier, M.H. Major facilitator superfamily. *Microbiol. Mol. Biol. Rev.* **1998**, *62*, 1–34. [PubMed]
17. Decottignies, A.; Grant, A.M.; Nichols, J.W.; de Wet, H.; McIntosh, D.B.; Goffeau, A. ATPase and multidrug transport activities of the overexpressed yeast ABC protein Yor1p. *J. Biol. Chem.* **1998**, *273*, 12612–12622. [CrossRef] [PubMed]
18. Goffeau, A.; Barrell, B.G.; Bussey, H.; Davis, R.W.; Dujon, B.; Feldmann, H.; Galibert, F.; Hoheisel, J.D.; Jacq, C.; Johnston, M.; et al. Life with 6000 genes. *Science* **1996**, *274*, 546–567. [CrossRef] [PubMed]
19. Bauer, B.E.; Wolfger, H.; Kuchler, K. Inventory and function of yeast ABC proteins: About sex, stress, pleiotropic drug and heavy metal resistance. *Biochim. Biophys. Acta* **1999**, *1461*, 217–236. [CrossRef]
20. Costa, C.; Dias, P.J.; Sá-Correia, I.; Teixeira, M.C. MFS multidrug transporters in pathogenic fungi: Do they have real clinical impact? *Front. Physiol.* **2014**, *5*, 197. [CrossRef] [PubMed]

21. Franz, R.; Michel, S.; Morschhäuser, J. A fourth gene from the *Candida albicans CDR* family of ABC transporters. *Gene* **1998**, *220*, 91–98. [CrossRef]
22. Balan, I.; Alarco, A.M.; Raymond, M. The *Candida albicans CDR3* gene codes for an opaque-phase ABC transporter. *J. Bacteriol.* **1997**, *179*, 7210–7218. [CrossRef] [PubMed]
23. Sanglard, D.; Ischer, F.; Monod, M.; Bille, J. Cloning of *Candida albicans* genes conferring resistance to azole antifungal agents: Characterization of *CDR2*, a new multidrug ABC transporter gene. *Microbiology* **1997**, *143*, 405–416. [CrossRef] [PubMed]
24. Costa, C.; Nunes, J.; Henriques, A.; Mira, N.P.; Nakayama, H.; Chibana, H.; Teixeira, M.C. *Candida glabrata* drug: H^+ antiporter CgTpo3 (ORF CAGL0I10384g): Role in azole drug resistance and polyamine homeostasis. *J. Antimicrob. Chemother.* **2014**, *69*, 1767–1776. [CrossRef] [PubMed]
25. Costa, C.; Pires, C.; Cabrito, T.R.; Renaudin, A.; Ohno, M.; Chibana, H.; Sá-Correia, I.; Teixeira, M.C. *Candida glabrata* drug: H^+ antiporter CgQdr2 confers imidazole drug resistance, being activated by transcription factor CgPdr1. *Antimicrob. Agents Chemother.* **2013**, *57*, 3159–3167. [CrossRef] [PubMed]
26. Torelli, R.; Posteraro, B.; Ferrari, S.; La Sorda, M.; Fadda, G.; Sanglard, D.; Sanguinetti, M. The ATP-binding cassette transporter—Encoding gene CgSNQ2 is contributing to the CgPDR1-dependent azole resistance of *Candida glabrata*. *Mol. Microbiol.* **2008**, *68*, 186–201. [CrossRef] [PubMed]
27. Costa, C.; Henriques, A.; Pires, C.; Nunes, J.; Ohno, M.; Chibana, H.; Sá-Correia, I.; Teixeira, M.C. The dual role of *Candida glabrata* drug: H^+ antiporter CgAqr1 (ORF CAGL0J09944g) in antifungal drug and acetic acid resistance. *Front. Microbiol.* **2013**, *4*, 170. [CrossRef] [PubMed]
28. Tobin, M.B.; Peery, R.B.; Skatrud, P.L. Genes encoding multiple drug resistance-like proteins in *Aspergillus fumigatus* and *Aspergillus flavus*. *Gene* **1997**, *200*, 11–23. [CrossRef]
29. Slaven, J.W.; Anderson, M.J.; Sanglard, D.; Dixon, G.K.; Bille, J.; Roberts, I.S.; Denning, D.W. Increased expression of a novel *Aspergillus fumigatus* ABC transporter gene, *atrF*, in the presence of itraconazole in an itraconazole resistant clinical isolate. *Fungal Genet. Biol.* **2002**, *36*, 199–206. [CrossRef]
30. Thornewell, S.J.; Peery, R.B.; Skatrud, P.L. Cloning and characterization of *CneMDR1*: A *Cryptococcus neoformans* gene encoding a protein related to multidrug resistance proteins. *Gene* **1997**, *201*, 21–29. [CrossRef]
31. Posteraro, B.; Sanguinetti, M.; Sanglard, D.; La Sorda, M.; Boccia, S.; Romano, L.; Morace, G.; Fadda, G.; Cassette, B. Identification and characterization of a *Cryptococcus neoformans* ATP binding cassette (ABC) transporter-encoding gene, *CnAFR1*, involved in the resistance to fluconazole. *Mol. Microbiol.* **2003**, *47*, 357–371. [CrossRef] [PubMed]
32. Gaur, M.; Choudhury, D.; Prasad, R. Complete inventory of ABC proteins in human pathogenic yeast, *Candida albicans*. *J. Mol. Microbiol. Biotechnol.* **2005**, *9*, 3–15. [CrossRef] [PubMed]
33. Dujon, B.; Sherman, D.; Fischer, G.; Durrens, P.; Casaregola, S.; Lafontaine, I.; de Montigny, J.; Marck, C.; Neuvéglise, C.; Talla, E.; et al. Genome evolution in yeasts. *Nature* **2004**, *430*, 35–44. [CrossRef] [PubMed]
34. Nierman, W.C.; Pain, A.; Anderson, M.J.; Wortman, J.R.; Kim, H.S.; Arroyo, J.; Berriman, M.; Abe, K.; Archer, D.B.; Bermejo, C.; et al. Genomic sequence of the pathogenic and allergenic filamentous fungus *Aspergillus fumigatus*. *Nature* **2005**, *438*, 1151–1156. [CrossRef] [PubMed]
35. Loftus, B.J.; Fung, E.; Roncaglia, P.; Rowley, D.; Amedeo, P.; Vamathevan, J.; Miranda, M.; Anderson, I.J.; Fraser, J.A.; Allen, J.E.; et al. The genome of the Basidiomycetous yeast and human pathogen *Cryptococcus neoformans*. *Science* **2005**, *307*, 1321–1324. [CrossRef] [PubMed]
36. Holmes, A.R.; Cardno, T.S.; Strouse, J.J.; Ivnitski-Steele, I.; Keniya, M.V.; Lackovic, K.; Monk, B.C.; Sklar, L.A.; Cannon, R.D. Targeting efflux pumps to overcome antifungal drug resistance. *Future Med. Chem.* **2016**, *8*, 1485–1501. [CrossRef] [PubMed]
37. K Redhu, A.; Shah, A.H.; Prasad, R. MFS transporters of *Candida* species and their role in clinical drug resistance. *FEMS Yeast Res.* **2016**, *16*. [CrossRef] [PubMed]
38. Lupetti, A.; Danesi, R.; Campa, M.; Del Tacca, M.; Kelly, S. Molecular basis of resistance to azole antifungals. *Trends Mol. Med.* **2002**, *8*, 76–81. [CrossRef]
39. Sanguinetti, M.; Posteraro, B.; La Sorda, M.; Torelli, R.; Fiori, B.; Santangelo, R.; Delogu, G.; Fadda, G. Role of AFR1, an ABC transporter-encoding gene, in the in vivo response to fluconazole and virulence of *Cryptococcus neoformans*. *Infect. Immun.* **2006**, *74*, 1352–1359. [CrossRef] [PubMed]
40. Cannon, R.D.; Lamping, E.; Holmes, A.R.; Niimi, K.; Baret, P.V.; Keniya, M.V.; Tanabe, K.; Niimi, M.; Goffeau, A.; Monk, B.C. Efflux-mediated antifungal drug resistance. *Clin. Microbiol. Rev.* **2009**, *22*, 291–321. [CrossRef] [PubMed]

41. Prasad, R.; De Wergifosse, P.; Goffeau, A.; Balzi, E. Molecular cloning and characterization of a novel gene of *Candida albicans, CDR1*, conferring multiple resistance to drugs and antifungals. *Curr. Genet.* **1995**, *27*, 320–329. [CrossRef] [PubMed]
42. Siikala, E.; Rautemaa, R.; Richardson, M.; Saxen, H.; Bowyer, P.; Sanglard, D. Persistent *Candida albicans* colonization and molecular mechanisms of azole resistance in autoimmune polyendocrinopathy-candidiasis-ectodermal dystrophy (APECED) patients. *J. Antimicrob. Chemother.* **2010**, *65*, 2505–2513. [CrossRef] [PubMed]
43. Moran, G.P.; Sanglard, D.; Donnelly, S.M.; Shanley, D.B.; Sullivan, D.J.; Coleman, D.C. Identification and expression of multidrug transporters responsible for fluconazole resistance in *Candida dubliniensis*. *Antimicrob. Agents Chemother.* **1998**, *42*, 1819–1830. [PubMed]
44. Berkow, E.L.; Manigaba, K.; Parker, J.E.; Barker, K.S.; Kelly, S.L.; Rogers, P.D. Multidrug transporters and alterations in sterol biosynthesis contribute to azole antifungal resistance in *Candida parapsilosis*. *Antimicrob. Agents Chemother.* **2015**, *59*, 5942–5950. [CrossRef] [PubMed]
45. Souza, A.C.R.; Fuchs, B.B.; Pinhati, H.M.S.; Siqueira, R.A.; Hagen, F.; Meis, J.F.; Mylonakis, E.; Colombo, A.L. *Candida parapsilosis* resistance to fluconazole: Molecular mechanisms and in vivo impact in infected *Galleria mellonella* larvae. *Antimicrob. Agents Chemother.* **2015**, *59*, 6581–6587. [CrossRef] [PubMed]
46. Choi, M.J.; Won, E.J.; Shin, J.H.; Kim, S.H.; Lee, W.G.; Kim, M.N.; Lee, K.; Shin, M.G.; Suh, S.P.; Ryang, D.W.; et al. Resistance mechanisms and clinical features of fluconazole-nonsusceptible *Candida tropicalis* isolates compared with fluconazole-less-susceptible isolates. *Antimicrob. Agents Chemother.* **2016**, *60*, 3653–3661. [CrossRef] [PubMed]
47. Sanglard, D.; Ischer, F.; Bille, J. Role of ATP-binding-cassette transporter genes in high-frequency acquisition of resistance to azole antifungals in *Candida glabrata*. *Antimicrob. Agents Chemother.* **2001**, *45*, 1174–1183. [CrossRef] [PubMed]
48. Vermitsky, J.-P.; Earhart, K.D.; Smith, W.L.; Homayouni, R.; Edlind, T.D.; Rogers, P.D. Pdr1 regulates multidrug resistance in *Candida glabrata*: Gene disruption and genome-wide expression studies. *Mol. Microbiol.* **2006**, *61*, 704–722. [CrossRef] [PubMed]
49. Katiyar, S.K.; Edlind, T.D. Identification and expression of multidrug resistance-related ABC transporter genes in *Candida krusei*. *Med. Mycol.* **2001**, *39*, 109–116. [CrossRef] [PubMed]
50. Lamping, E.; Ranchod, A.; Nakamura, K.; Tyndall, J.D.A.; Niimi, K.; Holmes, A.R.; Niimi, M.; Cannon, R.D. Abc1p is a multidrug efflux transporter that tips the balance in favor of innate azole resistance in *Candida krusei*. *Antimicrob. Agents Chemother.* **2009**, *53*, 354–369. [CrossRef] [PubMed]
51. Lamping, E.; Monk, B.C.; Niimi, K.; Holmes, A.R.; Tsao, S.; Tanabe, K.; Niimi, M.; Uehara, Y.; Cannon, R.D. Characterization of three classes of membrane proteins involved in fungal azole resistance by functional hyperexpression in *Saccharomyces cerevisiae*. *Eukaryot. Cell* **2007**, *6*, 1150–1165. [CrossRef] [PubMed]
52. He, X.; Zhao, M.; Chen, J.; Wu, R.; Zhang, J.; Cui, R.; Jiang, Y.; Chen, J.; Cao, X.; Xing, Y.; et al. Overexpression of both *ERG11* and *ABC2* genes might be responsible for itraconazole resistance in clinical isolates of *Candida krusei*. *PLoS ONE* **2015**, *10*, e0136185. [CrossRef] [PubMed]
53. Meneau, I.; Coste, A.T.; Sanglard, D. Identification of *Aspergillus fumigatus* multidrug transporter genes and their potential involvement in antifungal resistance. *Med. Mycol.* **2016**, *54*, 616–627. [CrossRef] [PubMed]
54. Abad, A.; Victoria Fernández-Molina, J.; Bikandi, J.; Ramírez, A.; Margareto, J.; Sendino, J.; Luis Hernando, F.; Pontón, J.; Garaizar, J.; Rementeria, A. What makes *Aspergillus fumigatus* a successful pathogen? Genes and molecules involved in invasive aspergillosis. *Rev. Iberoam. Micol.* **2010**, *27*, 155–182. [CrossRef] [PubMed]
55. Nascimento, A.M.; Goldman, G.H.; Park, S.; Marras, S.A.E.; Delmas, G.; Oza, U.; Lolans, K.; Dudley, M.N.; Mann, P.A.; Perlin, D.S. Multiple resistance mechanisms among *Aspergillus fumigatus* mutants with high-level resistance to itraconazole. *Antimicrob. Agents Chemother.* **2003**, *47*, 1719–1726. [CrossRef] [PubMed]
56. Da Silva Ferreira, M.E.; Malavazi, I.; Savoldi, M.; Brakhage, A.A.; Goldman, M.H.S.; Kim, H.S.; Nierman, W.C.; Goldman, G.H. Transcriptome analysis of *Aspergillus fumigatus* exposed to voriconazole. *Curr. Genet.* **2006**, *50*, 32–44. [CrossRef] [PubMed]
57. Chang, M.; Sionov, E.; Khanal Lamichhane, A.; Kwon-Chung, K.J.; Chang, Y.C. Roles of three *Cryptococcus neoformans* and *Cryptococcus gattii* efflux pump-coding genes in response to drug treatment. *Antimicrob. Agents Chemother.* **2018**, *62*. [CrossRef] [PubMed]

58. Basso, L.R.; Gast, C.E.; Bruzual, I.; Wong, B. Identification and properties of plasma membrane azole efflux pumps from the pathogenic fungi *Cryptococcus gattii* and *Cryptococcus neoformans*. *J. Antimicrob. Chemother.* **2015**, *70*, 1396–1407. [CrossRef] [PubMed]
59. Wirsching, S.; Michel, S.; Morschhäuser, J. Targeted gene disruption in *Candida albicans* wild-type strains: The role of the *MDR1* gene in fluconazole resistance of clinical *Candida albicans* isolates. *Mol. Microbiol.* **2000**, *36*, 856–865. [CrossRef] [PubMed]
60. Wirsching, S.; Moran, G.P.; Sullivan, D.J.; Coleman, D.C.; Morschhäuser, J. *MDR1*-mediated drug resistance in *Candida dubliniensis*. *Antimicrob. Agents Chemother.* **2001**, *45*, 3416–3421. [CrossRef] [PubMed]
61. Silva, A.P.; Miranda, I.M.; Guida, A.; Synnott, J.; Rocha, R.; Silva, R.; Amorim, A.; Pina-Vaz, C.; Butler, G.; Rodrigues, A.G. Transcriptional profiling of azole-resistant *Candida parapsilosis* strains. *Antimicrob. Agents Chemother.* **2011**, *55*, 3546–3556. [CrossRef] [PubMed]
62. Bizerra, F.C.; Nakamura, C.V.; De Poersch, C.; Estivalet Svidzinski, T.I.; Borsato Quesada, R.M.; Goldenberg, S.; Krieger, M.A.; Yamada-Ogatta, S.F. Characteristics of biofilm formation by *Candida tropicalis* and antifungal resistance. *FEMS Yeast Res.* **2008**, *8*, 442–450. [CrossRef] [PubMed]
63. Calabrese, D.; Bille, J.; Sanglard, D. A novel multidrug efflux transporter gene of the major facilitator superfamily from *Candida albicans (FLU1)* conferring resistance to fluconazole. *Microbiology* **2000**, *146*, 2743–2754. [CrossRef] [PubMed]
64. Park, S.; Perlin, D.S. Establishing surrogate markers for fluconazole resistance in *Candida albicans*. *Microb. Drug Resist.* **2005**, *11*, 232–238. [CrossRef] [PubMed]
65. Pais, P.; Costa, C.; Pires, C.; Shimizu, K.; Chibana, H.; Teixeira, M.C. Membrane proteome-wide response to the antifungal drug clotrimazole in *Candida glabrata*: role of the transcription factor CgPdr1 and the drug: H^+ antiporters CgTpo1_1 and CgTpo1_2. *Mol. Cell. Proteom.* **2016**, *15*, 57–72. [CrossRef] [PubMed]
66. Pais, P.; Pires, C.; Costa, C.; Okamoto, M.; Chibana, H.; Teixeira, M.C. Membrane proteomics analysis of the *Candida glabrata* response to 5-flucytosine: Unveiling the role and regulation of the drug efflux transporters CgFlr1 and CgFlr2. *Front. Microbiol.* **2016**, *7*, 2045. [CrossRef] [PubMed]
67. Tsai, H.-F.; Krol, A.A.; Sarti, K.E.; Bennett, J.E. *Candida glabrata PDR1*, a transcriptional regulator of a pleiotropic drug resistance network, mediates azole resistance in clinical isolates and petite mutants. *Antimicrob. Agents Chemother.* **2006**, *50*, 1384–1392. [CrossRef] [PubMed]
68. Paul, S.; Schmidt, J.A.; Moye-Rowley, W.S. Regulation of the CgPdr1 transcription factor from the pathogen *Candida glabrata*. *Eukaryot. Cell* **2011**, *10*, 187–197. [CrossRef] [PubMed]
69. Coste, A.; Turner, V.; Ischer, F.; Morschhäuser, J.; Forche, A.; Selmecki, A.; Berman, J.; Bille, J.; Sanglard, D. A mutation in Tac1p, a transcription factor regulating *CDR1* and *CDR2*, is coupled with loss of heterozygosity at chromosome 5 to mediate antifungal resistance in *Candida albicans*. *Genetics* **2006**, *172*, 2139–2156. [CrossRef] [PubMed]
70. Coste, A.; Selmecki, A.; Forche, A.; Diogo, D.; Bougnoux, M.E.; D'Enfert, C.; Berman, J.; Sanglard, D. Genotypic evolution of azole resistance mechanisms in sequential *Candida albicans* isolates. *Eukaryot. Cell* **2007**, *6*, 1889–1904. [CrossRef] [PubMed]
71. Morschhäuser, J.; Barker, K.S.; Liu, T.T.; BlaB-Warmuth, J.; Homayouni, R.; Rogers, P.D. The transcription factor Mrr1p controls expression of the *MDR1* efflux pump and mediates multidrug resistance in *Candida albicans*. *PLoS Pathog.* **2007**, *3*, e164. [CrossRef] [PubMed]
72. Dunkel, N.; Blaß, J.; Rogers, P.D.; Morschhäuser, J. Mutations in the multi-drug resistance regulator *MRR1*, followed by loss of heterozygosity, are the main cause of *MDR1* overexpression in fluconazole-resistant *Candida albicans* strains. *Mol. Microbiol.* **2008**, *69*, 827–840. [CrossRef] [PubMed]
73. Liu, T.T.; Znaidi, S.; Barker, K.S.; Xu, L.; Homayouni, R.; Saidane, S.; Morschhäuser, J.; Nantel, A.; Raymond, M.; Rogers, P.D. Genome-wide expression and location analyses of the *Candida albicans* Tac1p regulon. *Eukaryot. Cell* **2007**, *6*, 2122–2138. [CrossRef] [PubMed]
74. Znaidi, S.; De Deken, X.; Weber, S.; Rigby, T.; Nantel, A.; Raymond, M. The zinc cluster transcription factor Tac1p regulates *PDR16* expression in *Candida albicans*. *Mol. Microbiol.* **2007**, *66*, 440–452. [CrossRef] [PubMed]
75. Schubert, S.; Barker, K.S.; Znaidi, S.; Schneider, S.; Dierolf, F.; Dunkel, N.; Aïd, M.; Boucher, G.; Rogers, P.D.; Raymond, M.; et al. Regulation of efflux pump expression and drug resistance by the transcription factors Mrr1, Upc2, and Cap1 in *Candida albicans*. *Antimicrob. Agents Chemother.* **2011**, *55*, 2212–2223. [CrossRef] [PubMed]

76. Coste, A.T.; Karababa, M.; Ischer, F.; Bille, J.; Sanglard, D. *TAC1*, transcriptional activator of *CDR* genes, is a new transcription factor involved in the regulation of *Candida albicans* ABC transporters *CDR1* and *CDR2*. *Eukaryot. Cell* **2004**, *3*, 1639–1652. [CrossRef] [PubMed]
77. Caudle, K.E.; Barker, K.S.; Wiederhold, N.P.; Xu, L.; Homayouni, R.; Rogers, P.D. Genomewide expression profile analysis of the *Candida glabrata* Pdr1 regulon. *Eukaryot. Cell* **2011**, *10*, 373–383. [CrossRef] [PubMed]
78. Tsai, H.-F.; Sammons, L.R.; Zhang, X.; Suffis, S.D.; Su, Q.; Myers, T.G.; Marr, K.A.; Bennett, J.E. Microarray and molecular analyses of the azole resistance mechanism in *Candida glabrata* oropharyngeal isolates. *Antimicrob. Agents Chemother.* **2010**, *54*, 3308–3317. [CrossRef] [PubMed]
79. Selmecki, A.; Forche, A.; Berman, J. Genomic plasticity of the human fungal pathogen *Candida albicans*. *Eukaryot. Cell* **2010**, *9*, 991–1008. [CrossRef] [PubMed]
80. Poláková, S.; Blume, C.; Zárate, J.A.; Mentel, M.; Jørck-Ramberg, D.; Stenderup, J.; Piskur, J. Formation of new chromosomes as a virulence mechanism in yeast *Candida glabrata*. *Proc. Natl. Acad. Sci. USA* **2009**, *106*, 2688–2693. [CrossRef] [PubMed]
81. Sionov, E.; Lee, H.; Chang, Y.C.; Kwon-Chung, K.J. *Cryptococcus neoformans* overcomes stress of azole drugs by formation of disomy in specific multiple chromosomes. *PLoS Pathog.* **2010**, *6*, e1000848. [CrossRef] [PubMed]
82. Hagiwara, D.; Miura, D.; Shimizu, K.; Paul, S.; Ohba, A.; Gonoi, T.; Watanabe, A.; Kamei, K.; Shintani, T.; Moye-Rowley, W.S.; et al. A novel Zn_2-Cys_6 transcription factor AtrR plays a key role in an azole resistance mechanism of *Aspergillus fumigatus* by Co-regulating *cyp51A* and *cdr1B* expressions. *PLoS Pathog.* **2017**, *13*. [CrossRef] [PubMed]
83. Paul, S.; Doering, T.L.; Moye-Rowley, W.S. *Cryptococcus neoformans* Yap1 is required for normal fluconazole and oxidative stress resistance. *Fungal Genet. Biol.* **2015**, *74*, 1–9. [CrossRef] [PubMed]
84. Lev, S.; Desmarini, D.; Chayakulkeeree, M.; Sorrell, T.C.; Djordjevic, J.T. The Crz1/Sp1 transcription factor of *Cryptococcus neoformans* is activated by calcineurin and regulates cell wall integrity. *PLoS ONE* **2012**, *7*, e51403. [CrossRef] [PubMed]
85. Noble, S.M.; Gianetti, B.A.; Witchley, J.N. *Candida albicans* cell-type switching and functional plasticity in the mammalian host. *Nat. Rev. Microbiol.* **2017**, *15*, 96–108. [CrossRef] [PubMed]
86. Brown, A.J.P.; Brown, G.D.; Netea, M.G.; Gow, N.A.R. Metabolism impacts upon *Candida* immunogenicity and pathogenicity at multiple levels. *Trends Microbiol.* **2014**, *22*, 614–622. [CrossRef] [PubMed]
87. Levitz, S.M. The Ecology of *Cryptococcus neoformans* and the epidemiology of cryptococcosis. *Rev. Infect. Dis.* **1991**, *13*, 1163–1169. [CrossRef] [PubMed]
88. Chen, S.C.-A.; Meyer, W.; Sorrell, T.C. *Cryptococcus gattii* Infections. *Clin. Microbiol. Rev.* **2014**, *27*, 980–1024. [CrossRef] [PubMed]
89. Latgé, J.-P. *Aspergillus fumigatus* and Aspergillosis. *Clin. Microbiol. Rev.* **1999**, *12*, 310–350. [CrossRef] [PubMed]
90. Polke, M.; Hube, B.; Jacobsen, I.D. Candida survival strategies. In *Advances in Applied Microbiology*; Elsevier Ltd.: New York, NY, USA, 2015; Volume 91, pp. 139–235, ISBN 9780128022504.
91. Villar, C.C.; Dongari-Bagtzoglou, A. Immune defence mechanisms and immunoenhancement strategies in oropharyngeal candidiasis. *Expert Rev. Mol. Med.* **2008**, *10*. [CrossRef] [PubMed]
92. Mathews, M.; Jia, H.P.; Guthmiller, J.M.; Losh, G.; Graham, S.; Johnson, G.K.; Tack, B.F.; McCray, P.B. Production of β-defensin antimicrobial peptides by the oral mucosa and salivary glands. *Infect. Immun.* **1999**, *67*, 2740–2745. [PubMed]
93. Wunder, D.; Dong, J.; Baev, D.; Edgerton, M. Human Salivary Histatin 5 Fungicidal action does not induce programmed cell death pathways in *Candida albicans*. *Antimicrob. Agents Chemother.* **2004**, *48*, 110–115. [CrossRef] [PubMed]
94. Taylor-Smith, L.M. *Cryptococcus*—Epithelial interactions. *J. Fungi* **2017**, *3*, 53. [CrossRef] [PubMed]
95. Heung, L.J. Innate immune responses to *Cryptococcus*. *J. Fungi* **2017**, *3*, 35. [CrossRef] [PubMed]
96. Leopold Wager, C.M.; Hole, C.R.; Wozniak, K.L.; Wormley, F.L. *Cryptococcus* and phagocytes: Complex interactions that influence disease outcome. *Front. Microbiol.* **2016**, *7*, 105. [CrossRef] [PubMed]
97. Serrano-Gomez, D.; Dominguez-Soto, A.; Ancochea, J.; Jimenez-Heffernan, J.A.; Leal, J.A.; Corbi, A.L. Dendritic cell-specific intercellular adhesion molecule 3-grabbing nonintegrin mediates binding and internalization of *Aspergillus fumigatus* conidia by dendritic cells and macrophages. *J. Immunol.* **2018**, *173*, 5635–5643. [CrossRef]

98. Ellett, F.; Jorgensen, J.; Frydman, G.H.; Jones, C.N.; Irimia, D. Neutrophil interactions stimulate evasive hyphal branching by *Aspergillus fumigatus*. *PLoS Pathog.* **2017**, *13*, e1006154. [CrossRef] [PubMed]
99. O'Hanlon, D.E.; Moench, T.R.; Cone, R.A. Vaginal pH and microbicidal lactic acid when lactobacilli dominate the microbiota. *PLoS ONE* **2013**, *8*, e80074. [CrossRef] [PubMed]
100. Chaudry, A.N.; Travers, P.J.; Yuenger, J.; Colletta, L.; Evans, P.; Zenilman, J.M.; Tummon, A. Analysis of vaginal acetic acid in patients undergoing treatment for bacterial vaginosis. *J. Clin. Microbiol.* **2004**, *42*, 5170–5175. [CrossRef] [PubMed]
101. Fidel, P.L., Jr. Immunity in vaginal candidiasis. *Curr. Opin. Infect. Dis.* **2005**, *18*, 107–111. [CrossRef] [PubMed]
102. Niu, X.X.; Li, T.; Zhang, X.; Wang, S.X.; Liu, Z.H. *Lactobacillus crispatus* modulates vaginal epithelial cell innate response to *Candida albicans*. *Chin. Med. J.* **2017**, *130*, 273–279. [CrossRef] [PubMed]
103. Sipos, G.; Kuchler, K. Fungal ATP-binding cassette (ABC) transporters in drug resistance & detoxification. *Curr. Drug Targets* **2006**, *7*, 471–481. [PubMed]
104. Krishnamurthy, S.; Gupta, V.; Snehlata, P.; Prasad, R. Characterisation of human steroid hormone transport mediated by Cdr1p, a multidrug transporter of *Candida albicans*, belonging to the ATP binding cassette super family. *FEMS Microbiol. Lett.* **1998**, *158*, 69–74. [CrossRef] [PubMed]
105. Krishnamurthy, S.; Chatterjee, U.; Gupta, V.; Prasad, R.; Das, P.; Snehlata, P.; Hasnain, S.E.; Prasad, R. Deletion of transmembrane domain 12 of *CDR1*, a multidrug transporter from *Candida albicans*, leads to altered drug specificity: Expression of a yeast multidrug transporter in baculovirus expression system. *Yeast* **1998**, *14*, 535–550. [CrossRef]
106. Bauters, T.G.M.; Dhont, M.A.; Temmerman, M.I.L.; Nelis, H.J. Prevalence of vulvovaginal candidiasis and susceptibility to fluconazole in women. *Am. J. Obstet. Gynecol.* **2002**, *187*, 569–574. [CrossRef] [PubMed]
107. Spinillo, A.; Bernuzzi, A.M.; Cevini, C.; Gulminetti, R.; Luzi, S.; De Santolo, A. The relationship of bacterial vaginosis, *Candida* and *Trichomonas* infection to symptomatic vaginitis in postmenopausal women attending a vaginitis clinic. *Maturitas* **1997**, *27*, 253–260. [CrossRef]
108. Spinillo, A.; Capuzzo, E.; Nicola, S.; Baltaro, F.; Ferrari, A.; Monaco, A. The impact of oral contraception on vulvovaginal candidiasis. *Contraception* **1995**, *51*, 293–297. [CrossRef]
109. Fidel, P.L.; Cutright, J.; Steele, C. Effects of reproductive hormones on experimental vaginal candidiasis. *Infect. Immun.* **2000**, *68*, 651–657. [CrossRef] [PubMed]
110. White, S.; Larsen, B. *Candida albicans* morphogenesis is influenced by estogen. *Cell. Mol. Life Sci.* **1997**, *53*, 744–749. [CrossRef] [PubMed]
111. Cheng, G.; Yeater, K.M.; Hoyer, L.L. Cellular and molecular biology of *Candida albicans* estrogen response. *Eukaryot. Cell* **2006**, *5*, 180–191. [CrossRef] [PubMed]
112. Li, Y.; Prinz, W.A. ATP-binding Cassette (ABC) transporters mediate nonvesicular, raft-modulated sterol movement from the plasma membrane to the endoplasmic reticulum. *J. Biol. Chem.* **2004**, *279*, 45226–45234. [CrossRef] [PubMed]
113. Wilcox, L.J.; Balderes, D.A.; Wharton, B.; Tinkelenberg, A.H.; Rao, G.; Sturley, S.L. Transcriptional profiling identifies two members of the ATP-binding cassette transporter superfamily required for sterol uptake in yeast. *J. Biol. Chem.* **2002**, *277*, 32466–32472. [CrossRef] [PubMed]
114. Yang, M.L.; Uhrig, J.; Vu, K.; Singapuri, A.; Dennis, M.; Gelli, A.; Thompson, G.R. Fluconazole susceptibility in *Cryptococcus gattii* is dependent on the ABC transporter Pdr11. *Antimicrob. Agents Chemother.* **2016**, *60*, 1202–1207. [CrossRef] [PubMed]
115. Nagi, M.; Tanabe, K.; Ueno, K.; Nakayama, H.; Aoyama, T.; Chibana, H.; Yamagoe, S.; Umeyama, T.; Oura, T.; Ohno, H.; et al. The *Candida glabrata* sterol scavenging mechanism, mediated by the ATP-binding cassette transporter Aus1p, is regulated by iron limitation. *Mol. Microbiol.* **2013**, *88*, 371–381. [CrossRef] [PubMed]
116. Bard, M.; Sturm, A.M.; Pierson, C.A.; Brown, S.; Rogers, K.M.; Nabinger, S.; Eckstein, J.; Barbuch, R.; Lees, N.D.; Howell, S.A.; et al. Sterol uptake in *Candida glabrata*: Rescue of sterol auxotrophic strains. *Diagn. Microbiol. Infect. Dis.* **2005**, *52*, 285–293. [CrossRef] [PubMed]
117. Hazen, K.C.; Stei, J.; Darracott, C.; Breathnach, A.; May, J.; Howell, S.A. Isolation of cholesterol-dependent *Candida glabrata* from clinical specimens. *Diagn. Microbiol. Infect. Dis.* **2005**, *52*, 35–37. [CrossRef] [PubMed]
118. Li, Q.Q.; Tsai, H.F.; Mandal, A.; Walker, B.A.; Noble, J.A.; Fukuda, Y.; Bennett, J.E. Sterol uptake and sterol biosynthesis act coordinately to mediate antifungal resistance in *Candida glabrata* under azole and hypoxic stress. *Mol. Med. Rep.* **2018**, *17*, 6585–6597. [CrossRef] [PubMed]

119. Shah, A.H.; Singh, A.; Dhamgaye, S.; Chauhan, N.; Vandeputte, P.; Suneetha, K.J.; Kaur, R.; Mukherjee, P.K.; Chandra, J.; Ghannoum, M.A.; et al. Novel role of a family of major facilitator transporters in biofilm development and virulence of *Candida albicans*. *Biochem. J.* **2014**, *460*, 223–235. [CrossRef] [PubMed]
120. Nunes, P.A.; Tenreiro, S.; Sá-Correia, I. Resistance and adaptation to quinidine in *Saccharomyces cerevisiae*: role of *QDR1* (YIL120w), encoding a plasma membrane transporter of the major facilitator superfamily required for multidrug resistance. *Antimicrob. Agents Chemother.* **2001**, *45*, 1528–1534. [CrossRef] [PubMed]
121. Vargas, R.C.; Tenreiro, S.; Teixeira, M.C.; Fernandes, A.R.; Sá-correia, I. *Saccharomyces cerevisiae* multidrug transporter Qdr2p (Yil121wp): Localization and function as a quinidine resistance determinant. *Antimicrob. Agents Chemother.* **2004**, *48*, 2531–2537. [CrossRef] [PubMed]
122. Tenreiro, S.; Vargas, R.C.; Teixeira, M.C.; Magnani, C.; Sá-Correia, I. The yeast multidrug transporter Qdr3 (Ybr043c): Localization and role as a determinant of resistance to quinidine, barban, cisplatin, and bleomycin. *Biochem. Biophys. Res. Commun.* **2005**, *327*, 952–959. [CrossRef] [PubMed]
123. Santos, R.; Costa, C.; Mil-Homens, D.; Romão, D.; de Carvalho, C.C.C.R.; Pais, P.; Mira, N.P.; Fialho, A.M.; Teixeira, M.C. The multidrug resistance transporters CgTpo1_1 and CgTpo1_2 play a role in virulence and biofilm formation in the human pathogen *Candida glabrata*. *Cell. Microbiol.* **2017**, *19*, 1–13. [CrossRef] [PubMed]
124. Lin, X.; Qi, Y.; Yan, D.; Liu, H.; Chen, X.; Liu, L. *CgMED3* changes membrane sterol composition to help *Candida glabrata* tolerate. *Appl. Environ. Microbiol.* **2017**, *83*, 1–15. [CrossRef] [PubMed]
125. Li, R.; Kumar, R.; Tati, S.; Puri, S.; Edgerton, M. *Candida albicans* Flu1-Mediated efflux of salivary histatin 5 reduces its cytosolic concentration and fungicidal activity. *Antimicrob. Agents Chemother.* **2013**, *57*, 1832–1839. [CrossRef] [PubMed]
126. Kuchler, K.; Sterne, R.E.; Thorner, J. *Saccharomyces cerevisiae STE6* gene product: A novel pathway for protein export in eukaryotic cells. *EMBO J.* **1989**, *8*, 3973–3984. [CrossRef] [PubMed]
127. Raymond, M.; Dignard, D.; Alarco, A.M.; Mainville, N.; Magee, B.B.; Thomas, D.Y. A Ste6p/P-glycoprotein homologue from the asexual yeast *Candida albicans* transports the a-factor mating pheromone in *Saccharomyces cerevisiae*. *Mol. Microbiol.* **1998**, *27*, 587–598. [CrossRef] [PubMed]
128. Hsueh, Y.P.; Shen, W.C. A homolog of Ste6, the a-factor transporter in *Saccharomyces cerevisiae,* is required for mating but not for monokaryotic fruiting in *Cryptococcus neoformans*. *Eukaryot. Cell* **2005**, *4*, 147–155. [CrossRef] [PubMed]
129. Gibbons, J.G.; Beauvais, A.; Beau, R.; McGary, K.L.; Latgé, J.P.; Rokas, A. Global transcriptome changes underlying colony growth in the opportunistic human pathogen *Aspergillus fumigatus*. *Eukaryot. Cell* **2012**, *11*, 68–78. [CrossRef] [PubMed]
130. Kragl, C.; Schrettl, M.; Abt, B.; Sarg, B.; Lindner, H.H.; Haas, H. EstB-mediated hydrolysis of the siderophore triacetylfusarinine C optimizes iron uptake of *Aspergillus fumigatus*. *Eukaryot. Cell* **2007**, *6*, 1278–1285. [CrossRef] [PubMed]
131. Schrettl, M.; Kim, H.S.; Eisendle, M.; Kragl, C.; Nierman, W.C.; Heinekamp, T.; Werner, E.R.; Jacobsen, I.; Illmer, P.; Yi, H.; et al. SreA-mediated iron regulation in *Aspergillus fumigatus*. *Mol. Microbiol.* **2008**, *70*, 27–43. [CrossRef] [PubMed]
132. Weiss, G. Iron and immunity: A double-edged sword. *Eur. J. Clin. Investig.* **2002**, *32*, 70–78. [CrossRef]
133. Albertsen, M.; Bellahn, I.; Krämer, R.; Waffenschmidt, S. Localization and function of the yeast multidrug transporter Tpo1p. *J. Biol. Chem.* **2003**, *278*, 12820–12825. [CrossRef] [PubMed]
134. Tomitori, H.; Kashiwagi, K.; Asakawa, T.; Kakinuma, Y.; Michael, A.J.; Igarashi, K. Multiple polyamine transport systems on the vacuolar membrane in yeast. *Biochem. J.* **2001**, *353*, 681–688. [CrossRef] [PubMed]
135. Teixeira, M.C.; Cabrito, R.; Hanif, Z.M.; Vargas, R.C.; Tenreiro, S.; Sá-Correia, I. Yeast response and tolerance to polyamine toxicity involving the drug: H^+ antiporter Qdr3 and the transcription factors Yap1 and Gcn4. *Microbiology* **2011**, *157*, 945–956. [CrossRef] [PubMed]
136. Tyms, A. Polyamines and the growth of bacteria and viruses. In *The Physiology of Polyamines*; Bachrach, U., Heime, Y., Eds.; CRC Press: Boca Raton, FL, USA, 1989.
137. Tenreiro, S.; Nunes, P.A.; Viegas, C.A.; Neves, M.S.; Teixeira, M.C.; Cabral, G.; Sá-Correia, I. *AQR1* gene (ORF YNL065w) encodes a plasma membrane transporter of the major facilitator superfamily that confers resistance to short-chain monocarboxylic acids and quinidine in *Saccharomyces cerevisiae*. *Biochem. Biophys. Res. Commun.* **2002**, *292*, 741–748. [CrossRef] [PubMed]

138. Velasco, I.; Tenreiro, S.; Calderon, I.L.; André, B. *Saccharomyces cerevisiae* Aqr1 is an internal-membrane transporter involved in excretion of amino acids. *Eukaryot. Cell* **2004**, *3*, 1492–1503. [CrossRef] [PubMed]
139. Romão, D.; Cavalheiro, M.; Mil-Homens, D.; Santos, R.; Pais, P.; Costa, C.; Takahashi-Nakaguchi, A.; Fialho, A.M.; Chibana, H.; Teixeira, M.C. A New determinant of *Candida glabrata* virulence: The acetate exporter CgDtr1. *Front. Cell. Infect. Microbiol.* **2017**, *7*, 473. [CrossRef] [PubMed]
140. Bernardo, R.T.; Cunha, D.V.; Wang, C.; Pereira, L.; Silva, S.; Salazar, S.B.; Schröder, M.S.; Okamoto, M.; Takahashi-Nakaguchi, A.; Chibana, H.; et al. The CgHaa1-Regulon Mediates Response and Tolerance to Acetic Acid Stress in the Human Pathogen *Candida glabrata*. *G3: Genes Genomes Genet.* **2017**, *7*, 1–18. [CrossRef] [PubMed]
141. Smriti; Krishnamurthy, S.; Dixit, B.L.; Gupta, C.M.; Milewski, S.; Prasad, R. ABC transporters Cdr1p, Cdr2p and Cdr3p of a human pathogen *Candida albicans* are general phospholipid translocators. *Yeast* **2002**, *19*, 303–318. [CrossRef]
142. Fox, L.M.; Cox, D.G.; Lockridge, J.L.; Wang, X.; Chen, X.; Scharf, L.; Trott, D.L.; Ndonye, R.M.; Veerapen, N.; Besra, G.S.; et al. Recognition of lyso-phospholipids by human natural killer T lymphocytes. *PLoS Biol.* **2009**, *7*, e1000228. [CrossRef] [PubMed]
143. Cox, D.; Fox, L.; Tian, R.; Bardet, W.; Skaley, M.; Mojsilovic, D.; Gumperz, J.; Hildebrand, W. Determination of cellular lipids bound to human CD1d molecules. *PLoS ONE* **2009**, *4*, e5325. [CrossRef] [PubMed]
144. De Libero, G.; Mori, L. Recognition of lipid antigens by T cells. *Nat. Rev. Immunol.* **2005**, *5*, 485–496. [CrossRef] [PubMed]
145. Netea, M.G.; Joosten, L.A.B.; van der Meer, J.W.M.; Kullberg, B.-J.; van de Veerdonk, F.L. Immune defence against *Candida* fungal infections. *Nat. Rev. Immunol.* **2015**, *15*, 630–642. [CrossRef] [PubMed]
146. Brown, G.D. Innate antifungal immunity: The key role of phagocytes. *Annu. Rev. Immunol.* **2011**, *29*, 1–21. [CrossRef] [PubMed]
147. Miramón, P.; Kasper, L.; Hube, B. Thriving within the host: *Candida* spp. interactions with phagocytic cells. *Med. Microbiol. Immunol.* **2013**, *202*, 183–195. [CrossRef] [PubMed]
148. Seider, K.; Brunke, S.; Schild, L.; Jablonowski, N.; Wilson, D.; Majer, O.; Barz, D.; Haas, A.; Kuchler, K.; Schaller, M.; et al. the facultative intracellular pathogen *Candida glabrata* subverts macrophage cytokine production and phagolysosome maturation. *J. Immunol.* **2011**, *187*, 3072–3086. [CrossRef] [PubMed]
149. Orsi, C.F.; Colombari, B.; Ardizzoni, A.; Peppoloni, S.; Neglia, R.; Posteraro, B.; Morace, G.; Fadda, G.; Blasi, E. The ABC transporter-encoding gene *AFR1* affects the resistance of *Cryptococcus neoformans* to microglia-mediated antifungal activity by delaying phagosomal maturation. *FEMS Yeast Res.* **2009**, *9*, 301–310. [CrossRef] [PubMed]
150. Goulart, L.; Silva, L.K.R.E.; Chiapello, L.; Silveira, C.; Crestani, J.; Masih, D.; Vainstein, M.H. *Cryptococcus neoformans* and *Cryptococcus gattii* genes preferentially expressed during rat macrophage infection. *Med. Mycol.* **2010**, *48*, 932–941. [CrossRef] [PubMed]
151. Fontes, A.C.L.; Oliveira, D.B.; Santos, J.R.A.; Carneiro, H.C.S.; De Queiroz Ribeiro, N.; De Oliveira, L.V.N.; Barcellos, V.A.; Paixão, T.A.; Abrahão, J.S.; Resende-Stoianoff, M.A.; et al. A subdose of fluconazole alters the virulence of *Cryptococcus gattii* during murine cryptococcosis and modulates type I interferon expression. *Med. Mycol.* **2017**, *55*, 203–212. [CrossRef] [PubMed]
152. Paul, S.; Diekema, D.; Moye-Rowley, W.S. Contributions of *Aspergillus fumigatus* ATP-binding cassette transporter proteins to drug resistance and virulence. *Eukaryot. Cell* **2013**, *12*, 1619–1628. [CrossRef] [PubMed]
153. White, T.C. Increased mRNA Levels of *ERG16*, *CDR*, and *MDR1* correlate with increases in azole resistance in *Candida albicans* isolates from a patient infected with human immunodeficiency virus. *Antimicrob. Agents Chemother.* **1997**, *41*, 1482–1487. [PubMed]
154. Hiller, D.; Sanglard, D.; Morschhauser, J. Overexpression of the *MDR1* gene is sufficient to confer increased resistance to toxic compounds in *Candida albicans*. *Antimicrob. Agents Chemother.* **2006**, *50*, 1365–1371. [CrossRef] [PubMed]
155. Becker, J.M.; Henry, L.K.; Jiang, W.; Koltin, Y. Reduced virulence of *Candida albicans* mutants affected in multidrug resistance. *Infect. Immun.* **1995**, *63*, 4515–4518. [PubMed]
156. Yamada-Okabe, T.; Yamada-Okabe, H. Characterization of the *CaNAG3*, *CaNAG4*, and *CaNAG6* genes of the pathogenic fungus *Candida albicans*: Possible involvement of these genes in the susceptibilities of cytotoxic agents. *FEMS Microbiol. Lett.* **2002**, *212*, 15–21. [CrossRef] [PubMed]

157. Cavalheiro, M.; Teixeira, M.C. *Candida* biofilms: Threats, challenges, and promising strategies. *Front. Med.* **2018**, *5*, 28. [CrossRef] [PubMed]
158. Rajendran, R.; Mowat, E.; McCulloch, E.; Lappin, D.F.; Jones, B.; Lang, S.; Majithiya, J.B.; Warn, P.; Williams, C.; Ramage, G. Azole resistance of *Aspergillus fumigatus* biofilms is partly associated with efflux pump activity. *Antimicrob. Agents Chemother.* **2011**, *55*, 2092–2097. [CrossRef] [PubMed]
159. Ferrari, S.; Sanguinetti, M.; Torelli, R.; Posteraro, B.; Sanglard, D. Contribution of *CgPDR1*-regulated genes in enhanced virulence of azole-resistant *Candida glabrata*. *PLoS ONE* **2011**, *6*, e17589. [CrossRef] [PubMed]
160. Vale-Silva, L.A.; Moeckli, B.; Torelli, R.; Posteraro, B.; Sanglard, D. Upregulation of the adhesin gene *EPA1* mediated by *PDR1* in *Candida glabrata* leads to enhanced host colonization. *mSphere* **2016**, *1*, 1–16. [CrossRef] [PubMed]
161. Monteiro, P.T.; Pais, P.; Costa, C.; Manna, S.; Sa-Correia, I.; Teixeira, M.C. The PathoYeastract database: An information system for the analysis of gene and genomic transcription regulation in pathogenic yeasts. *Nucleic Acids Res.* **2017**, *45*, D597–D603. [CrossRef] [PubMed]
162. Alonso-Monge, R.; Román, E.; Arana, D.M.; Prieto, D.; Urrialde, V.; Nombela, C.; Pla, J. The Sko1 protein represses the yeast-to-hypha transition and regulates the oxidative stress response in *Candida albicans*. *Fungal Genet. Biol.* **2010**, *47*, 587–601. [CrossRef] [PubMed]
163. Zhang, X.; De Micheli, M.; Coleman, S.T.; Sanglard, D.; Moye-Rowley, W.S. Analysis of the oxidative stress regulation of the *Candida albicans* transcription factor, Cap1p. *Mol. Microbiol.* **2000**, *36*, 618–629. [CrossRef] [PubMed]
164. Davis, D.; Wilson, R.B.; Mitchell, A.P. *RIM101*-dependent and-independent pathways govern pH responses in *Candida albicans*. *Mol. Cell. Biol.* **2000**, *20*, 971–978. [CrossRef] [PubMed]
165. Davis, D.; Edwars John, J.; Mitchell, A.P.; Ibrahim, A.S. *Candida albicans RIM101* pH response pathway is required for host-pathogen interactions. *Infect. Immun.* **2000**, *68*, 5953–5959. [CrossRef] [PubMed]
166. Nicholls, S.; Leach, M.D.; Priest, C.L.; Brown, A.J.P. Role of the heat shock transcription factor, Hsf1, in a major fungal pathogen that is obligately associated with warm-blooded animals. *Mol. Microbiol.* **2009**, *74*, 844–861. [CrossRef] [PubMed]
167. Leach, M.D.; Cowen, L.E. to sense or die: mechanisms of temperature sensing in fungal pathogens. *Curr. Fungal Infect. Rep.* **2014**, *8*, 185–191. [CrossRef]
168. Bruno, V.M.; Kalachikov, S.; Subaran, R.; Nobile, C.J.; Kyratsous, C.; Mitchell, A.P. Control of the *C. albicans* cell wall damage response by transcriptional regulator Cas5. *PLoS Pathog.* **2006**, *2*, e21. [CrossRef] [PubMed]
169. Vasicek, E.M.; Berkow, E.L.; Bruno, V.M.; Mitchell, A.P.; Wiederhold, N.P.; Barker, K.S.; Rogers, P.D. Disruption of the transcriptional regulator Cas5 results in enhanced killing of *Candida albicans* by Fluconazole. *Antimicrob. Agents Chemother.* **2014**, *58*, 6807–6818. [CrossRef] [PubMed]
170. Nobile, C.J.; Fox, E.P.; Nett, J.E.; Sorrells, T.R.; Mitrovich, Q.M.; Hernday, A.D.; Tuch, B.B.; Andes, D.R.; Johnson, A.D. A Recently evolved transcriptional network controls biofilm development in *Candida albicans*. *Cell* **2013**, *148*, 126–138. [CrossRef] [PubMed]
171. Mukherjee, P.K.; Chandra, J.; Kuhn, D.M.; Ghannoum, M.A. Mechanism of fluconazole resistance in *Candida albicans* biofilms: Phase-specific role of efflux pumps and membrane sterols. *Infect. Immun.* **2003**, *71*, 4333–4340. [CrossRef] [PubMed]
172. Lepak, A.; Nett, J.; Lincoln, L.; Marchillo, K.; Andes, D. Time course of microbiologic outcome and gene expression in *Candida albicans* during and following in vitro and in vivo exposure to fluconazole. *Antimicrob. Agents Chemother.* **2006**, *50*, 1311–1319. [CrossRef] [PubMed]
173. Fox, E.P.; Bui, C.K.; Nett, J.E.; Hartooni, N.; Mui, M.C.; Andes, D.R.; Nobile, C.J.; Johnson, A.D. An expanded regulatory network temporally controls *Candida albicans* biofilm formation. *Mol. Microbiol.* **2015**, *96*, 1226–1239. [CrossRef] [PubMed]
174. Nobile, C.J.; Mitchell, A.P. Genetics and genomics of *Candida albicans* biofilm formation. *Cell. Microbiol.* **2006**, *8*, 1382–1391. [CrossRef] [PubMed]
175. Lane, S.; Birse, C.; Zhou, S.; Matson, R.; Liu, H. DNA array studies demonstrate convergent regulation of virulence factors by Cph1, Cph2, and Efg1 in *Candida albicans*. *J. Biol. Chem.* **2001**, *276*, 48988–48996. [CrossRef] [PubMed]
176. Ha, K.C.; White, T.C. Effects of azole antifungal drugs on the transition from yeast cells to hyphae in susceptible and resistant isolates of the pathogenic yeast *Candida albicans*. *Antimicrob. Agents Chemother.* **1999**, *43*, 763–768. [PubMed]

177. Mogavero, S.; Tavanti, A.; Senesi, S.; Rogers, P.D.; Morschhäuser, J. Differential requirement of the transcription factor Mcm1 for activation of the *Candida albicans* multidrug efflux pump *MDR1* by its regulators Mrr1 and Cap1. *Antimicrob. Agents Chemother.* **2011**, *55*, 2061–2066. [CrossRef] [PubMed]
178. Znaidi, S.; Nesseir, A.; Chauvel, M.; Rossignol, T.; D'Enfert, C. A comprehensive functional portrait of two heat shock factor-type transcriptional regulators involved in *Candida albicans* morphogenesis and virulence. *PLoS Pathog.* **2013**, *9*, e1003519. [CrossRef] [PubMed]
179. Silver, P.M.; Oliver, B.G.; White, T.C. Role of *Candida albicans* Transcription factor Upc2p in Drug resistance and sterol metabolism. *Eukaryot. Cell* **2004**, *3*, 1391–1397. [CrossRef] [PubMed]
180. Lavoie, H.; Hogues, H.; Mallick, J.; Sellam, A.; Nantel, A.; Whiteway, M. Evolutionary tinkering with conserved components of a transcriptional regulatory network. *PLoS Biol.* **2010**, *8*, e1000329. [CrossRef] [PubMed]
181. Dogra, S.; Krishnamurthy, S.; Gupta, V.; Dixit, B.L.; Gupta, C.M.; Sanglard, D.; Prasad, R. Asymmetric distribution of phosphatidylethanolamine in *C. albicans*: Possible mediation by *CDR1*, a multidrug transporter belonging to ATP binding cassette (ABC) superfamily. *Yeast* **1999**, *15*, 111–121. [CrossRef]
182. Noble, J.A.; Tsai, H.-F.; Suffis, S.D.; Su, Q.; Myers, T.G.; Bennett, J.E. *STB5* is a negative regulator of azole resistance in *Candida glabrata*. *Antimicrob. Agents Chemother.* **2013**, *57*, 959–967. [CrossRef] [PubMed]
183. Roetzer, A.; Klopf, E.; Gratz, N.; Marcet-Houben, M.; Hiller, E.; Rupp, S.; Gabaldón, T.; Kovarik, P.; Schüller, C. Regulation of *Candida glabrata* oxidative stress resistance is adapted to host environment. *FEBS Lett.* **2011**, *585*, 319–327. [CrossRef] [PubMed]
184. Chen, K.H.; Miyazaki, T.; Tsai, H.F.; Bennett, J.E. The bZip transcription factor Cgap1p is involved in multidrug resistance and required for activation of multidrug transporter gene *CgFLR1* in *Candida glabrata*. *Gene* **2007**, *386*, 63–72. [CrossRef] [PubMed]
185. Merhej, J.; Thiebaut, A.; Blugeon, C.; Pouch, J.; Ali Chaouche, M.E.A.; Camadro, J.-M.; Le Crom, S.; Lelandais, G.; Devaux, F. A network of paralogous stress response transcription factors in the human pathogen *Candida glabrata*. *Front. Microbiol.* **2016**, *7*, 645. [CrossRef] [PubMed]

10

The Transcription Factor ZafA Regulates the Homeostatic and Adaptive Response to Zinc Starvation in *Aspergillus fumigatus*

Rocío Vicentefranqueira [1], Jorge Amich [2], Laura Marín [1], Clara Inés Sánchez [1], Fernando Leal [1] and José Antonio Calera [1,*]

1 Instituto de Biología Funcional y Genómica (IBFG-CSIC), Departamento de Microbiología y Genética, Universidad de Salamanca, 37007 Salamanca, Spain; rvrdew@usal.es (R.V.); lauramarin@usal.es (L.M.); cisanchezs@usal.es (C.I.S.); fleal@usal.es (F.L.)

2 Manchester Fungal Infection Group (MFIG), Faculty of Biology, Medicine and Health, University of Manchester, Manchester M13 9NT, UK; jorge.amichelias@manchester.ac.uk

* Correspondence: jacalera@usal.es

Abstract: One of the most important features that enables *Aspergillus fumigatus* to grow within a susceptible individual and to cause disease is its ability to obtain Zn^{2+} ions from the extremely zinc-limited environment provided by host tissues. Zinc uptake from this source in *A. fumigatus* relies on ZIP transporters encoded by the *zrfA*, *zrfB* and *zrfC* genes. The expression of these genes is tightly regulated by the ZafA transcription factor that regulates zinc homeostasis and is essential for *A. fumigatus* virulence. We combined the use of microarrays, Electrophoretic Mobility Shift Assays (EMSA) analyses, DNase I footprinting assays and in silico tools to better understand the regulation of the homeostatic and adaptive response of *A. fumigatus* to zinc starvation. We found that under zinc-limiting conditions, ZafA functions mainly as a transcriptional activator through binding to a zinc response sequence located in the regulatory regions of its target genes, although it could also function as a repressor of a limited number of genes. In addition to genes involved in the homeostatic response to zinc deficiency, ZafA also influenced, either directly or indirectly, the expression of many other genes. It is remarkable that the expression of many genes involved in iron uptake and ergosterol biosynthesis is strongly reduced under zinc starvation, even though only the expression of some of these genes appeared to be influenced directly or indirectly by ZafA. In addition, it appears to exist in *A. fumigatus* a zinc/iron cross-homeostatic network to allow the adaptation of the fungus to grow in media containing unbalanced Zn:Fe ratios. The adaptive response to oxidative stress typically linked to zinc starvation was also mediated by ZafA, as was the strong induction of genes involved in gliotoxin biosynthesis and self-protection against endogenous gliotoxin. This study has expanded our knowledge about the regulatory and metabolic changes displayed by *A. fumigatus* in response to zinc starvation and has helped us to pinpoint new ZafA target genes that could be important for fungal pathogens to survive and grow within host tissues and, hence, for virulence.

Keywords: *Aspergillus fumigatus*; zinc; transcription; regulation

---

1. Introduction

Zinc is an essential nutrient element that plays a critical role in many different biological processes as a structural and/or as a catalytic component of many different enzymes [1,2]. Indeed, zinc is required, in both pathogens and their hosts, for the normal functioning of hundreds of enzymes and regulatory proteins in all cells. For this reason, zinc uptake and distribution are subjected to a strict homeostatic control. This is critical to ensure an appropriate steady supply of zinc and to prevent the noxious effects that both excess and deficiency of zinc may have on cell growth and differentiation.

Free-living, mutualist and commensal microorganisms obtain zinc from non-living matter such as water, soil or organic compounds present in their surrounding environment. In contrast, microbial pathogens have to obtain zinc from the tissues of the host they parasitize. However, zinc in living tissues is subjected to a strict homeostatic control that restricts the access of pathogens to it. Indeed, intracellular eukaryotic zinc proteins bind zinc tightly with pK_d stability constants (i.e., $-\log K_d$) of 10–12 [3]. As a consequence, although the concentration of total zinc within most eukaryotic cells is in the micromolar range (100–500 μM) [4,5], the amount of intracellular free Zn^{2+} ions is commensurately about six to seven orders of magnitude lower than the overall cellular zinc concentration. It has been estimated that the concentration of free Zn^{2+} ions in different types of mammalian cells and tissues range from tens to hundreds of picomoles per liter [6]. For instance, the concentration of free Zn^{2+} ions reported in human red blood cells is 24 pM [7], which indicates that a single red blood cell (90 fL volume) should have 1–2 atoms of free Zn^{2+} ions [8].

Aspergillus fumigatus is a saprophyte filamentous fungus that usually grows on organic decaying matter. However, it is also able to grow as a parasite in the lungs of immunosuppressed individuals and cause invasive pulmonary aspergillosis (IPA), which is one of the fungal infectious diseases with the highest mortality rate among immunosuppressed patients [9]. One of the most important features that enables *A. fumigatus* to grow within a susceptible host and causes disease is its ability to obtain Zn^{2+} ions from the hostile environment provided by host tissues [10]. *A. fumigatus* zinc uptake from host tissues relies on transporters of the ZIP family encoded by the *zrfA*, *zrfB* and *zrfC* genes [11,12]. The ZrfC transporter seems to be well adapted to function under the alkaline zinc-limiting conditions of mammals' bodies and plays a major role in zinc uptake from host tissues. Interestingly, the ZrfA and ZrfB zinc transporters, despite their expression are higher in acidic than in alkaline zinc-limiting media, also play a relevant role in virulence. Thus, the virulence of a Δ*zrfA*Δ*zrfB*Δ*zrfC* mutant is fully abrogated in a murine model of invasive pulmonary aspergillosis [13], as is that of a Δ*zafA* mutant [14], which lacks the gene encoding the zinc-responsiveness transcriptional factor ZafA that regulates zinc homeostasis in *A. fumigatus*. Hence, the ZafA-mediated induction of the zinc uptake system under zinc-limiting conditions is a key homeostatic function required for optimal fungal growth within host tissues.

The most investigated ZafA orthologue is the Zap1 transcription factor of *Saccharomyces cerevisiae* [15]. Several genome-wide transcriptional profiling studies in *S. cerevisiae* have shown that Zap1 influences the expression of many genes required to implement properly the adaptive and homeostatic responses to zinc deficiency [16–18]. Similar studies on Zap1-regulated genes have been also performed in the pathogenic yeasts *Candida albicans* and *Cryptococcus gattii* [19,20]. These Zap1-like yeast transcription factors have 3–4 canonical zinc fingers domains (ZFDs) of the C2H2-type and four ZFDs of the CWCH2-type. The latter are typically clustered in pairs forming two tandem motifs (tCWCH2) [21] (Figure 1). Interestingly, in transcription factors carrying tCWCH2 motifs, only the CWCH2 zinc finger of the tCWCH2 motif closer to a canonical C2H2 zinc finger interacts with the DNA backbone, whereas its partner CWCH2 zinc finger is dedicated to protein-protein interactions and does not interact with the DNA [22–24]. Actually, it has been proposed that the tCWCH2 motifs are involved in inter-ZFD interactions and influence both the recognition and binding capacities of their neighboring canonical C2H2 domains to DNA [21]. Since the activity of the transcription factors having tCWCH2 motifs appear to be largely influenced by this type of ZFDs, it is very likely that the transcriptional profile under zinc starvation in yeast carrying Zap1-like factors with two tCWCH2 motifs differs to a certain extent from that observed in *A. fumigatus* and other filamentous fungi carrying ZafA-like factors with a unique tCWCH2 motif [14] (Figure 1). To discover new ZafA target genes essential for fungal virulence other than those encoding ZIP transporters, we performed a genome-wide transcription profiling in *A. fumigatus* grown in vitro under alkaline zinc-limiting conditions to mimic those found by the fungus in the lungs of a susceptible host. In addition, we analyzed the promoter regions of the genes that exhibited the highest differential expression levels between zinc-replete and zinc-limiting conditions. To this purpose, we used a combination of in vitro and in silico procedures to identify the consensus DNA zinc response motif to which ZafA binds under zinc-limiting conditions.

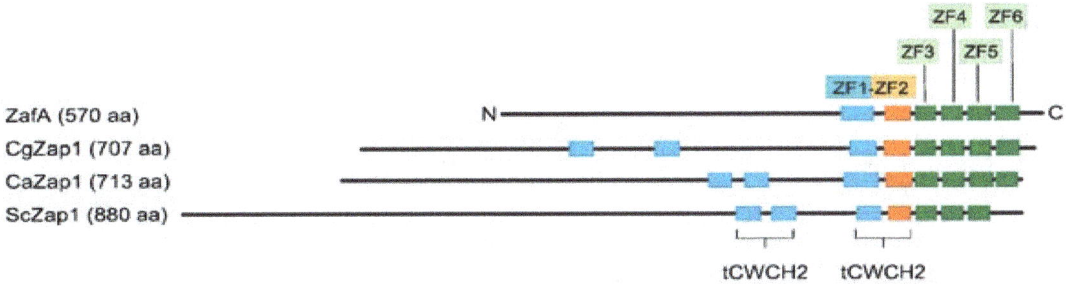

Figure 1. Schematic representation of the transcriptional regulators of zinc homeostasis from *Aspergillus fumigatus* (ZafA), *Cryptococcus gattii* (CgZap1), *Candida albicans* (CaZap1) and *Saccharomyces cerevisiae* (ScZap1). Green boxes indicate canonical zinc finger (ZF) domains of the C2H2-type. Blue and orange boxes indicate ZFs of the CWCH2-type. These ZFs are typically arranged in pairs forming tandem CWCH2 motifs (tCWCH2). The ZF of the CWCH2-type that is presumably able to bind DNA is indicated as an orange box. Protein sequences were aligned taking as reference the ZF of the C2H2-type located towards the N-terminus in ZafA (i.e., ZF3).

2. Materials and Methods

2.1. Strains and Culture Media

The *A. fumigatus* strains used in this study are listed in Table 1. These fungal strains were routinely grown in either the PDA complex medium (20 g/L potato dextrose agar, 20 g/L sucrose, 2.5 g/L $MgSO_4$-$7H_2O$) or in the liquid synthetic dextrose nitrate zinc-limiting medium (SDN–Zn, pH 7.2) (1.7 g/L YNB without amino acids, without ammonium sulphate and without zinc [CYN2401, Formedium], 20 g/L Dextrose, 3 g/L $NaNO_3$, 12 μM $FeSO_4$-7 H_2O, 6 μM $CuSO_4$-5 H_2O, 10 μM Na_2MoO_4-2 H_2O), which was supplemented with zinc as specified using a sterile stock solution of 1 mM $ZnSO_4$-$7H_2O$ in ultrapure water.

Table 1. *Aspergillus fumigatus* strains used in this study. Genes in brackets were reintroduced into the *A. fumigatus* genome by targeting them at the intergenic region between the AFUA_2G08360 (*pyrG*) and AFUA_2G08350 genes.

Strain	Detailed Genotype	Reference
CEA17	*pyrG1* (auxotrophic $PyrG^-$)	[11]
AF14	Wild-type (isogenic to CEA17)	[12]
AF171	Δ*zafA::hisG* (isogenic to CEA17)	[14]
AFZR0	Wild-type [*luc* ← $PzrfC^{wt}$ → *gfp*] (isogenic to CEA17)	This study
AFZR1	Wild-type [*luc* ← $PzrfC^{ZR123}$ → *gfp*] (isogenic to CEA17)	This study

2.2. Culture of *Aspergillus fumigatus* for RNA Isolation

To obtain RNA under zinc-limiting culture conditions to be used for both microarray analyses and Real Time quantitative PCR (RT-qPCR) experiments, the wild-type and Δ*zafA* mutant strain were inoculated to a density of 1.5×10^6 spores/mL in 200 mL of the SDN–Zn zinc limiting medium and incubated at 37 °C with shaking at 200 rpm for 20 h. Similarly, to obtain RNA under zinc-replete culture conditions, the wild-type strain was inoculated and incubated as described previously in the SDN–Zn zinc limiting medium supplemented with 100 μM zinc. In all cases, spores grown in PDA were used as inoculum.

The mycelia were harvested by filtration on filter paper, washed twice with sterile water and snap-frozen in liquid nitrogen. After grinding the mycelia in the presence of liquid nitrogen, the RNA was extracted using the RNeasy Plant Mini Kit (74904, QIAGEN, Hilden, Germany) according to manufacturer's instructions. RNA was eluted in 50 μL of RNase-free water. The concentration and quality of RNA was determined by UV spectrometry (Nanodrop ND1000 spectrophotometer, Thermo Fisher Scientific, Waltham, MA, USA) and checked on 0.8% agarose gels stained with ethidium bromide. RNA samples were stored at −80 °C until use.

2.3. Microarray Experiments

The *A. fumigatus* Af293 DNA microarray slides (version 4) with 2× replicate 70-mer oligonucleotide printings used in this study were obtained (April 2010) through the Pathogen Functional Genomics Resource Center of the National Institute of the Allergy and Infectious Diseases/National Institute of Health (NIAID/NIH), managed and funded by the Division of Microbiology and Infectious Diseases (DMID) and operated by the J. Craig Venter Institute.

Total RNA was treated with RNase DNase-free and 2 μg of total RNA DNA-free was used for cDNA synthesis, which was performed using SuperScript III RT and a dNTP/5-(3-aminoallyl)-dUTP labelling mix. Upon elimination of unincorporated aa-dUTP, either the Cy5 or Cy3 dye was coupled to the aminoallyl-labelled cDNA by incubation for 1 h at room temperature in 0.1 M sodium carbonate (pH 9.3). Free dyes were removed using the QIAGEN PCR purification kit and were calculated for the total picomoles of dyes incorporation and the pmol cDNA/pmol Cy dye ratios upon measuring spectrophotometrically the cDNA concentration, $OD_{650\ nm}$ for Cy5 and $OD_{550\ nm}$ for Cy3. Microarray experiments were performed in duplicate with dye labels reversed. Each slide was hybridized with 1:1 mix of two differentially labeled probes Cy3 and Cy5 (1100 pmoles of each one) in a HS 4800 Pro™ Hybridization Station (Tecan Group Ltd., Männedorf, Switzerland) and scanned using the Axon GenePix 4000B microarray scanner. The TIFF images generated were analyzed using Spotfinder 321a to obtain relative transcript levels. Data were normalized with MIDAS using LOWESS (Locally Weighted Scatterplot Smoothing) and the dye-swap procedure (all softwares were developed by the J. Craig Venter Institute to be used for DNA microarray slides provided by the NIAID/NIH). The resulting data were averaged from duplicated genes on each array and from duplicate flip-dye arrays for each experiment, taking a total of four intensity data points for each gene. A volcano-plot algorithm was used to identify genes that exhibited statistical significance ($p < 0.05$) with a change in expression levels $\geq$ 1.5-fold. Differentially expressed genes at the 95% confidence level were determined using T-test implemented in the MEV program of the TM4 microarray software suite (http://www.tm4.org). The microarray data have been deposited in the GEO database under accession number GSE109389.

2.4. RT-qPCR

The concentration of total RNA in all samples were brought to a final concentration of 150 ng/μL. To remove genomic DNA, 1.5 μg of total RNA were treated with RQ1 DNase I (M610, Promega, Madison, WI, USA) and checked by conventional PCR for the complete absence of gDNA. Next, 1 μg of DNase-treated RNA was reversed transcribed using the SuperScript II Reverse Transcriptase (18064-014, Invitrogen, ThermoFisher Scientific) and oligo $(dT)_{15}$ (C1101, Promega) or random hexamers (SO142, ThermoFisher Scientific) as primers. Prior to the qPCR reactions, the cDNA samples were diluted 1:3 in water (except for reactions against the 18S rRNA that were diluted 1:1200 in water). Quantitative real time PCR (qPCR) reactions were performed in a BioRad CFX96 equipment. A typical qPCR reaction mixture (10 μL) contained 13.5 ng cDNA (32 pg when the qPCR was for 18S rRNA), a specific pair of primers (150 nM final concentration) and the SYBR Premix ExTaq (Tli RNaseH Plus) (RR420A, Takara). The amount of cDNA used per reaction was calculated on the basis that all RNA had been reversed transcribed into cDNA, including the rRNAs. Primers used for qPCR are listed in Table S1. PCRs were carried out for 40 cycles, denaturation at 95 °C for 10 s, annealing at 59 °C for 20 s and extension at 72 °C for 20 s. The relative expression level with respect to 18S rRNA (REL/18S) was calculated by the $2^{-\Delta Ct}$ method. The relative expression ratio (rER) was calculated by the $2^{-\Delta\Delta Ct}$ method using the expression level of the 18S rRNA as internal reference.

2.5. *Expression and Purification of the Recombinant* ZafA *Protein*

An *Eco*RI-flanked DNA fragment (482 bp) carrying the coding sequence for the C-terminal 140 amino acids of ZafA (residues 434–570) was obtained by high-fidelity PCR using as template the plasmid pZAF14, which carried the complete cDNA for the ZafA coding sequence [14], and the pair of oligonucleotides JA181/JA182 (Table S2). This fragment was digested with *Eco*RI and ligated to the *Eco*RI site of the pGEX-5X-3 plasmid (GE Healthcare, Little Chalfont, UK) to generate the pGEX-5X-ZafA plasmid. The ZafA coding sequence inserted into the pGEX-5X-ZafA plasmid was confirmed by sequencing. The pGEX-5X-ZafA plasmid was used to transform *Escherichia coli* BL21-DE3. The resulting strain was able to synthesize high amounts of the four C-terminal zinc fingers of ZafA (ZF3-6) fused to the C-terminus of GST upon induction with IPTG (0.25 mM). Although the GST-ZafA$^{ZF3\text{-}6}$ protein aggregated into inclusion bodies, it was easily solubilized using a slightly acidic lysis buffer (20 mM Tris-HCl, 150 mM NaCl, 100 mM $ZnCl_2$, 0.1% Triton X-100, 5 mM DTT [pH 6.7]), instead of the most standard lysis buffer at pH 7.5. The GST-ZafA$^{ZF3\text{-}6}$ protein was purified using Glutathione Sepharose 4B (GE Healthcare, Cat. 17075601) and eluted with elution buffer (50 mM Tris-ClH [pH 8.0], 150 mM NaCl, 0.1% Triton X-100, 10 mM reduced glutathione). The eluted GST-ZafA$^{ZF3\text{-}6}$ protein was concentrated with an Amicon Ultra-15 3K device (Millipore, Burlington, MA, USA) and dialyzed in a D-Tube Dialyzer Maxi unit (MWCO 3.5 kDa) (Merck-Millipore, Novagen, Temecula, CA, USA) against the factor Xa buffer (20 mM Tris-Cl, pH 6.5, 50 mM NaCl, 1 mM $CaCl_2$). Upon optimizing the cleavage conditions of the GST-ZafA$^{ZF3\text{-}6}$ protein with factor Xa, the purified GST-ZafA$^{ZF3\text{-}6}$ protein was treated with 25 ng factor Xa (NEB, P8010, Ipswich, MA, USA) per 260 ng of protein for 6 h at room temperature to achieve 100% cleavage of GST-ZafA$^{ZF3\text{-}6}$ protein, as judged in SDS-PAGE gels stained with coomassie blue. The factor Xa was removed from the cleavage reaction with Xarrest™ Agarose (Merck-Millipore, cat. 69038). Following the capture of Factor Xa, the agarose was removed by spin-filtration. The cleavage reaction without factor Xa, which contained equimolar amounts of GST and ZafA$^{ZF3\text{-}6}$, was dialyzed against binding buffer (25 mM Tris-HCl, pH 8.0, 50 mM KCl, 10 μM $ZnCl_2$, 1 mM $MgCl_2$, 1 mM DTT). Proteins were stored at −20 °C until use.

The GST protein that was used as control was expressed from plasmid pGEX-5X-3, purified, digested with factor Xa and dialyzed as described for the GST-ZafA$^{ZF3\text{-}6}$ protein.

Protein concentrations were estimated by measuring A280 nm in a NanoDrop spectrophotometer (ThermoFisher) and taking into consideration that the extinction molar coefficients for the GST and ZafA$^{ZF3\text{-}6}$ moieties of the GST-ZafA$^{ZF3\text{-}6}$ protein were 1.632 and 0.1811 $mg^{-1} \times mL \times cm^{-1}$, respectively.

2.6. *Construction of Plasmids to Obtain Probes for Electrophoretic Mobility Shift Assays and DNase I Footprinting Experiments*

Two overlapping DNA fragments of the *zafA* promoter (P*zafA*) of 397 bp and 233 bp were obtained by PCR using as template gDNA from the wild-type AF14 strain and the pair of oligonucleotides JA204/JA394 and JA375/JA204, respectively (Table S2). The PCR products were ligated to the pGEM-T vector (Promega, cat. A1360) to generate the pZAF151 and pZAF91 plasmids.

The complete sequence of the bidirectional promoter P*aspf2-zrfC* that drives the expression of the *aspf2* and *zrfC* genes (abbreviated as P*zrfC*, 884 bp) was amplified by PCR using as template gDNA from the wild-type AF14 strain and the pair of oligonucleotides JA194/JA196. The PCR product was ligated to the pGEM-T easy vector (A1360, Promega) to generate the pASFP2-ZRF31 plasmid. Similarly, a 215-bp DNA fragment of P*zrfC* right next to the *zrfC* coding sequence was amplified using the pair of oligonucleotides JA376/JA377 and the PCR product was ligated to the pGEM-T vector to generate the pASFP2-ZRF311 plasmid. Finally, 539 bp of P*zrfC* right next to the *zrfC* coding sequence were excised from the pASFP2-ZRF31 plasmid following an *Eco*RV/*Msc*I digestion-religation to generate the pASFP2-ZRF312 plasmid, which only carried 349 bp of P*zrfC* right next to the *aspf2* coding sequence.

A 222-bp DNA fragment of the *zrfA* promoter (P*zrfA*) was amplified by PCR using as template gDNA from the wild-type AF14 strain and the pair of oligonucleotides JA378/JA379. The PCR product was ligated to the pGEM-T vector to generate the pZRF10 plasmid.

A 256-bp DNA fragment of the *zrfB* promoter (P*zrfB*) was amplified by PCR using as template gDNA from the wild-type AF14 strain and the pair of oligonucleotides JA380/JA381. The PCR product was ligated to the pGEM-T vector to generate the pZRF261 plasmid.

A 191 bp-DNA fragment of the *alcA* promoter of *Aspergillus nidulans* (P*alcA*) was amplified by high-fidelity PCR using the pair of oligonucleotides JA261/JA388 and as template gDNA from the *A. nidulans* strain G1059 [25]. The PCR product was ligated to the pGEM-T vector to generate plasmid pALC3.

All subcloned PCR products were sequenced to verify the absence of any mutation that could have been introduced during PCR.

2.7. Preparation of Probes for Electrophoretic Mobility Shift Assays

DNA probes for different promoters (P*zafA*, P*zrfC*, P*zrfA*, P*zrfB* and P*alcA*) were amplified by high-fidelity PCR using Pfu polymerase and purified using the QIAquick PCR Purification Kit (QIAGEN). The oligonucleotides used as primers (Table S2) and plasmids used as templates for DNA amplification by PCR were the following: For P*zafA* EMSA assays we used a 233-bp DNA fragment amplified by PCR using a dilution of the pZAF91 plasmid as template and the pair of oligonucleotides JA375/JA204 as primers; For P*zrfC* EMSA assays we used a 221-bp DNA fragment amplified by PCR using a dilution of the pASFP2-ZRF311 plasmid as template and the pair of oligonucleotides JA376/JA377; For P*zrfA* EMSA assays we used a 222-bp DNA fragment amplified by PCR using a dilution of the pZRF10 plasmid as template and the pair of oligonucleotides JA378/JA379 as primers; For P*zrfB* EMSA assays we used a 256-bp DNA fragment amplified by PCR using a dilution of the pZRF261 plasmid as template and the pair of oligonucleotides JA380/JA381 as primers; For P*alcA* EMSA assays we used a 213-bp DNA fragment amplified by PCR using a dilution of the pALC3 plasmid as template and the pair of oligonucleotides JA261/JA388 as primers.

2.8. Preparation of Probes for DNase I Footprinting Assays

6-FAM-5′-labelled DNA probes for different promoters (P*zafA*, P*zrfC*, P*zrfA*, P*zrfB* and P*alcA*) were amplified by high-fidelity PCR using Pfu polymerase and purified using the QIAquick PCR Purification Kit (QIAGEN). The oligonucleotides used as primers (Table S2) and plasmids used as templates in DNA amplification by PCR are described next.

Four different probes were used for the P*zafA* DNase I footprinting assays: (i) Two 432 bp DNA fragments amplified by PCR using the pZAF91 plasmid as template and the pair of oligonucleotides FAM-Rv/Fw and Rv/FAM-Fw as primers to get them labelled in 5′-ends of the sense and antisense strands respectively (these probes carried 229 bp of P*zafA* plus two flanking sequences corresponding to the MCS of the vector); (ii) A536 bp DNA fragment amplified by PCR using the pZAF151 plasmid as template and the pair of oligonucleotides FAM-Rv/JA204 as primers to get it labelled in the 5′-end of the sense strand (this probe carried 396 bp of P*zafA* plus one flanking sequence corresponding to the MCS of the vector); (iii) A 435 bp DNA fragment amplified by PCR using the pZAF151 plasmid as template and the pair of oligonucleotides Rv/FAM-JA439 as primers to get it labelled in the 5′-end of the antisense strand (this probe carried 295 bp of P*zafA*).

Four different probes were used for the P*zrfC* DNase I footprinting assays: (i) A 322 bp DNA fragment amplified by PCR using the pASPF2-ZRF311 plasmid as template and the pair of oligonucleotides FAM-Fw/JA377 as primers to get it labelled in the 5′-end of the sense strand for *zrfC* (this probe carried 215 bp of P*zrfC* plus one flanking sequence corresponding to the MCS of the vector); (ii) A 347 bp DNA fragment amplified by PCR using the pASFP2-ZRF311 plasmid as a template and the pair of oligonucleotides JA376/FAM-Rv as primers to get it labelled in the 5′-end of the antisense strand for *zrfC* (this probe carried 215 bp of P*zrfC* plus one flanking sequence corresponding to the MCS of the vector); (iii) A 393 bp DNA fragment amplified by PCR using the pASPF2-ZRF312 plasmid as template and the pair of oligonucleotides FAM-Fw/JA7 as primers to get it labelled in the 5′-end of the sense strand for *zrfC* (this probe carried 349 bp of P*zrfC* plus one flanking sequence corresponding to the MCS of the vector); (iv) A 504 bp DNA fragment amplified by PCR using the pASPF2-ZRF312 plasmid as template and the pair of oligonucleotides JA194/FAM-Rv as primers to get it labelled in the 5′-end of the antisense strand for *zrfC* (this probe carried 349 bp of P*zrfC* plus one flanking sequence corresponding to the MCS of the vector).

Two different probes were used for the P*zrfB* DNase I footprinting assays: (i) A 456 bp DNA fragment amplified by PCR using the pZRF261 plasmid as template and the pair of oligonucleotides FAM-Fw/Rv as primers to get it labelled in the 5′-end of the sense strand; (ii) A 456 bp DNA fragment amplified by PCR using the pZRF261 plasmid as template and the pair of oligonucleotides Fw/FAM-Rv as primers to get it labelled in the 5′-end of the antisense strand. Both probes carried 256 bp of P*zrfB* plus two flanking sequences corresponding to the MCS of the vector.

One probe was used for the P*zrfA* DNase I footprinting assays. A 350 bp DNA fragment amplified by PCR using the pZRF10 as template and the pair of oligonucleotides JA378/FAM-Rv as primers to get it labelled in the 5′-end of the antisense strand (this probe carried 217 bp of P*zrfA* plus one flanking sequence corresponding to the MCS of the vector).

One probe was used for the P*alcA* DNase I footprinting assays. A 413 bp DNA fragment of the pALC3 plasmid carrying 213 bp of P*alcA* plus two flanking sequences corresponding to the MCS of the vector were amplified by high-fidelity PCR and the pair of oligonucleotides FAM-Fw/Rv or Fw/FAM-Rv.

2.9. Electrophoretic Mobility Shift Assays and DNase I Footprinting Assays Reactions and Analyses

Reactions for EMSA experiments (20 μL) were assembled in 0.5-mL microtubes and carried out in EMSA buffer (25 mM Tris-HCl [pH 8], 50 mM KCl, 1 mM $MgCl_2$, 12.5% glycerol, 1 mM DTT), containing 1 μL BSA (0.2 mg/mL), 0.25–0.75 pmoles of the target DNA and the amount of the equimolar mixture of GST and $ZafA^{ZF3\text{-}6}$ required to add 0.125–24 pmoles $ZafA^{ZF3\text{-}6}$. Reactions were incubated for 1 h at 30 °C before adding 4 μL of loading buffer (20% sucrose, 0.002% bromophenol blue). Reactions were loaded in a polyacrylamide 5% EMSA gel that had been pre-run in TBE 1× for 10 min at 4 °C in a cold room. Gels were run at 100 V for approximately 75 min, stained with a solution of ethidium bromide (5 μg/mL) for 20 min at room temperature, washed for 10 min with distilled water and photographed on a UV transilluminator in a gel documentation system.

Reactions for footprinting assays (60 μL) were assembled in 0.5-mL microtubes and carried out in an EMSA buffer containing 3 μL BSA (0.2 mg/mL), 0.5 pmoles of the desired 6-carboxyfluorescein (6-FAM)-labeled DNA fragment and 12 pmoles of $ZafA^{ZF3\text{-}6}$. Control reactions were assembled identically but omitting $ZafA^{ZF3\text{-}6}$. All DNA fragments used for footprinting assays were obtained by high-fidelity PCR using as primers both a 6-FAM-5′-labelled oligonucleotide and a non-labeled oligonucleotide, as described above. After incubating the footprinting reactions for 45 min at 30 °C, DNA was partially digested with 0.01 U of DNase I by adding 4 μL of a DNase I stock solution (0.0025 U/μL) per reaction and incubated at 25 °C for 1 min. The reaction was stopped immediately by adding 340 μL of stop buffer (9 mM Tris-HCl [pH 8], 40 mM EDTA). DNA was extracted with one volume of phenol:chloroform:isoamyl alcohol (25:24:1) followed by an extraction with one volume of chloroform:isoamyl alcohol (24:1). DNA in the aqueous phase was precipitated with 0.1 volumes of a non-buffered 3.0 M AcNa solution plus 2.5 volumes of ethanol. Precipitation of DNA was left to stand to proceed overnight at −20 °C. After centrifugation, the DNA pellet was washed twice with 70% ethanol, allowed to air dry at room temperature, suspended in 10 μL of Hi-Di formamide, denatured at 95 °C for 3 min and cooled on ice. All DNase I footprinting reactions were analyzed electrophoretically on an automated capillary DNA sequencer using the GeneScan™ 500 LIZ (Thermofisher) dye Size Standard as a calibrator. Each footprinting reaction was performed in parallel to four dideoxynucleotide-based sequencing reactions of the corresponding DNA probe, using as a primer the same 6-FAM 5′-labelled oligonucleotides utilized to amplify each DNA fragment by PCR.

2.10. Construction of Plasmids Used for *Aspergillus fumigatus* Transformation

The strains AFZR0 and AFZR1 of *A. fumigatus* used in this study were able to express the coding sequences of both the firefly luciferase (*luc*; as a reporter of *aspf2* expression) and the green fluorescent protein (*gfp*; as a reporter of *zrfC* expression) under control of either a wild-type version of the bidirectional *aspf2-zrfC* promoter ($\text{P}zrfC^{\text{wt}}$) or a mutant version of this promoter whose ZR motifs had been inactivated by site directed mutagenesis ($\text{P}zrfC^{\text{ZR123}}$).

The CEA17 uridine-uracil-auxotrophic *pyrG1* strain was transformed with two different EcoRI-EcoRI DNA fragments of 7286 bp, excised respectively from plasmids pPYRGQ191 and pPYRGQ193 to generate respectively the AFZR0 and AFZR1 strains (Figure S1).

The plasmids pPYRGQ191 and pPYRGQ193 were generated by ligating XbaI-FspI DNA fragments (4105 bp), which carried respectively the [$luc \leftarrow \text{P}zrfC^{\text{wt}} \rightarrow gfp$] and [$luc \leftarrow \text{P}zrfC^{\text{ZR123}} \rightarrow gfp$] constructs, to the pPYRGQ31 plasmid digested with XbaI/SmaI. The pPYRGQ31 plasmid was an improved version of the pPYRGQ3 plasmid that had been designed previously in our laboratory to revert specifically the *pyrG1* mutation (C756T) in the *A. fumigatus* CEA17 or in any PyrG^- CEA17 derivative strain and select PyrG^+ prototrophic strains bearing the DNA fragment of interest inserted between its AFUA_2G08360 (*pyrG*) and AFUA_2G08350 loci [11].

The plasmids used to transform *A. fumigatus* were linearized by digestion with *Eco*RI, extracted with phenol:chloroform:IAA, precipitated with acetate/isopropanol, washed in 70% ethanol, dissolved in 50% (*v*/*v*) of KC solution (0.6 M KCl, 50 mM CaCl; pH 6.0–6.5) and used for transformation as described below.

2.11. Generation of Protoplasts and Transformation of *Aspergillus fumigatus*

Protoplasts of *A. fumigatus* were prepared using a new protocol developed in our laboratory to obtain high-quality protoplasts that were very susceptible to transformation. In brief, to obtain protoplasts of the CEA17 PyrG^- strain we inoculated 5×10^8 conidia of this strain in the SDN medium supplemented with 0.05% (*w*/*v*) uracil, 0.12% (*w*/*v*) uridine and 20% (*v*/*v*) of a sterile conditioned medium that was produced by ourselves and contained a highly active α-glucanase. The culture was incubated at 37 °C for 14 h. Germlings were collected by filtration through a cell strainer unit (40 μm), suspended in 10 mL of protoplasting buffer (0.2 g VinoTaste, 0.75 M KCl, 25 mM citrate/phosphate; pH 5.8) (it had been previously sterilized by filtration through a 0.22 μm filter unit) and incubated at 35 °C with shaking at 120 rpm for 2 h. The protoplasting suspension was filtered through a miracloth (Merck-Millipore, Calbiochem Cat. 475855; 22–25 μm) and centrifuged at 1200× *g* for 10 min a 4 °C. The protoplast pellet was washed in 15 mL of a cold KC solution (0.6 M KCl, 50 mM CaCl; pH 6.0–6.5) by mixing gently and centrifuged at 1200× *g* for 10 min at 4 °C. The protoplast pellet was suspended into 0.4 mL of KC solution and used for transformation.

Aliquots of 0.2 mL of protoplast suspension were dispensed in 15-mL conical tubes to which were added sequentially the transforming DNA (~10 μg) and 0.5 mL of PEG buffer (30% PEG-6000 [*w*/*v*], 0.6 M KCl, 50 mM $CaCl_2$, 10 mM Tris-HCl; pH 7.5). The protoplast-DNA-PEG mixture was incubated on ice for 30 min and then at 25 °C for 30 min in a water bath. Next, 9.3 mL of KC solution was added to each protoplast-DNA-PEG solution, mixed by inversion, centrifuged at 1200× *g* for 10 min at 4 °C, suspended in 0.5 mL of KC solution, mixed with 6 mL of soft agar (AMM with 0.6 M KCl plus 0.4% [*w*/*v*] agarose) and poured onto two selective AMM plates. Plates were incubated at 37 °C until PyrG^+ fungal transformants had grown. Several independent transformants were isolated and re-isolated on AMM agar plates. The transformants that had undergone homologous recombination at the expected locus were confirmed by PCR. A sample of conidia scrapped with a cotton swab from a colony of each isolated was inoculated into 1 mL of AMM and incubated overnight at 37 °C to obtain minipreps of genomic DNA suitable for PCR analysis.

2.12. Detection of SOD Activity on PAGE Gels

After 20 h of incubation of a wild-type strain in liquid SDN–Zn medium, mycelium was harvested through filtration, washed with cold sterile water and snap-frozen on liquid N_2. Mycelium was ground in a mortar with a pestle in presence of liquid N_2 until it became a fine dust, suspended into 0.4 mL of native protein extraction buffer (36 mM KH_2PO_4/K_2HPO_4 [pH 7.8]; 1 mM EDTA; 0.1% Triton X-100; 5% [*v*/*v*] glycerol; 0.5% [*v*/*v*] Protease inhibitor cocktail-EDTA [Thermo Scientific, cat. 87785]) and clarified by centrifugation at 14,000 × *g* for 10 min at 4 °C. Proteins were separated by native PAGE (T = 8%) at 120 V at 4 °C and gels were washed twice with distilled water (10 min each). Gels were incubated for 20 min in 50 mL of an Nitro Blue Tetrazolium Chloride (NBT) solution (2.45 mM [N6876, Sigma-Aldrich, St. Louis, MO, USA] in 36 mM KH_2PO_4/K_2HPO_4 [pH 7.8]), transferred to the developing solution (28 μM riboflavin, 28 mM TEMED in 36 mM KH_2PO_4/K_2HPO_4 [pH 7.8]) and illuminated with white light until transparent bands were readily observed in a dark-blue background due to formazan generated after reduction of NBT with O_2^- formed by reduction of riboflavin in the presence of O_2.

3. Results

3.1. Under Zinc-Limiting Conditions ZafA Influences the Expression of Genes Related to Many Different Metabolic and Biosynthetic Processes in Addition to Those Required to Maintain Zinc Homeostasis

When *A. fumigatus* grows under zinc-limiting conditions, a significant change in the transcription level of the most direct ZafA-target genes is expected. In addition, other genes not targeted by ZafA may also change their expression levels as a side effect of the adaptation to the zinc-limiting conditions triggered by ZafA. To identify all the putative ZafA-target genes we designed an experimental approach based in the following theoretical assumptions: (i) Some genes that changed their expression level in a wild-type strain under zinc-limiting conditions would be regulated either directly or indirectly by ZafA, whereas other genes would change their expression level in response to zinc starvation in a ZafA-independent manner. We referred to the former genes as putative directly and indirectly ZafA-regulated (DZR and IZR) genes, whereas the later ones were referred to as non-ZafA-regulated (NZR) genes; (ii) The NZR genes could be either up-regulated or down-regulated both in the wild-type strain and Δ*zafA* mutant grown under zinc-limiting with respect to zinc-replete conditions; (iii) The expression level of the DZR genes in a Δ*zafA* strain should be similar under both zinc-limiting and zinc-replete conditions; (iv) The intrinsic lack of the appropriate homeostatic and adaptive responses to zinc starvation in the Δ*zafA* strain would result in a strain-specific adaptive response to relieve the lack of *zafA* in this mutant that might involve changes in the expression level of many genes that in a wild-type strain would not change under zinc starvation, and that we referred to as strain-specific adaptive (SSA) genes.

Therefore, by keeping these assumptions in mind we performed two independent microarray experiments (Exp#1 and Exp#2) (Figure 2). Exp#1 was aimed to determine genes expressed differentially in a wild-type strain grown under zinc-limiting conditions versus zinc-replete conditions (Results in Table S3). Exp#2 was aimed to determine the genes expressed differentially in a Δ*zafA* strain with respect to a wild-type strain, both grown under zinc-limiting conditions (Table S4). Upon comparing the differentially regulated genes detected in Exp#1 and Exp#2, 112 putative IZR genes (19 up-regulated and 93 down-regulated in both the wild-type strain and Δ*zafA* mutant) and 153 putative DZR genes were identified (Figure 2). More specifically, 118 DZR genes that were up-regulated in the wild-type strain according to Exp#1 emerged as down-regulated in the Δ*zafA* strain according to Exp#2, whereas 35 DZR genes that were down-regulated in the wild-type strain according to Exp#1 emerged as up-regulated in the Δ*zafA* strain according to Exp#2 (Table S5). It would be expected that the direct targets of ZafA were included among the DZR genes. It would be expected that the genes targeted indirectly by ZafA were included among the IZR genes.

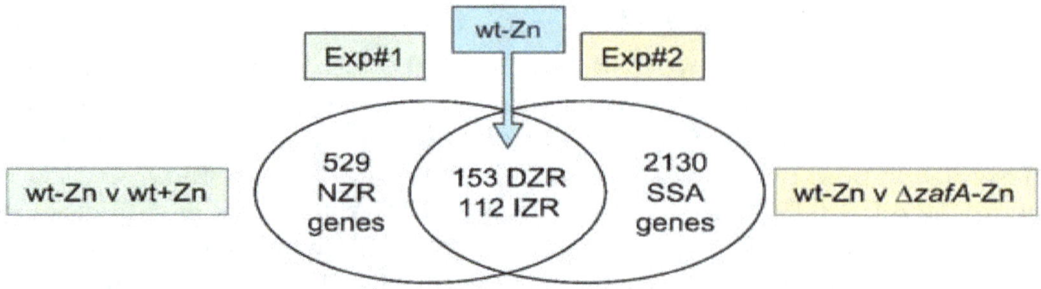

Exp#1	Subgroup of genes			Total number
	NZR	DZR	IZR	
Up-regulated	145	118	19	282
Down-regulated	384	35	93	512
Subtotal	529	153	112	794

Exp#2	Subgroup of genes			Total number
	SSA	DZR	IZR	
Up-regulated	1287	35	19	1424
Down-regulated	843	118	93	971
Subtotal	2130	153	112	2395

Figure 2. Quantitative summary of different types of genes detected in microarray experiments. SSA: strain-specific adapted (genes); DZR: directly ZafA regulated; IZR: indirectly ZafA regulated ; NZR: non-ZafA regulated.

To validate the microarray analysis, we measured by RT-qPCR the relative expression ratio of 56 genes whose expression changed significantly in a wild-type strain grown under zinc-limiting versus zinc-replete conditions. More precisely, we measured the relative expression of 10 IZR, 22 NZR and 24 DZR genes (Table 2). The expression levels of the *zafA*, *zrfA*, *zrfB* and *zrfC* genes, whose expression profiles had been well defined previously [11,12,14], were measured as positive controls. The expression of the actin gene (AFUA_6G04740/*actA*), whose expression did not change significantly under zinc starvation neither in a wild-type nor in a Δ*zafA* mutant [11,14], was measured as a negative control. In addition, the expression levels of six additional genes selected at random, whose expression did not change also under zinc starvation neither in a wild-type nor in a Δ*zafA* mutant, were also measured as negative controls (Table 2). The results obtained by both techniques were coincident and the correlation between microarray data and those measured by RT-qPCR were highly significant (Pearson's $r = 0.69$, $P < 0.0001$) in spite of the high difference in sensitivity and accuracy between these experimental procedures.

Table 2. Measurement by RT-qPCR of the expression levels of several genes of each group detected in microarrays, both in a wild-type strain grown in zinc-limiting versus zinc-replete conditions (as in Exp#1) and in a Δ*zafA* strain grown under zinc-limiting conditions with respect to a wild-type strain grown in the same culture conditions (i.e., as in Exp#2). ZafA can be formally considered as an inductor or repressor of the DZR genes, as indicated. The indicated genes (*) should be reallocated into the specified group according to RT-qPCR data, provided that the genes were considered (arbitrarily) to be expressed differentially when their transcription levels changed > 1.5-fold. Expression of genes in **red** and **blue** show induction or repression respectively.

Gene ID	Group of Genes	Gene Name	wt − Zn/wt + Zn rER ± SD	Δ*zafA* − Zn/wt − Zn rER ± SD	Predicted Effect of ZafA on Gene Expression	Reallocating Subgroup of Genes *
AFUA_1G01550	DZR	*zrfA*	231.3 ± 27.8	−207.7 ± 18.9	Induction	
AFUA_1G02150	Control	*gfdA*	−1.25 ± 0.15	1.17 ± 0.11		
AFUA_1G03150	DZR	*erg24A*	−49.9 ± 7.0	2.0 ± 0.2	Repression	
AFUA_1G04620	IZR	-	−4.9 ± 0.4	−1.9 ± 0.2		
AFUA_1G07480	NZR	*hem13*	−6.0 ± 0.8	−1.6 ± 0.1		IZR
AFUA_1G10060	NZR	-	3.1 ± 0.2	−1.2 ± 0.1		

Table 2. *Cont.*

Gene ID	Group of Genes	Gene Name	wt − Zn/wt + Zn rER ± SD	Δ*zafA* − Zn/wt − Zn rER ± SD	Predicted Effect of ZafA on Gene Expression	Reallocating Subgroup of Genes *
AFUA_1G10080	DZR	*zafA*	31.5 ± 3.0	−21582 ± 4316	Induction	
AFUA_1G10130	NZR	*sahA*	1.9 ± 0.1	1.1 ± 0.1		
AFUA_1G12830	IZR	*niaD*	−1.6 ± 0.1	−5.2 ± 0.7		
AFUA_1G13510	NZR	*facB*	4.6 ± 0.6	1.0 ± 0.1		
AFUA_1G14550	DZR	*sodC/sod3*	1698.7 ± 198.2	−1176.5 ± 142.4	Induction	
AFUA_1G15590	NZR	*cybS/sdh4*	2.9 ± 0.4	1.1 ± 0.1		
AFUA_1G17190	NZR	*sidI*	−92.5 ± 8.7	1.1 ± 0.1		
AFUA_2G00320	NZR	*erg3B*	−271.7 ± 31.7	−1.6 ± 0.2		IZR
AFUA_2G01260	DZR	*srbA*	−15.8 ± 2.1	2.1 ± 0.2	Repression	
AFUA_2G03010	NZR	-	−1.7 ± 0.2	−1.0 ± 0.1		
AFUA_2G03700	NZR	*hmg1*	−2.6 ± 0.2	−1.1 ± 0.1		
AFUA_2G03860	DZR	*zrfB*	33.0 ± 2.7	−79.3 ± 7.7	Induction	
AFUA_2G07680	IZR	*sidA*	−27.3 ± 3.3	−6.9 ± 0.6		
AFUA_2G08740	DZR	*zrfF*	24.8 ± 1.8	−16.0 ± 2.0	Induction	
AFUA_2G11120	DZR	*gtmA*	5.7 ± 0.7	−20.3 ± 1.8	Induction	
AFUA_2G14570	NZR	*zrcC*	−2.1 ± 0.2	−1.1 ± 0.1		
AFUA_2G15010	NZR	-	−1.5 ± 0.2	−1.2 ± 0.1		
AFUA_2G15290	DZR	-	−26.0 ± 3.6	3.2 ± 0.3	Repression	
AFUA_2G17550	IZR	*ayg1*	−2.7 ± 0.4	−103.5 ± 10.8		
AFUA_3G02270	DZR	*cat1*	18.9 ± 1.8	−2.0± 0.2	Induction	
AFUA_3G03640	IZR	*mirB*	−3225.8 ± 304.5	−10.0 ± 1.2		
AFUA_3G14440	NZR	-	−3.5 ± 0.5	−1.3 ± 0.1		
AFUA_4G03410	NZR	*fhpA*	−3.1 ± 0.3	−1.4 ± 0.2		
AFUA_4G03460	IZR	*srbB*	−50.4 ± 5.9	−1.1 ± 0.1		NZR
AFUA_4G03930	DZR	*cysX*	12786.9 ± 1492.2	−7751.9 ± 938.0	Induction	
AFUA_4G06530	NZR	*metR*	−1.6 ± 0.2	1.2 ± 0.1		
AFUA_4G09560	DZR	*zrfC*	1270.1 ± 108.0	−5377.1 ± 424.8	Induction	
AFUA_4G10730	Control	*rvb1*	1.1 ± 0.2	−1.2 ± 0.1		
AFUA_4G12840	IZR	-	−1.6 ± 0.2	−1.7 ± 0.1		
AFUA_5G01030	DZR	*gpdB*	−1.2 ± 0.1	77.7 ± 7.5		SSA
AFUA_5G01970	NZR	*gpdA*	1.8 ± 0.2	1.0 ± 0.1		
AFUA_5G02180	NZR	*cysB*	−2.6 ± 0.2	1.1 ± 0.1		
AFUA_5G03800	NZR	*ftrA*	−31.0 ± 2.2	1.4 ± 0.2		
AFUA_5G03920	NZR	*hapX*	−12.2 ± 1.5	−1.2 ± 0.1		
AFUA_5G04130	Control	*phoA*	1.1 ± 0.1	−1.3 ± 0.2		
AFUA_5G06240	DZR	*alcC*	−26.8 ± 1.9	3.8 ± 0.5	Repression	
AFUA_5G06270	NZR	*hemA*	1.8 ± 0.2	−1.0 ± 0.1		
AFUA_5G08090	DZR	*pyroA*	2.7 ± 0.3	−1.8 ± 0.2	Induction	
AFUA_5G09240	DZR	*sodA/sod1*	−4.7 ± 0.7	7.3 ± 0.8	Repression	
AFUA_5G09360	Control	*calA*	1.1 ± 0.1	1.1 ± 0.1		
AFUA_5G09680	NZR	*carC/sdh3*	3.9 ± 0.4	−1.0 ± 0.1		
AFUA_5G10560	Control	*cox5A*	−1.2 ± 0.2	1.0 ± 0.1		
AFUA_6G00690	DZR	-	−2.8 ± 0.3	5.2 ± 0.6	Repression	
AFUA_6G04430	NZR	-	2.0 ± 0.2	1.3 ± 0.2		
AFUA_6G04740	Control	*actA*	−1.0 ± 0.1	1.2 ± 0.1		
AFUA_6G05160	DZR	*azf1*	1.9 ± 0.2	−23.9 ± 2.9	Induction	
AFUA_6G07720	IZR	*acuF*	−2.2 ± 0.2	−1.7 ± 0.2		
AFUA_6G09630	DZR	*gliZ*	45.9 ± 6.0	−67.2 ± 5.3	Induction	
AFUA_6G09710	DZR	*gliA*	3548.5 ± 87.4	−3039.5 ± 294.8	Induction	
AFUA_6G09740	DZR	*gliT*	53.6 ± 3.9	−477.3 ± 59.7	Induction	
AFUA_7G00250	IZR	*tubB2*	−7.0 ± 0.5	−10.0 ± 1.2		
AFUA_7G02560	Control	*dld1*	−1.1 ± 0.1	1.0 ± 0.1		
AFUA_7G04730	IZR	*enb1*	−48.3 ± 5.8	−2.4 ± 0.2		
AFUA_7G05070	NZR	*frdA*	−56.5 ± 7.4	1.9 ± 0.1	Repression	DZR
AFUA_7G06570	DZR	*zrcA*	−5.9 ± 0.7	16.6 ± 1.5	Repression	
AFUA_7G06790	DZR	*yct1*	6039.9 ± 362.4	−5555.6 ± 577.8	Induction	
AFUA_8G02450	DZR	*gzbA*	84.8 ± 8.0	−275.5 ± 32.2	Induction	
AFUA_8G02620	DZR	*mchC*	1155.6 ± 134.9	−524.3 ± 63.4	Induction	

SSA: strain-specific adapted (genes); DZR: directly ZafA regulated; IZR: indirectly ZafA regulated ; NZR: non-ZafA regulated.

3.2. Zinc Starvation Influences the Expression of Genes Related to Many Different Biological Processes

A functional categorization of the 512 down-regulated and 282 up-regulated genes in a wild-type strain grown under zinc-limiting conditions was performed on the *Aspergillus fumigatus* AF293 (AspGD) genome using the gene ontology (GO) tool integrated in FungiFun2, which is an updated and easy-to-use online resource for functional enrichment analysis of fungal genes [26]. The functional categorization of the down-regulated genes revealed that 26.0% of the input genes were significantly categorized (i.e., 133/512). These genes were related to ergosterol biosynthesis ($p = 1.32 \times 10^{-9}$), cellular response to iron starvation ($p = 1.49 \times 10^{-9}$), fatty acid biosynthesis ($p = 3.65 \times 10^{-5}$), α(1,3)-glucan biosynthesis ($p = 0.00013$), calcium transport ($p = 0.00013$) and cellular response to hypoxia ($p = 0.0005$). The functional categorization of the up-regulated genes revealed that 18.8% of the genes were significantly categorized (i.e., 53/282). These genes were related to ascospore formation ($p = 1.74 \times 10^{-5}$), asexual development (conidia formation) ($p = 2.08 \times 10^{-4}$), mitochondrial respiratory chain complex I ($p = 8.5 \times 10^{-5}$), zinc transport ($p = 8.5 \times 10^{-5}$), cellular hyperosmotic response ($p = 0.00021$), and G1 cell cycle arrest in response to nitrogen starvation ($p = 0.00078$). Hence, by using FungiFun2 the functional categorization of 186 genes could be described. In a more careful manual revision we were able to functionally allocate 291 genes into 28 different biological processes and outline the major homeostatic and adaptive responses displayed by the fungus to deal with zinc starvation (Table S6) (see discussion). 247 genes encoded uncharacterized proteins that either were similar to characterized proteins in other organisms or harbored at least one catalytic domain with a predicted function, regardless of its putative subcellular location. Finally, there were also 256 genes that encoded either uncharacterized protein orthologues in other organisms or hypothetical proteins.

Thus, it became apparent that many genes were down regulated under zinc-limiting conditions, mainly those whose expression was induced under iron starvation or influenced by the intracellular calcium levels, those required for fatty acid and phospholipid biosynthesis, and those encoding enzymes involved in ergosterol biosynthesis and whose expression was also strongly co-regulated by iron and hypoxia. Other down-regulated genes encoded proteins related to ethanol metabolism, disulfide bond formation in the endoplasmatic reticulum (ER), enzymes of the citric acid cycle and glycolytic pathway, and components of the mitochondrial electron transport chain (ETC) (Table S6). On the other hand, it was overwhelming the predominance, under zinc-limiting conditions, of up-regulated genes involved in sexual and asexual development, hyphal growth and autophagy, ribosomal assembly and/or translation, response to hyperosmotic stress and regulating and maintaining zinc homeostasis (Table S6). Zinc starvation also influenced, either positively or negatively, the expression of genes that were typically regulated in response to hypoxia and oxidative stress. In addition, the expression of genes involved in biosynthesis of the cell wall, growth factors (riboflavin, thiamine and pyridoxin), heme group, detoxification of D-2-hydroxyglutarate coupled to D-lactate formation, acetate utilization, cytoskeleton and chromatin remodeling and regulation of the cell cycle were also influenced by zinc starvation. Finally, zinc starvation also noticeably influenced the expression levels of genes involved in NAD, sulfur, spermidine and nitrogen metabolism, and others involved in biosynthesis of some secondary metabolites (Table S6). In this regard, it was remarkable that the expression of genes related to gliotoxin biosynthesis was strongly induced under zinc-limiting conditions.

The analysis of the distribution of the 291 genes, categorized functionally based on the most likely role of ZafA in regulating their expression, as defined by their assignation to either the DZR/IZR or NZR group of genes (Table S6), indicated that ZafA influenced either directly or indirectly the expression of $\geq$60% of the genes involved in the homeostatic response to zinc starvation, fungal development, response to oxidative stress, nitrate assimilation, acetate utilization and in the functioning of the tricarboxylic acid cycle and mitochondrial electron transport chain.

3.3. The ZafA *Transcription Factor Binds to Promoter Regions of Homeostatic Genes Whose Transcription Is Induced under Zinc-Limiting Conditions*

We assumed that the DZR genes should be the ones most directly targeted by ZafA, such that in their promoter regions there would be at least a copy of a zinc responsive (ZR) consensus sequence to which ZafA might bind. Hence, we used the MEME algorithm as a first approach to identify potential regulatory elements and/or repeated patterns shared among the promoters of 67 genes that could be the most direct ZafA target genes [27]. These genes were chosen on the basis of their fold changes in Exp#1, such that the 54 genes more up-regulated and the 13 genes more down-regulated were selected (Table S5). Thus, we found two motifs (M1 and M2) that were found significantly distributed among the analyzed promoters (E-value for M1 = 3.6×10^{-37}; E-value for M2 = 1.7×10^{-17}) (Figure 3). The M1 motif showed two short CT-rich sequences flanking the 5′-CAAGGT-3′ core sequence and was present in a number of 1 to 5 copies in the promoter regions of 28 genes (i.e., 42.4% of the analyzed genes). The M2 motif corresponded to a relatively homogeneous long AG rich sequence and was present in a number of 1 to 6 copies in the promoters of 36 genes (i.e., 54.5% of the analyzed genes). However, a control MEME search for repeated patterns in the promoter regions of 71 genes (38 SSA genes plus 33 genes whose expression was not influenced by zinc starvation that were selected at random) (Table S7), also produced a M2-like AG-rich motif in 52.1% of the genes (E-value for the M2-like motif = 3.9×10^{-59}). Besides, the M2 motif was not detected in the promoter region of the genes *zrfA* and *zrfC*, whose transcription had been shown to be strongly and directly up-regulated by ZafA under zinc-limiting conditions [11,14]. In contrast, the M1 motif was found in a number of 3 to 5 copies in the promoter regions of the *zafA*, *zrfA*, *zrfB*, *zrfC* and *zrfF* genes, that encoded the major components of the zinc homeostatic system in *A. fumigatus*. Moreover, by using the RSAT algorithm [28], we found that one motif nearly identical to M1 was widely distributed among promoters of all DZR genes, whereas no motif detected among IZR genes showed any similarity with M1. Taken together, these findings suggested that the M1 motif could be a genuine DNA regulatory sequence for binding ZafA.

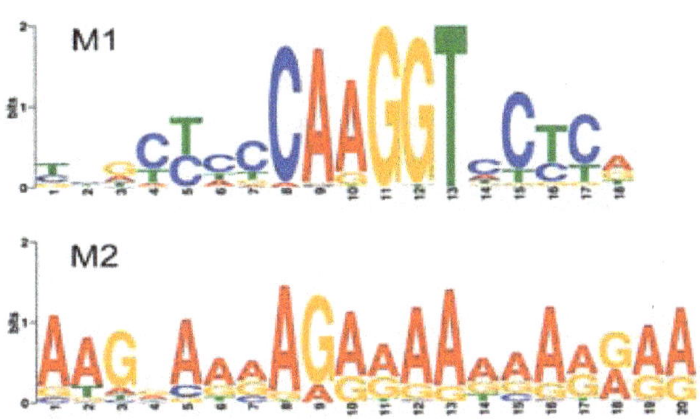

Figure 3. Overrepresented motifs in the promoter regions of the most DZR genes. These motifs were found using the MEME algorithm after analyzing DNA sequences expanding from −20 to −1000 bp from the predicted translation start codons of the ORFs of 67 DZR genes (for numbering purposes, we assigned position −1 to the nucleotide preceding the A of the ATG start codon).

To show whether ZafA was able to bind to the promoter regions of the homeostatic genes *zafA*, *zrfA*, *zrfB* and *zrfC*, we analyzed by EMSA the ability of ZafA to bind to short DNA fragments (210–260 bp) of these promoters harboring the previously identified M1 motif. All attempts to express the full-length ZafA protein in *E. coli* were unsuccessful. However, we had success in expressing a recombinant polypeptide corresponding to the C-terminal 140 amino acids of ZafA (residues 434–570 that included the four most C-terminal zinc fingers ZF3-6) fused to the C-terminus of GST. By using this polypeptide we confirmed the binding and observed that the mobility of all DNA-protein complexes in PAGE gels reduced stepwise as the ZafA:DNA ratio increased, which indicated that ZafA$^{ZF3\text{-}6}$ was able to bind, with different affinities, to more than one ZafA binding site in all DNA fragment tested

(Figure 4). Particularly, three steps were observed for the P*zrfA* DNA fragment (Figure 4A) and two for the P*zrfB*, P*zrfC* and P*zafA* DNA fragments (Figure 4B and left panels of C and D), which matched the number of M1-like motifs found in these promoters. Besides, given that at a ZafA:DNA molar ratio of 6.0 both the P*zrfC* and P*zafA* fragments were almost completely shifted (Figure 4C,D, left panels), we performed EMSAs assays at lower ZafA:DNA ratios (between 0.4 and 4.0, right panels). As shown, in both cases, a ZafA:DNA ratio of four was sufficient to shift most of the DNA. This suggested that in both fragments P*zafA* and P*zrfC* there were two ZR motifs to which two ZafA molecules would bind with similar affinities but stronger than those used to bind to the ZR motifs in the P*zrfA* and P*zrfB* fragments.

3.4. *The* ZafA *Transcription Factor Binds Specifically to a 15-bp Zinc-Response Consensus Sequence*

To identify the DNA sequence to which ZafA binds, we performed a fluorescent DNase I footprinting analysis by using fluorescently 6-FAM-labeled primers in parallel to dideoxynucleotide DNA sequencing. This procedure allows the accurate separation of 5′-end-labeled DNA fragments using a capillary-based automated DNA sequencer and to identify the nucleotide sequence of sites protected against DNase digestion [29]. To identify the DNA binding site for ZafA we used several 6-FAM-5′-labelled DNA probes carrying short fragments of the promoter regions from the homeostatic genes *zrfA*, *zrfB*, *zrfC* and *zafA* (see material and methods section) that harbored 1–2 copies of the M1 motif detected previously by MEME analyses. Thus, in the P*zafA* fragments used as probes, four different regions protected by ZafA from its enzymatic digestion with DNase I were found, that were called ZRR1-4 (for Zinc-Response motif located in the promoter region of gene encoding the Regulatory protein ZafA) (Figure 5 and Figure S2). Similarly, in the P*zrfA* and P*zrfC* fragments used as probes, three different ZafA-protected regions in each one were found, that were called ZRA1-3 and ZRC1-3 (for Zinc-Response motif located respectively in the promoter region of *zrfA* and *zrfC*). Besides, in the P*zrfB* fragments, two different ZafA-protected regions were found, that were called ZRB1-2 (for Zinc-Response motif located in the promoter region of *zrfB*) (Figure 5 and Figure S2). It is interesting to recall that in nearly all cases, highly hypersensitive regions to DNase I digestion were observed, that contrasted clearly with the adjacent ZafA-protected regions (Figure S2). The comparison of all ZafA-protected regions brought the ZR consensus sequence 5′-DYYVYCARGGTVYYY-3′ (D = A or G or T; V = A or G or C; R = A or G) (Figure 5), which strongly resembled the M1 motif detected after MEME analysis (Figure 3).

3.5. *The Highly Conserved 5′-CARGGT-3′ Core of the ZR Motif Is Essential for ZafA Binding*

The ZR consensus motif showed a highly conserved 5′-CARGGT-3′ hexanucleotide core that could be essential for ZafA to recognize and bind specifically to it, such that the replacement of a purine by a pyrimidine, or vice-versa, could reduce or impair the binding of ZafA. We thought that this hexanucleotide sequence, rather than the short CT-rich flanking sequences, was required for the specific binding of ZafA. To confirm this, we searched in the *Aspergillus* genome database for a DNA fragment corresponding to the promoter region of any gene with a relatively high number of short CT-rich sequences ($\geq$3 bp) and that contained just one ZR consensus motif, to be used as probe for both EMSA and DNase I footprinting assays. Thus, we selected a 191-bp DNA fragment, the *alcA* gene promoter from *A. nidulans* that met our requirements to be used as a probe. We confirmed by a DNase I footprinting assay that ZafA only protected a region of this DNA fragment that contained the ZR consensus motif (Figure 6A). To ascertain whether the 5′-CARGGT-3′ sequence was essential for ZafA binding, we created a mutated version of this probe in which its 5′-CAAGGT-3′ core had been changed to 5′-CTCAGT-3′. The binding of ZafA to the wild-type P*alcA* probe at ZafA:DNA ratios lower than 6.0 resulted in a retarded DNA:protein complex as shown by EMSA (Figure 6B). In contrast, ZafA did not bind to the P*alcA* probe in which the ZR motif had been mutated. These results showed that ZafA was able to bind to the ZR motif and that the 5′-CARGGT-3′ hexanucleotide core sequence was essential for ZafA to recognize such motif.

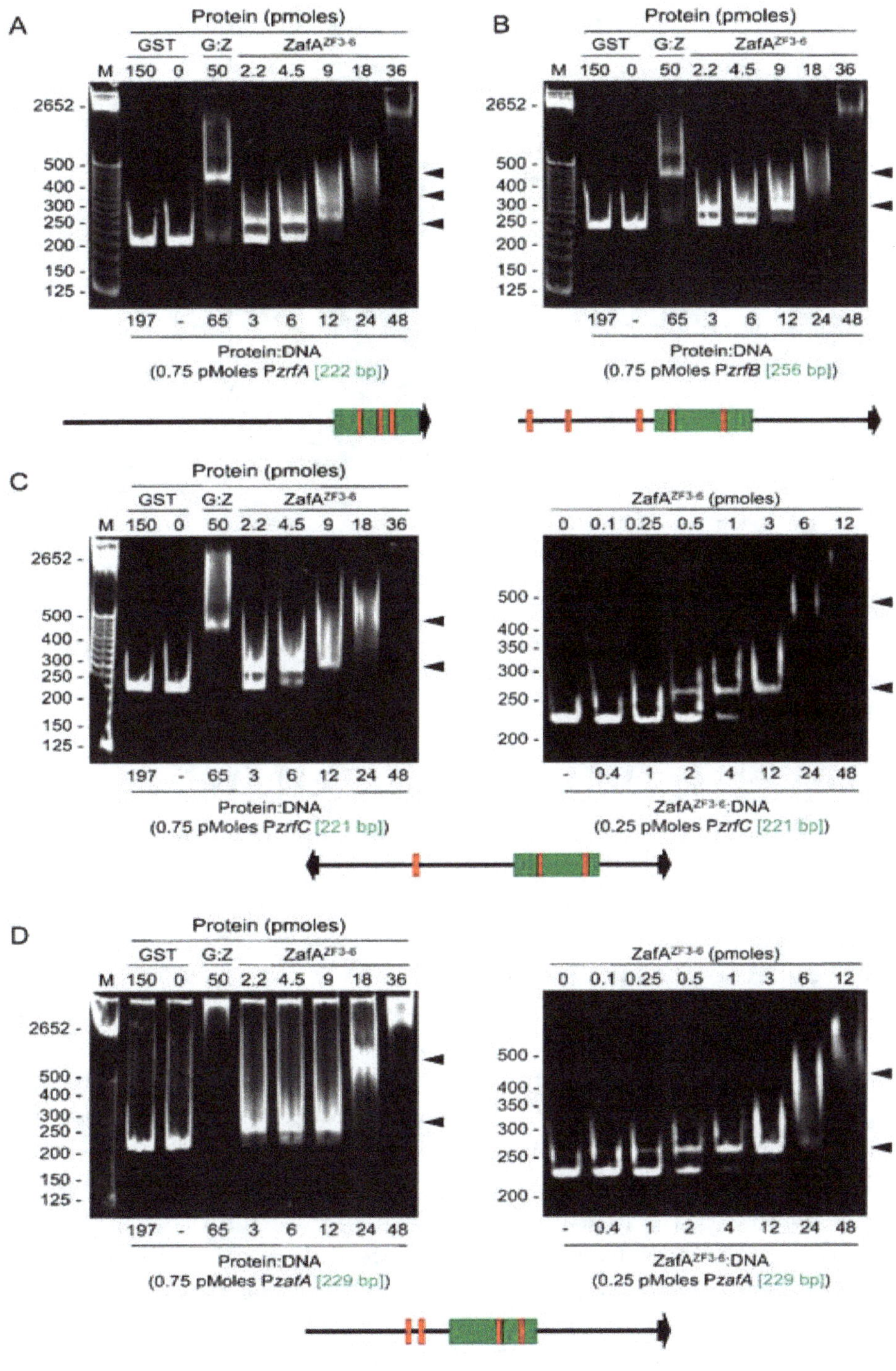

Figure 4. Analyses by Electrophoretic Mobility Shift Assays (EMSA) of the interaction of ZafA^{ZF3-6} with different DNA fragments. (**A**) Interaction of ZafA^{ZF3-6} with a DNA fragment from a promoter region of *zrfA* (green box) that carried three putative ZafA binding motifs (red boxes); (**B**) interaction of ZafA^{ZF3-6} with a DNA fragment from a promoter region of *zrfB* (green box) that carried two putative ZafA binding motifs (red boxes); (**C**) interaction of ZafA^{ZF3-6} with a DNA fragment from a promoter region of *zrfC* (green box) that carried two putative ZafA binding motifs (red boxes); (**D**) interaction of ZafA^{ZF3-6} with a DNA fragment from a promoter region of *zafA* (green box) that carried two putative ZafA binding motifs (red boxes). In the right panel of (C) and (D), reactions were analyzed with lower ZafA^{ZF3-6}:DNA ratios to gain resolution. All DNA fragments were also incubated without protein and in the presence of both 150 pmoles of purified GST and 50 pmoles of the fusion protein GST-ZafA^{ZF3-6} (as controls) to attain a GST:DNA ratio of 197 and a GST-ZafA^{ZF3-6}:DNA (G:Z) ratio 65. A 25-bp DNA ladder was used as a reference.

ZRA1	-82	tcagtgCGACCTCAAGGTACCCAGCATgccagcgc	-48
ZRA2′	-84	tcagtctACTGCCAAGGTCCTTCGCCTGGtcggtg	-118
ZRA3	-159	agaggTAGCTCACAAGGTGTgtctactctcgacca	-130
ZRB1	-372	aatcacGATCCTCAAGGTCCCTACAGGATTCactt	-338
ZRB2′	-503	tTGCCTTGCCACCAAGGTCCTCAATTGCGgattca	-469
ZRC1′	-175	CACACTAACTCCCAAGGTATCTGCGGCCaagagca	-209
ZRC2′	-292	gcttgttGCTCTCAAGGTCCTCGATCCAAGactct	-326
ZRC3′	-616	cttgatCGCTACCAAGGTGTCCTTGGCAtcctgta	-650
ZRR1	-368	gtGGGAAGCTCCCAAGGTCCTCTTGgatttgcaca	-334
ZRR2	-428	gcccctttCCCTCAAGTTGCtcgcacagatctgga	-394
ZRR3	-631	ggtgcTTGCTCGCAGGGTCCTCACTCTCCTTCTTG	-597
ZRR4	-664	cgcttTTTCCCCCAGGGTCCTCATTAAAgaatagg	-630
Consensus		-------DYYVYCARGGTVYYY-------------	

Figure 5. Alignment of DNA sequences protected against DNase I digestion from the DNA fragments used for EMSA analyses. Protected sequences are in capital letters whereas the surrounding sequences are indicated in gray lower case letters (D = A or G or T; V = A or G or C; R = A or G). ZR motifs labelled with a prime symbol indicate that the DNA sequence shown in the picture corresponded to that in the antiparallel strand.

3.6. ZafA *Induces Gene Expression in vivo through Binding to the ZR Motifs*

Although mutations within the 5′-CARGGT-3′ hexanucleotide core prevented the binding of the recombinant ZafA$^{ZF3\text{-}6}$ protein to the ZR motifs in vitro, it could be possible that in vivo the wild-type ZafA protein binds to a DNA sequence different from the ZR motif determined in vitro. Hence, to ascertain whether ZafA truly bound to the ZR motifs in the fungus growing in zinc-limiting media, we analyzed in vivo the effect of the inactivation of the three ZR motifs (ZR1, ZR2 and ZR3) present in the divergent promoter that drives the transcription of both *aspf2* and *zrfC* (P*zrfC*) on the transcription of these genes [11]. To test this, we introduced, at the *pyrG* locus of a uridine-uracil-auxotrophic strain (CEA17), the coding sequences of both the luciferase (*luc*) and green fluorescent protein (*gfp*) arranged divergently and separated by a P*zrfC* mutant version (P*zrfC*^{ZR123}) whose three ZR motifs had been inactivated by replacing each 5′-CAAGGT-3′ hexanucleotide core by the mutated 5′-ACATGT-3′ sequence (Figure S1). It must be noted that, in this construction, the ORF of *aspf2* and *zrfC* had been replaced respectively by that of *luc* and *gfp*. Hence, this construction was devised in such a way that the transcription level of *luc* and *gfp* would indicate the functionality of the mutant promoter (P*zrfC*^{ZR123}) in a wild-type genetic background, while the expression levels of the endogenous *aspf2* and *zrfC* genes could be used as internal controls of the transcriptional promoter activity of P*zrfC*^{wt}. We expected that if these ZR motifs were truly recognized by ZafA in vivo, the mutation of their conserved hexanucleotide cores should prevent the binding of ZafA to P*zrfC*^{ZR} and the expression of both *luc* and *gfp*. As shown, the transcription of both reporter genes driven by P*zrfC*^{ZR123} in the AFZR1 strain grown under zinc-limiting conditions collapsed as if the fungus was growing in zinc-replete conditions (Figure 7). More precisely, the relative expression ratio (rER) of the *luc* and *gfp* transcripts in AFZR1 was reduced respectively by 523- and 611-fold as measured by RT-qPCR, whereas the relative expression ratios (rERs) of *asfp2* and *zrfC*, which were used as endogenous controls, were identical to that in the control AFZR0 strain that carried the P*zrfC*^{wt}. These results undoubtedly showed that ZafA has to bind to the ZR motifs in vivo to induce gene expression under physiological conditions of zinc starvation.

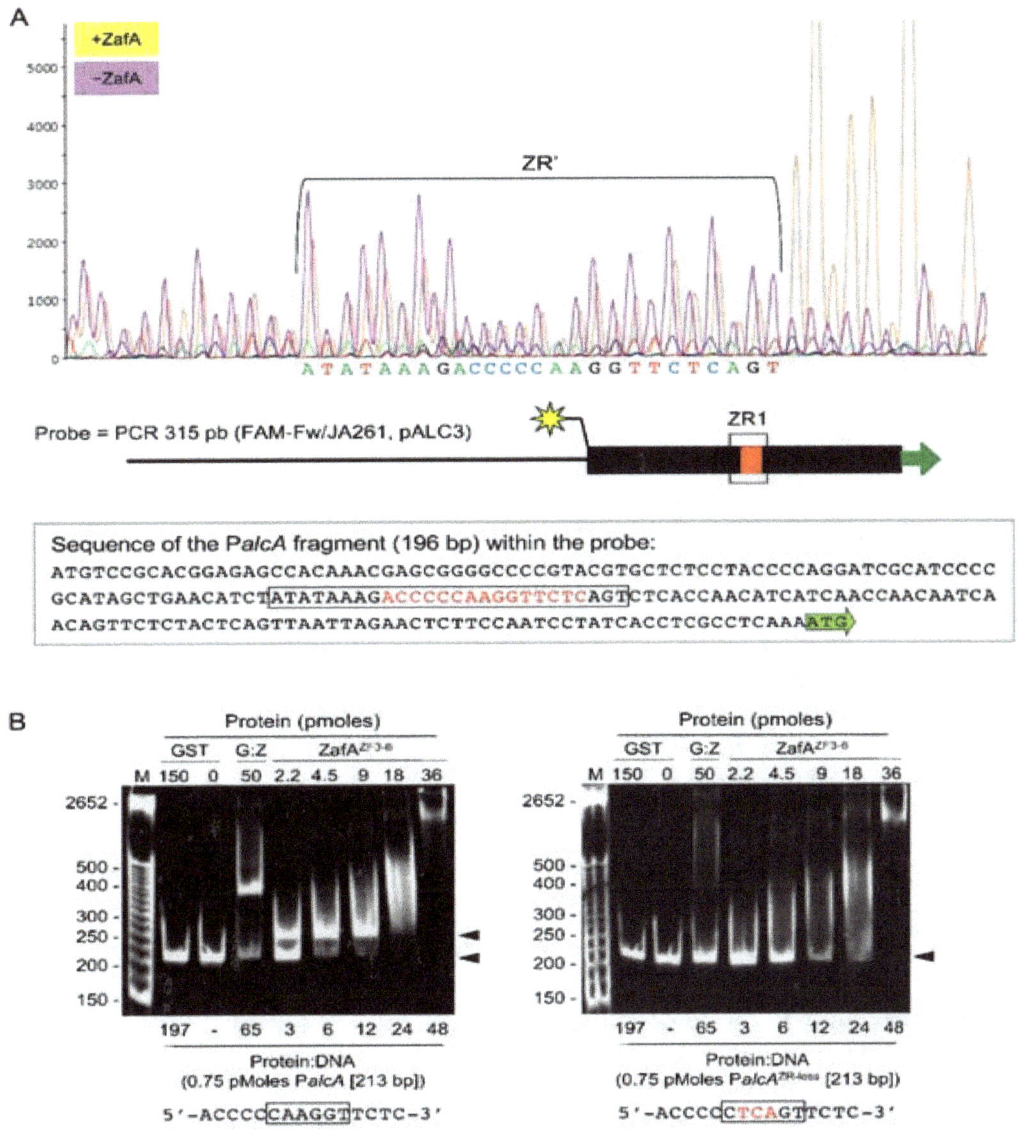

Figure 6. Effect of mutations in the conserved hexanucleotide core of the ZR consensus motif on ZafA binding in vitro. (**A**) Binding of ZafA$^{ZF3\text{-}6}$ to a DNA fragment carrying a single ZR consensus motif in a CT-rich context as shown by a DNase I protection assay. The purple chromatogram was obtained upon incubating the DNA fragment in the absence of ZafA$^{ZF3\text{-}6}$, such that the DNA remained naked and, hence, unprotected from DNase I digestion. The yellow chromatogram was obtained upon incubating the DNA in the presence of ZafA$^{ZF3\text{-}6}$. ZafA bound to DNA prevented its digestion with DNase I resulting in a stretch of yellow peaks lower in high than purple peaks. A short stretch of high yellow peaks at the right side of the chromatogram indicated a hypersensitive region to DNase I digestion. The protected region is delimited by a bracket. Below the chromatogram is shown a schematic representation of the whole intergenic region of the *alcA* gene with the beginning of the ORF located at the right side (green arrow). The sequence of the DNA fragment corresponding to the P*alcA* used in the assay is located in the scheme as a black rectangle with the ZR consensus motif in red. The protected region has been squared in the scheme and sequence. The yellow star indicates the end 6-FAM labeled strand detected by the capillary-based automated DNA sequencer; (**B**) Analysis by EMSA of binding of ZafA$^{ZF3\text{-}6}$ to a DNA fragment in which the 5′-CAAGGT-3′ hexanucleotide core of its only ZR motif (left panel) had been mutated to 5′-CTCAGT-3′ (right panel). The DNA fragments were also incubated without protein and in the presence of both 150 pmoles of purified GST and 50 pmoles of the fusion protein GST-ZafA$^{ZF3\text{-}6}$ (as controls) to attain a GST:DNA ratio of 197 and a GST-ZafA$^{ZF3\text{-}6}$:DNA (G:Z) ratio 65. A 25-bp DNA ladder was used as a reference.

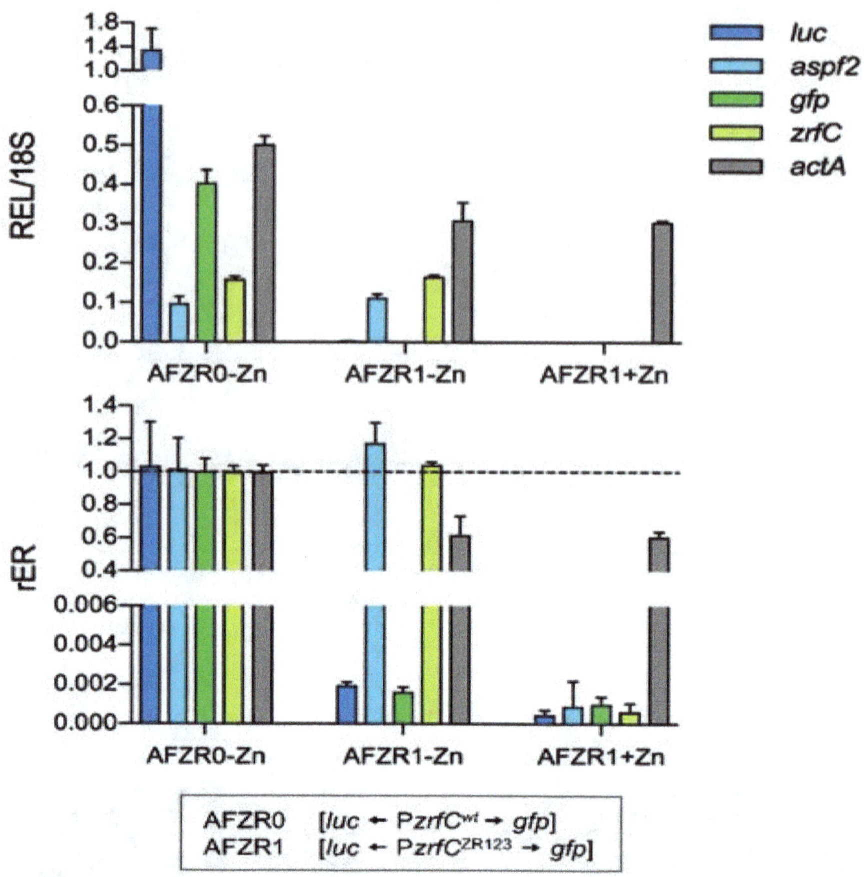

Figure 7. Effect of mutations in the conserved hexanucleotide core of the ZR consensus motif on ZafA binding in vivo. (Upper panel) Relative expression levels (REL) of endogenous *aspf2* and *zrfC* genes and their corresponding reporter genes (*luc* and *gfp*) driven by a wild-type (in the AFZR0 strain) and mutant version (in the AFZR1 strain) or the divergent *aspf2-zrfC* promoter (abbreviated as P*zrfC*). In the mutant version of this promoter the three ZR motifs present in it (P*zrfC*^{ZR123}) had been inactivated by site-directed mutagenesis. Both strains were cultured under zinc-limiting conditions in SDN–Zn for 20 h at 37 °C. The AFZR1 strain was also grown under zinc-replete conditions in SDN + 100 μM Zn to be used as a control of the effect of zinc on the transcriptional activity of ZafA on P*zrfC*^{wt}. (Lower panel) Relative expression ratio (rER) of data represented in the upper panel after their normalization with respect to the expression level in the AFZR0 strain grown under zinc-limiting conditions. The expression level of the actin gene was also measured by RT-qPCR as an additional control. The 18S rRNA was used as an internal reference for all relative quantifications.

3.7. The ZR Motifs Appear to Function as Transcriptional Regulatory Sequences When Located within 1.2 Kb Upstream from the Predicted Translation Start Codon of the ORFs Whose Expression Is Influenced by Zinc

Although the highly conserved 5′-CARGGT-3′ core of the ZR motif was essential for ZafA binding, it exhibited a relatively high degree of variability in the 5′ and 3′-end sequences that flanked the conserved core. This fact could influence the affinity of ZafA binding to the different ZR motifs in the DNA. In addition, it would not be unexpected that ZafA was able to bind also to ZR motifs harboring a certain degree of sequence degeneration. Thus, it could be possible that microarray data under the tested culture conditions had not revealed all ZafA potential targets if the expression of an unknown number of genes were influenced, in addition to zinc starvation, by other environmental signals. Hence, to obtain further evidence on the role of the ZR motif as a regulatory sequence of gene expression under zinc-limiting conditions, we performed a genome-scale search for ZR motifs in the *A. fumigatus* genome by utilizing the RSAT web server [28]. To perform this search, we used as a query pattern the ZR consensus sequence or ZR0 motif, while admitting one substitution out of the conserved hexanucleotide core. Hence, nine additional different degenerated ZR-like motifs (ZR1-9) were possible (Table S8). Since there is one gene every 2938 bp in the genome of *A. fumigatus* and the mean gene length is 1431 bp [30], it can be deducted that the average intergenic sequence is 1482 bp. In order to identify most of the genes harboring ZR-like motifs in their promoter regions, the search for them was extended up to −3000 bp upstream of the predicted translation start codon (TSC) of the open reading frames (ORFs) (i.e., about 2× the size of an average intergenic sequence). By enabling and disabling the overlapping with upstream coding sequences we differentiated two sets of ZR motifs: (1) Non-overlapping ZRs, which were located in the intergenic sequences corresponding to the promoter regions of genes regulated presumably by ZafA; and (2) Overlapping ZRs, which were located either within an upstream ORF or in an intergenic sequence that would correspond to the promoter region of an upstream gene.

A detailed analysis of the non-overlapped ZRs at a genome-scale indicated that there were 545 different ZR motifs distributed among 499 different intergenic sequences harboring the promoter regions that drive the expression of 671 different coding sequences (since 51.3% of such coding sequences were arranged as divergent pairs of genes in the genome). About 91.4% of all genes, including both non-divergent and divergent arranged genes, had in their upstream intergenic regions only one ZR motif, 7.4% had 2 ZRs and 1.2% showed ≥3 ZRs. The most abundant ZR motifs in promoter regions were ZR0, ZR7 and ZR9 (103.3 ± 3.2 per ZR motif). The next most abundant ZR motifs in the promoter regions were ZR2, ZR3, ZR5 and ZR8 (83.5 ± 6.9 per ZR motif). The less abundant ZR motifs were ZR1, ZR4 and ZR6 (31.7 ± 6.7 per ZR motif), as would be expected for the ZR motifs with the lowest variability. Upon analyzing the distribution in the intergenic regions of the most abundant ZRs depending on both the type of ZR and their distance to their correspondent ORFs, it was determined that the overall distribution of the most abundant ZR motifs was influenced very significantly by their distance to the TSC of the ORFs (2-way ANOVA, $p < 0.0001$) but not by the type of ZR motif (2-way ANOVA, $p = 0.322$). Similarly, the overall distribution in the intergenic regions of the less abundant ZR motifs (ZR1, ZR4 and ZR6) was also influenced significantly by their distance to the TSC of the ORFs (2-way ANOVA, $p = 0.0021$) but not by the type of ZR motif (2-way ANOVA, $p = 0.36$). Taken together, these findings suggested that the distance of the ZR motifs to the TSC of the ORFs appeared to be an important factor that determined their distribution in the intergenic promoter regions.

We then analyzed the distribution of all ZR motifs (i.e., non-overlapped plus overlapped ZRs) with respect to their distance to the ORFs. The results revealed that, as expected for a random distribution of ZRs along the DNA, the percentage of ZR motifs within each 200 bp DNA fraction, in which was arbitrarily divided the DNA sequences of 3000 bp located upstream the ORFs, maintained constant between 5.8–7.7% (Figure 8A; blue symbols). Accordingly, the cumulative percent of all ZR motifs (i.e., including both non-overlapped and overlapped ZR motifs) increased directly proportional to the distance to the ORFs ($R^2 = 0.999$), as would be expected for a random distribution (Figure 8B; blue symbols). However, when the distribution of both non-overlapped and overlapped ZR motifs were analyzed separately, they showed opposite distribution patterns. Thus, within each 200 bp DNA fraction, the percent of non-overlapped ZR motifs (Figure 8A; black symbols) reduced exponentially ($R^2 = 0.963$) from 15.3% to 2.2%, whereas that of the overlapped ZR motifs (Figure 8A; red symbols) increased exponentially ($R^2 = 0.955$) as their distance to the ORFs increased from 0.3% to 11.0%. Accordingly, the increase of the cumulative percent of non-overlapped ZR motifs reduced gradually with the distance to the ORFs at a rate that was proportional to the amount of the remaining ZR motifs, i.e., according to an exponential one phase decay relationship ($R^2 = 0.999$) (Figure 8B; black symbols), as would be expected if the ZR motifs were required to be located in a relatively close proximity to the ORFs for them to function as regulatory motifs. In contrast, within the analyzed range (i.e., between −1 to −3000 bp upstream of the ORFs) the increase in the cumulative percent of the overlapped ZR motifs increased with the distance to the ORFs according to a third order polynomial relationship ($R^2 = 0.999$) (Figure 8B; red symbols). Interestingly, the graphical representation of this function showed two phases:

An initial exponential increase of the cumulative percent of the overlapped ZR motifs (until is reached 1200 bp upstream the ORFs) followed by an increase in the cumulative percent of overlapped ZR motifs that was directly proportional to the distance to the ORFs. The exponential part of this representation reflected the distribution of regulatory ZRs located in the intergenic promoter sequences of upstream genes with very short ORFs that were located in the near vicinity of the reference gene; whereas the arithmetic part of the representation reflected the random distribution of the ZR motifs 1200 bp upstream the TSCs. Besides, this distance matched perfectly the average size of the upstream distance to ORFs that was defined by the highest difference between the cumulative percent of overlapped and non-overlapped ZRs located within the 3000 bp upstream the ORFs (Figure 8B).

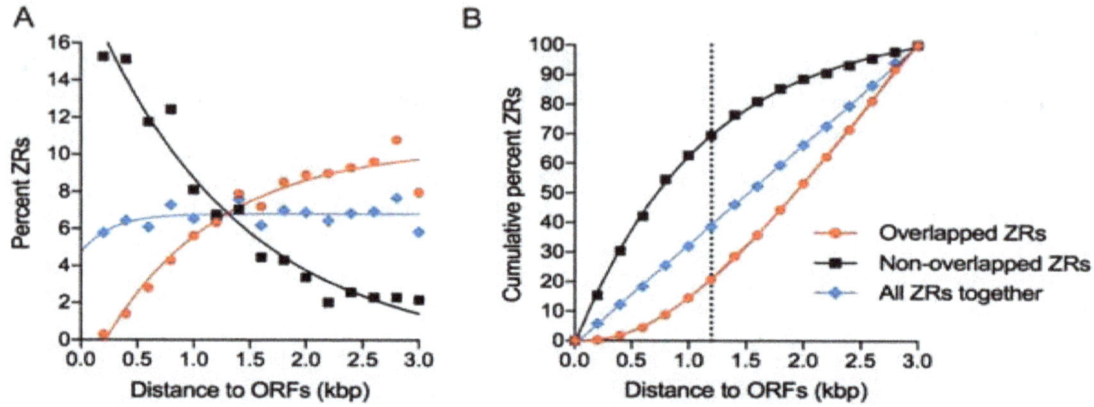

Figure 8. Distribution of ZR motifs at a genome scale in the upstream regions of the predicted open reading frames (ORFs). (**A**) Representation of the percentage of ZR motifs (overlapped, non-overlapped and all together) with respect to their distance to the predicted translation start codons (TSC) of the ORFs; (**B**) representation of the cumulative percent of ZR motifs with respect to their distance to the predicted translation start codons of the ORFs. The dotted line indicates the average size of the DNA sequence that is located upstream of the predicted TSCs containing the ZR motifs with the highest probability of being involved in regulating gene expression (i.e., the functionally relevant ZR motifs). In both graphs, the distance of the ZR motifs to the ORFs represented on the x-axes was divided into 15 fractions of 200 bp each.

Interestingly, the same tendency was observed for pairs of genes arranged divergently whose intergenic regions contained ZR motifs. Thus, the gene having most of the ZR motifs located at less than 1200 bp from the predicted TSC had a higher probability of being regulated by ZafA than the gene that had the ZR motifs at a distance >1200 bp of its TSC. For instance, in the intergenic region of the divergent pair of genes AFUA_1G01560/AFUA_1G01550 there were three motifs located respectively at −75, −105 and −157 bp from the TSC of AFUA_1G01550 (*zrfA*) and at −1784, −1754 and −1702 bp from the TSC of AFUA_1G01560. However, only the AFUA_1G01550 gene (*zrfA*) was induced by ZafA. In contrast, those genes arranged divergently and separated by intergenic sequences < 1200 bp are co-regulated simultaneously by ZafA (e.g., gene pairs AFUA_4G09560/AFUA_4G09580, AFUA_4G03920/AFUA_4G03930 or AFUA_8G02450/AFUA_8G02460). These results suggest that the ZR motifs located within 1200 bp upstream of the TSC of an ORF appear to be functionally relevant in the ZafA-mediated regulation of gene expression under zinc-limiting conditions.

Finally, a comparison of genes detected by microarrays in a wild-type strain as differentially regulated under zinc starvation with that found in silico harboring, non-overlapping ZR motifs in their promoter regions revealed that 31 DZR genes (i.e., 20.3% of the 153 DZR genes) and 55 non-DZR genes (i.e., 8.6% of 641 non-DZR genes) had ZR motifs in their promoters. Interestingly, 150 SSA genes (i.e., 7.0% of 2130 SSA genes) also had non-overlapping ZR motifs in their promoter regions. In addition, 30 DZR genes had their ZR motifs located within 1200 bp from their predicted TSC (i.e., 96.8% of all DZR genes with ZRs). In contrast, the weighted average percent of the non-DZR genes with ZR motifs located within 1200 bp from their predicted TSC was 71.2%. Taken together, these results indicated that ZR motifs predicted to be functionally relevant were located in the promoters of 19.6% of the DZR genes but only in 5.4% of genes not regulated directly by ZafA.

3.8. Putative Role of ZafA *as a Repressor under Zinc-Limiting Conditions and Identification of the Most Likely Direct Target Genes of* ZafA

The data obtained from the microarray experiments showed that, of all genes from a wild-type strain of *A. fumigatus* whose transcription level was influenced under zinc-limiting conditions, 64.5% were down-regulated whereas 35.5% were up-regulated (Figure 2). In contrast, 22.9% of the DZR genes were down-regulated whereas 77.1% were up-regulated. These results suggested that ZafA functioned mainly as a transcriptional activator rather than as a repressor.

In the microarray version used in this study, the AFUA_7G06570 gene (*zrcA*) had not been included. However, this gene encodes an important putative vacuolar zinc transporter of the CDF family likely involved in the homeostatic response to zinc excess [10]. Besides, it harbors one copy of the ZR consensus motif in its promoter region. Thus, we investigated whether the *zrcA* transcription was also influenced by ZafA under zinc-limiting conditions. It was shown by RT-qPCR that the expression level of *zrcA* reduced by about 6-fold in a wild-type strain grown in a zinc-limiting versus a zinc-replete medium, while it increased by 16-fold in a Δ*zafA* mutant grown in a zinc-limiting medium compared to a wild-type strain grown in the same conditions, i.e., ZafA was formally a repressor of *zrcA* under zinc-limiting conditions (Table 2). Hence, it would be theoretically possible that ZafA also down-regulated the expression of other DZR genes. In this regard, we confirmed by RT-qPCR that ZafA could also be formally considered as a repressor of the genes AFUA_2G01260/*srbA* [ZR3], AFUA_2G15290 [ZR5], AFUA_5G06240/*alcC* [ZR8] and AFUA_6G00690 [ZR5] under zinc-limiting conditions (Table 2). Importantly, all of these genes carried ZR motifs with one substitution in their promoter regions.

On the other hand, it was shown previously through a combination of in vitro and in silico analyses that at least 30 DZR genes with ZR motifs located within 1200 bp from their predicted TSC were putative direct ZafA targets. However, we also observed under zinc-limiting conditions, that some induced (e.g., *gtmA*, *pyroA*, *azf1*, *gliA*, *gliT*) and repressed genes (e.g., *sod1*, *erg24A*) (Table 2), which according to their expression profiles should be formally considered as direct ZafA targets, did not have obvious ZR motifs in their promoter sequences. However, after a search for non-overlapping ZR motifs with two substitutions in the promoter regions (until 1200 bp upstream of the predicted TSCs) using the RSAT software and the ZR consensus motif (ZR0) as a query sequence, 18 additional DZR genes harboring ZR degenerated motifs were found. Interestingly, among these genes were AFUA_6G09310 and AFUA_5G09240/*sodA*, which were ZafA-repressed genes, and *gliA*, which was one of the most strongly induced genes under zinc-limiting conditions. More importantly, this research also allowed us to detect additional ZR motifs in the promoter regions of genes encoding both important zinc homeostatic proteins (e.g., one additional site was detected in *zrfA* and *zafA* thus bringing the total number of ZRs in the promoters of these genes to 3 and 4 respectively) and other genes of unknown function but whose expression was also strongly induced by ZafA under zinc-limiting conditions (e.g., one additional ZR motif was detected in the AFUA_7G06810/*sarA* promoter and the AFUA_8G02460-AFUA_8G02450/*gzbA* divergent promoter; two additional ZR motifs were detected in the AFUA_8G02620/*mchC* promoter and the AFUA_4G03920-AFUA_4G03930/*cysX* divergent promoter).

Finally, it is interesting to recall that unlike the expression level of genes encoding zinc-independent enzymes typically involved in defense against reactive oxygen species (ROS), such as *cat1*, *cat2* and *sodC*; increases under zinc-limiting conditions, the expression level of *sodA*, which encodes a cytosolic Zn/Cu-superoxide dismutase, is reduced most likely as a mechanism to reduce the biosynthesis of the enzyme, since its functionality is strongly reduced under zinc-limiting conditions (Figure 9).

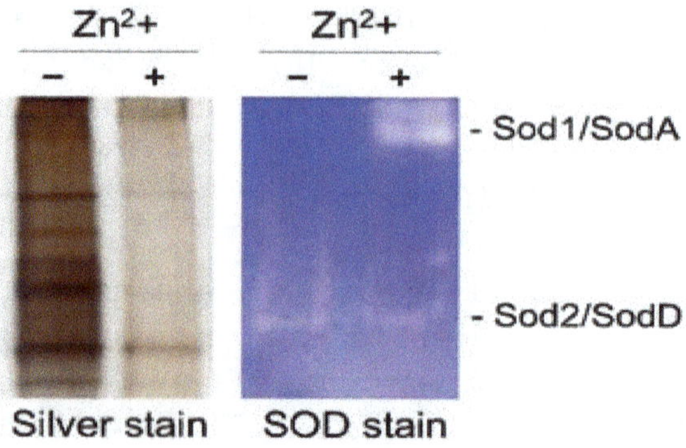

Figure 9. Detection of superoxide activity onto PAGE gels. Total extracts of native proteins were obtained from a wild-type strain of *A. fumigatus* grown under zinc-limiting (SDN–Zn) and zinc-replete conditions (SDN + 100 μM Zn), separated in a PAGE gel (T = 8%) and stained as described in the materials and methods section. Sod1/SodA is a cytosolic Cu/Zn-dependent superoxide dismutase whereas Sod2/SodD is a mitochondrial Mn-dependent superoxide dismutase.

In summary, these results supported the notion that the ZR consensus motif and other ZR motifs with different degeneration degrees out of the 5′-CARGGT-3′ hexanucleotide core, could function as regulatory sequences to which ZafA would bind under zinc-limiting conditions, and be brought to 49, the total number of DZR genes with ZR motifs (i.e., 31.8% of DZR genes) whose expression was regulated directly by ZafA, including 20 confirmed and 29 predicted genes (Table 3).

Table 3. Genes regulated or that were predicted to be regulated by ZafA. The expression of genes in **red** and **blue** was shown to be induced and repressed respectively by ZafA, as confirmed by RT-qPCR and/or northern-blot. The expression of genes in **black** and **green** was predicted to be induced and repressed respectively by ZafA. Start and end positions of the ZR motifs were numbered taking as reference that the base preceding the A nucleotide of the ATG translation start codon is at position −1. Motifs labeled with an asterisk (*) had two substitutions with respect to the ZR consensus motif out of the hexanucleotide core sequence 5′-CARGGC-3′ (ZR0*).

Gene ID	Gene Name	Strand	Start	End	Sequence ZR Motif	Type of ZR Motif
AFUA_1G01550	*zrfA*	D	−75	−61	GACCTCAAGGTACCC	ZR2
		R	−105	−91	ACTGCCAAGGTCCTT	ZR0
		D	−157	−143	GCTCACAAGGTGTGT	ZR0*
AFUA_1G05900	-	D	−393	−379	TTCGTCAAGGTTGTT	ZR0*
AFUA_1G09810	-	R	−168	−154	ACTCCCAGGGTACTT	ZR0
AFUA_1G10080	*zafA*	D	−361	−347	GCTCCCAAGGTCCTC	ZR0
		D	−448	−434	CCCCTCAGGGTATTA	ZR0*
		D	−624	−610	GCTCGCAGGGTCCTC	ZR5
		D	−657	−643	TCCCCCAGGGTCCTC	ZR0
AFUA_1G12170	-	R	−364	−350	ATTACCAAGGTGATA	ZR0*
AFUA_1G12850	*crnA*	R	−500	−486	TGTCCCAGGGTGTAC	ZR0*
AFUA_1G14550	*sodC/sod3*	R	−123	−109	AGCATCAAGGTCCTC	ZR2
		D	−160	−146	GATCCCAAGGTCCCC	ZR2
AFUA_1G14560	*msdS*	D	−664	−650	TCTACCAGGGTATAT	ZR8
		D	−928	−914	ATCGCCAGGGTCTTA	ZR9
AFUA_1G14700	-	R	−181	−167	GCACACAAGGTACTC	ZR0*
AFUA_2G01260	*srbA*	D	−886	−872	TTGGTCAAGGTCCTT	ZR3
AFUA_2G01610	-	D	−841	−827	GTCAGCAGGGTCATC	ZR0*
AFUA_2G02950	-	D	−160	−146	GTCTCCAAGGTCTCC	ZR4
AFUA_2G03860	*zrfB*	R	−359	−345	ATCCTCAAGGTCCCT	ZR0
		D	−496	−482	GCCACCAAGGTCCTT	ZR0
		D	−794	−780	TCTCCCAAGGTCCCC	ZR0
		D	−893	−879	ACTCCCAAGGTCCTC	ZR0
AFUA_2G06140	-	R	−461	−447	GTTCCCAAGGTCTCC	ZR0

Table 3. *Cont.*

Gene ID	Gene Name	Strand	Start	End	Sequence ZR Motif	Type of ZR Motif
AFUA_2G07810	-	D	−756	−742	GTAGGCAAGGTGCCT	ZR0*
AFUA_2G08280	*maeA*	R	−910	−896	TTCACCAGGGTAGAC	ZR0*
AFUA_2G08740	*zrfF*	R	−329	−315	TCTCCCAAGGTCCGC	ZR8
		R	−616	−602	ATAGCCAAGGTAGCT	ZR0*
AFUA_2G15290	-	R	−68	−54	GTCAACAGGGTGCTC	ZR5
AFUA_3G02270	*cat1*	D	−1052	−1038	TTGACCAGGGTCTCT	ZR3
AFUA_3G10680	-	R	−179	−165	GATCCCAAGGTCCTT	ZR2
		D	−233	−219	TCCCCCAGGGTCCCC	ZR0
AFUA_3G13100	-	D	−581	−567	TTCGTCAAGGTTTCA	ZR0*
AFUA_3G13940	-	D	−1073	−1059	TTTTCCAAGGTGTTG	ZR0 *
AFUA_4G03920	-	R	−307	−293	CTCACCAAGGTCCCC	ZR1
		D	−438	−424	ACCTCCAAGGTCCTG	ZR0*
		R	−576	−562	TCTATCAAGGTAATT	ZR7
		R	−605	−591	GCCTCCAAGGTAGTC	ZR0*
AFUA_4G03930	*cysX*	D	−272	−258	GCCTCCAAGGTAGTC	ZR0*
		D	−301	−287	TCTATCAAGGTAATT	ZR1
		R	−439	−425	ACCTCCAAGGTCCTG	ZR0*
		D	−570	−556	CTCACCAAGGTCCCC	ZR7
AFUA_4G09560	*zrfC*	R	−196	−182	ACTCCCAAGGTATCT	ZR0
		R	−313	−299	GCTCTCAAGGTCCTC	ZR0
		R	−637	−623	GCTACCAAGGTGTCC	ZR0
		D	−749	−735	GCCATCAGGGTAGAC	ZR0*
AFUA_4G09580	*aspf2*	R	−149	−135	GCCATCAGGGTAGAC	ZR0*
		D	−261	−247	GCTACCAAGGTGTCC	ZR0
		D	−585	−571	GCTCTCAAGGTCCTC	ZR0
		D	−702	−688	ACTCCCAAGGTATCT	ZR0
AFUA_4G10460	*hcsA*	R	−538	−524	ATCGGCAAGGTACAT	ZR0*
AFUA_5G02010	-	D	−122	−108	TTCTCCAGGGTCTTA	ZR0*
AFUA_5G03060	-	R	−807	−793	GCGCGCAAGGTACTT	ZR0*
AFUA_5G05710	-	R	−100	−86	TTCACCAAGGTTTTG	ZR0*
AFUA_5G06240	*alcC*	D	−595	−581	TCCCCCAGGGTACAT	ZR8
AFUA_5G09240	*sodA/sod1*	R	−198	−184	ATTCACAGGGTATTA	ZR0*
AFUA_5G12780	-	D	−99	−85	ACTCCCAAGGTACTC	ZR0
AFUA_5G13940	-	R	−231	−217	TCTGTCAGGGTCTGT	ZR8
AFUA_6G00690	-	D	−77	−63	GTCCACAAGGTCTTC	ZR5
AFUA_6G08580	*fkbp4*	D	−134	−120	GCCCTCAAGGTTCCT	ZR6
AFUA_6G09310	-	D	−1068	−1054	AGTGACAAGGTATTC	ZR0*
AFUA_6G09630	*gliZ*	D	−790	−776	TCTAACAAGGTCCTC	ZR5
		D	−836	−822	GCCCCCAAGGTGCCT	ZR0
AFUA_6G09710	*gliA*	R	−469	−455	GTTTGCAAGGTACTC	ZR0*
		R	−522	−508	TCCCCCAAGGTCACA	ZR0*
AFUA_6G10260	*akr1*	D	−180	−166	GTCGTCAAGGTTCCC	ZR6
AFUA_7G02360	-	R	−323	−309	TCGATCAAGGTGCTT	ZR3
AFUA_7G03970	-	D	−396	−382	TGTACCAAGGTATGT	ZR0*
AFUA_7G06570	*zrcA*	D	−915	−901	GTCCCCAAGGTACTC	ZR0
AFUA_7G06790	*yct1*	D	−224	−210	GTTCACAAGGTTCTT	ZR0*
		D	−305	−291	TCTACCAAGGTCCTT	ZR0
AFUA_7G06810	*sarA*	R	−187	−173	TCCAACAAGGTACCT	ZR5
		R	−276	−262	CCTCCCAGGGTTCTC	ZR0*
AFUA_8G01930	-	R	−603	−589	GCCATCAAGGTCGAT	ZR0*
AFUA_8G02450	*gzbA*	R	−165	−151	GTCTTCAAGGTTCTC	ZR0*
		D	−401	−387	GTCCCCAAGGTTCTC	ZR6
AFUA_8G02460	-	R	−617	−603	GTCCCCAAGGTTCTC	ZR6
		D	−853	−839	GTCTTCAAGGTTCTC	ZR0*
AFUA_8G02620	*mchC*	R	−65	−51	ACCCCCAAGGTTCGC	ZR0*
		R	−172	−158	ACTCCCAAGGTACCT	ZR0
		R	−192	−178	GGGCTCAAGGTCCTC	ZR0*

4. Discussion

The effect of zinc-deficiency on the regulation of gene expression and the homeostatic and adaptive response to zinc starvation has been extensively analyzed at a genome-wide scale in the yeast *Saccharomyces cerevisiae* [16–18]. In this yeast, the regulatory response to zinc starvation at the transcriptional level relies on the Zap1 transcription factor [31]. We described for the first time that regulation of zinc homeostasis in a fungal pathogen is essential for virulence [13,14]. Similar studies, conducted later in different *Candida* and *Cryptococcus* species, *Histoplasma capsulatum* and *Blastomyces dermatitidis*, have also highlighted the importance of maintaining zinc homeostasis for the virulence of these pathogenic yeast [19,20,32–36]. In this paper, we report the transcriptional profiling of *A. fumigatus* under zinc starvation and show that ZafA regulates the expression of its most direct target genes through binding to one or more ZR consensus motifs located in their promoter regions.

In both *S. cerevisiae* and the pathogenic fungi studied thus far, the genes more strongly induced by the ZafA/Zap1 orthologues encode membrane transporters of the ZIP family, involved in zinc uptake from zinc-limiting media. Besides, it has been observed that zinc-deficiency increases ROS production [20,33,37] while it reduces sulfate assimilation as a putative mechanism to alleviate oxidative stress under zinc-limiting conditions [38]. In this regard, the adaptive response to zinc deficiency is well mirrored at the transcriptional level by changes in the expression of genes encoding proteins involved in ROS detoxification and assimilation of inorganic sulfur both in *S. cerevisiae* [18] and in all pathogenic yeasts [19,20]. Similarly, in *A. fumigatus* grown under zinc-limiting conditions, genes encoding zinc-independent proteins involved in ROS detoxification (e.g., *cat1*, *cat2* and *sodC*) are up-regulated, while *metR* [39], which is the major regulator of inorganic sulfur assimilation, is down-regulated (Table 2 and Table S6). There are, however, some remarkable differences between species regarding specific aspects. Among the most noteworthy are those related to iron metabolism, ergosterol biosynthesis and protection against oxidative stress, which appears to be linked to the production of certain secondary metabolites.

The major difference between *A. fumigatus* and the yeasts *S. cerevisiae*, *C. albicans* and *C. gatti* regarding iron metabolism is that only *A. fumigatus* is able to synthesize and secrete siderophores for iron uptake under iron-limiting conditions [40]. The only gene related to iron homeostasis that has been reported to be induced by Zap1 in *S. cerevisiae* under zinc-limiting conditions is *FET4* [16,18], which encodes a low-affinity $Zn^{2+}/Fe^{2+}/Cu^{+}$ transporter [41]. In *C. albicans* grown under zinc-limiting conditions, the expression of some genes encoding proteins of the reductive pathway (e.g., *FRE2* and *FET34*) is up-regulated, whereas the expression of others is down-regulated (e.g., *FRE5*, *FRE7*, *FRE10*, *FET3* and *FTH1*). In *C. gatti* grown under zinc-limiting conditions, the expression of the genes CNBG_3602 and CNBG_2036 is down-regulated [20]. They encode proteins similar to FtrA and MirB of *A. fumigatus* that function respectively in the reductive and non-reductive/siderophore-mediated iron uptake system. In *A. fumigatus* are down-regulated, under zinc-limiting conditions, several genes encoding proteins that are involved in iron uptake, including the FetC/FrtA oxidase/permease complex of the reductive iron uptake system and several non-reductive siderophore transporters of *A. fumigatus* (Table 2 and Table S6). In addition, genes encoding regulators of iron homeostasis (e.g., *hapX* and *srbA*) and siderophore biosynthesis are also down-regulated in *A. fumigatus* under zinc starvation (Table 2 and Table S6). Therefore, provided that all transcriptional profiling studies performed thus far in fungal pathogens have been done under non-iron-limiting conditions, it is concluded that the expression of genes encoding proteins required for iron uptake appear to be reduced under zinc-limiting conditions, which indicates that a reduction of iron intake from non-iron-limiting media appears to be an adaptive response to zinc deficiency. Whether Zap1 plays a direct or indirect role in regulating the expression of genes involved in iron homeostasis in yeast has not been reported [19]. However, it appears that in *A. fumigatus* growing under zinc-limiting conditions, only the expression of some genes related to iron homeostasis is directly or indirectly regulated by ZafA (e.g., *srbA*, *enb1*, *mirB* and *sidA*), whereas most of them appear to be regulated in a ZafA-independent manner (Table 2 and Table S6). On the other hand, the transcriptional profiling of *A. fumigatus* grown in zinc-replete media following a shift from iron-limiting to iron-replete conditions has revealed that the expression of genes typically involved in the homeostatic response to zinc deficiency (e.g., *zafA*, *zrfA* and *zrfB*) is up-regulated whereas that of genes involved in the homeostatic response to zinc excess is down-regulated (e.g., *zrcA*) [42]. The expression profile of these ZafA-regulated genes in the referred conditions has been interpreted as a homeostatic mechanism to prevent zinc excess and zinc toxicity under iron starvation [43]. In addition, in a wild-type strain growing in zinc-replete media under iron-replete conditions HapX mediates both the up-regulation of genes typically involved in the homeostatic response to zinc deficiency (e.g., *zafA* and *zrfB*) and the down-regulation of genes involved in the homeostatic response to zinc excess (e.g., *zrcA* and *zrcC*) [44]. However, it is known that the expression of *hapX* is reduced dramatically under iron-replete conditions [44], which indicates that the predicted action of HapX on the expression of the aforementioned genes must be exerted by the low basal amount of HapX that is synthesized under iron-replete conditions [45]. It is difficult to understand that the HapX-mediated increase of the transcription level of *zafA*, which encodes the key major regulator of zinc homeostasis, only reflects changes in the expression level of *zrfB* and *zrcA* (of all putative direct targets of ZafA). Nevertheless, this could be explained upon considering that *zrfB* is the zinc homeostatic gene with the highest number of ZR motifs in its promoter, whereas *zrcA* is one of the few genes whose expression is strongly repressed by ZafA that harbors one ZR consensus motif in its promoter region (Table 3). Hence, it could be possible that the low increase in the expression level of *zafA* detected in a wild-type strain versus a Δ*hapX* strain (about 1.8-fold) [44], allows synthesizing a little (although sufficient) amount of ZafA. This regulator could bind preferentially to the promoters of *zrfB* and *zrcA* to induce the former and repress the later. The *zrcC* gene does not have ZR motifs in its promoter region and most likely its repression under zinc-limiting conditions is not directly mediated by ZafA. The HapX-mediated co-regulation of the *zrfB*, *zrcA* and *zrcC* expression in *A. fumigatus* might have evolved as an adaptive response to iron excess caused by a sudden iron supplement under zinc-replete conditions. This response would prevent the rapid storage into the vacuole (mediated by ZrcA and ZrcC) of the zinc taken up by ZrfB. The most likely reason would be that a concentration of cytosolic zinc higher than usual is required to prevent iron toxicity during a transient iron excess. This adaptive response recalls the proactive mechanism that operates in *S. cerevisiae* to protect cells against a sudden high increase of zinc concentration in the medium or "zinc shock" [46]. This mechanism relies on the function of *ZRC1* that is the orthologue of the *zrcA* gene of *A. fumigatus*. *ZRC1* is up-regulated by Zap1 to enhance the storage into the vacuole of zinc that is incorporated by Zrt1 under zinc-limiting conditions [46,47]. Provided that these studies have been performed in media containing a relatively low amount of iron such as that present in the yeast nitrogen base (i.e., 0.74 μM) used to make the yeast synthetic minimum medium, it could be possible that zinc storage following a "zinc shock" is intended to prevent zinc toxicity due to iron insufficiency. In summary, a mutual relationship between regulation of homeostasis of zinc and iron appears to exist. This zinc/iron cross-homeostasis could be essential for fungal growth in zinc-replete media. It would not only prevent the excessive zinc uptake and zinc toxicity under iron starvation, as proposed previously [43], but also it might increase the cytosolic concentration of zinc to prevent iron toxicity under iron-replete conditions and/or prevent an excessive iron uptake from non-iron-limiting media and iron toxicity under zinc starvation. Consequently, the zinc/iron cross-homeostasis would allow the fungus to grow well in media containing unbalanced Zn:Fe ratios.

Some NZR genes are down-regulated, both in zinc-limiting media under iron-replete conditions and in zinc-replete media after a shift from iron-limiting to iron-replete conditions, such as *hmg1*, which encodes the enzyme of the committed step in ergosterol biosynthesis, and several genes related to siderophore biosynthesis (e.g., *sidC*, *sidF*, *sidG*, *amcA*) [44]. This finding suggests that the reduction of both iron uptake and ergosterol biosynthesis might also have co-evolved as part of the fungal adaptive response both to zinc starvation under non-iron-limiting conditions, and to iron excess under non-zinc-limiting conditions. In addition, a relatively high number of genes whose expression is regulated by the sterol-response element binding proteins (SREPBs), SrbA and SrbB, are also influenced by zinc starvation [48,49]. For instance, several genes involved in ergosterol biosynthesis (i.e., *erg1*, *erg3A/B*, *erg5*, *erg13B*, *erg24A/B*, *erg25A/B* and *hmg1*), ethanol catabolism (*alcC*), heme biosynthesis (*hem13* and *hem14*) and nitrate assimilation (*niiA* and *niaD*), are up-regulated by SREPBs in hypoxia and down-regulated under (normoxic) zinc-limiting conditions (Table 2). Similarly, the own expression of *srbA* and *srbB* is strongly reduced under (normoxic) zinc-limiting conditions (Table 2). On the other hand, it is known that the transcription of *srbB* is autoinduced by SrbB and starts earlier (and is stronger) than that of *srbA*, which is autoinduced by SrbA [49]. Besides, the RNAseq data for the wild-type, Δ*srbA* and Δ*srbB* strains, after 2 h in hypoxia, revealed that the expression level of *srbB* in the Δ*srbA* mutant is lower than in the wild-type strain; whereas the expression level of *srbA* in the Δ*srbB* mutant is higher than in the wild-type strain, i.e., SrbA is formally an inductor of *srbB* whereas SrbB is a repressor of *srbA* [49]. Since *srbA* can be formally considered as a direct ZafA target (Table 2), it could be possible that *srbA* repression initiated by ZafA, under normoxic zinc-limiting conditions, triggers a cascade of transcriptional events that ultimately results in the strong down-regulation of *srbA* and *srbB* (and that of their target genes) under sustained zinc-limiting conditions. However, the same RNAseq experiment also indicated that SrbA and SrbB are formally positive regulators of *zrfA*, *zrfB* and *zrfC* but negative regulators of *zafA* [49]. In addition, SrbA is a positive regulator of *zrcA* and *zrcC* whereas SrbB is a negative regulator of these genes [49]. Hence, provided that these studies have been performed in zinc-replete media, the positive regulation of *zrfA*, *zrfB* and *zrfC* by SrbA and SrbB, along with the early negative regulation of *zrcA* and *zrcC* by SrbB, this suggests that a cytoplasmic zinc concentration higher than usual may be beneficial for fungal growth in hypoxia. Of note, this regulatory mechanism for the adaptive response to hypoxia resembles the one involved in preventing iron toxicity during iron excess under zinc-replete conditions. In addition, it has been reported that the fungal zinc content is about 3-fold higher in mycelium grown in hypoxia than in normoxia [50]. However, the SREPB-mediated down-regulation of *zafA* by SrbA and SrbB under hypoxic zinc-replete conditions suggests that the expression *zrfA*, *zrfB* and *zrfC* should be induced directly by these factors instead of being induced by ZafA.

S. cerevisiae and *C. albicans* lack SREPBs orthologues and appear to have evolved different regulatory mechanism [51]. In either case, under hypoxic (zinc-replete) conditions the expression of the *ERG* genes is down-regulated in *S. cerevisiae* [52], but up-regulated in *C. albicans* [53] and *A. fumigatus* [48]. This suggests that the sterol content in *S. cerevisiae* under hypoxic conditions is largely sufficient to sustain growth whereas in *C. albicans* and *A. fumigatus* it is largely insufficient, thus requiring the increase of the expression of the ergosterol biosynthetic genes encoding enzymes that catalyze oxygen-dependent reactions (Erg1, Erg11, Erg25 and Erg3). However, it has been reported that the expression of the *ERG* genes is down-regulated in a *S. cerevisiae* Δ*zap1* mutant [16], which indicates the ScZap1 is formally a positive regulator of the *ERG* genes. In contrast, in a *C. albicans* Δ*zap1* mutant the expression of the *ERG* genes is up-regulated [19], which indicates the CaZap1 is formally a negative regulator of the *ERG* genes. However, the *ERG* genes in *S. cereviasie* and *C. albicans* lack Zap1 binding motifs in their promoter regions, which suggests that both ScZap1 and CaZap1 regulate indirectly the expression of these genes [19]. Similarly, the *erg* genes of *A. fumigatus* lack ZR motifs in their promoters and, under zinc-limiting conditions, only a few *erg* genes (e.g., *erg5*, *erg13B*, *erg24A*, *erg24B* and *erg3B*) are likely repressed either directly or indirectly by ZafA, whereas it is likely that the expression of other genes (e.g., *hmg1*, *erg1*, *erg3A*, *erg25A* and *erg25B*) are down-regulated in a ZafA-independent manner (Table 2 and Table S6). In either case, one possibility is that the repression of the *erg* genes under normoxic zinc-limiting conditions is an indirect consequence of *srbA* repression by ZafA.

Zinc starvation increases the expression level of genes encoding components of the electron acceptor complexes I-III of the mitochondrial electron transport chain (ETC) (e.g., *sdh3* and *sdh4* that encode the inner-membrane-anchored subunits of the succinate deshydrogenase), while it reduces the encoding of the mitochondrial fumarate reductase (FrdA) and some genes encoding components of complex IV of the ETC (e.g., AFUA_2G03010 and AFUA_3G14440). The *frdA* gene, which is one of the most strongly induced genes during hypoxia in *A. fumigatus* [54], encodes a FAD-dependent enzyme similar to the yeast Frd1 enzyme that couples the reduction [fumarate → succinate] to the oxidation [ubiquinol → ubiquinone] (i.e., the reverse reaction that is catalyzed by the succinate deshydrogenase) [55]. The complexes I and III are considered as major sites of ROS generation in mitochondria [56]. Thus, it is tempting to speculate that the imbalance between the expression of genes encoding components of the electron acceptor complexes I/II and electron donor complex IV under zinc-limiting conditions may disturb the normal electron flux through the ETC in normoxia. In this scenario, not all electrons that enter the ETC are finally used for O_2 reduction, at the same time that the intracellular partial pressure of O_2 in the fungus growing under zinc-limiting conditions becomes relatively higher than in the fungus growing in zinc-replete media. As a consequence, the intracellular O_2 may reach a slightly hyperbaric concentration while it increases the probability of adventitious reactions of reduced flavins with O_2 leading to the formation of (ROS) [57]. It is known that enzymes of the succinate/fumarate oxidoreductase family, which include the succinate dehydrogenases and fumarate reductases, are prone to react adventitiously with O_2 and autoxidation resulting in the formation of superoxide anion and/or H_2O_2 (because they contain flavins that appear to be the primary site of electron transfer to O_2) [57,58]. For instance, the *E. coli* NadB flavoprotein, which is structurally and evolutionary related to succinate/fumarate oxidoreductases, accounts for about 25% of all H_2O_2 generated endogenously during aerobic growth [59]. Thus, the reduction of the expression level of *frdA* could be interpreted as a mechanism to prevent an excess of ROS formation under zinc-limiting conditions.

Interestingly, the adaptive response against oxidative stress displayed by *A. fumigatus* appears to differ significantly from that displayed by the yeast *S. cerevisiae*, in which only two gene-encoding enzymes for protection against ROS, *SOD1* and *TSA1*, appear to be critical for growth in low zinc [37,60]. The expression level of *SOD1* in *S. cerevisiae*, which encodes the orthologue to the *A. fumigatus* SodA Cu/Zn-superoxide dismutase, is similar under both zinc-replete and zinc-limiting conditions [60]. In contrast, in *A. fumigatus* the expression level of *sodA* reduced significantly under zinc-limiting conditions, most likely as a mechanism to reduce the biosynthesis of the Cu/Zn-SOD whose functionality is strongly reduced under zinc-limiting conditions (Figure 9). Besides, *A. fumigatus* lacks an obvious orthologous of *TSA1*, which encodes a protein with a dual peroxiredoxin-chaperone function that enables yeast cells to adapt both oxidative stress and deficient folding caused by zinc starvation [37,61]. In summary, the adaptive response against oxidative stress in *A. fumigatus* under zinc-limiting conditions might rely on a dual regulatory mechanism that involves both the down-regulation of genes encoding ROS generating enzymes and the up-regulation of genes encoding ROS detoxifying, zinc-independent enzymes.

Unlike pathogenic yeast, *A. fumigatus* has at least 26 biosynthetic gene clusters (named as BGC1-26) that enables it to produce a great diversity of secondary metabolites and mycotoxins [62]. Interestingly, the expression level of 17 genes belonging to 11 different BGCs are differentially regulated under zinc-limiting conditions (Table S6). The BGC-20 dedicated to gliotoxin (GT) biosynthesis appear to be the most largely influenced by zinc starvation, as revealed by the high expression level of *gliZ*, *gliT*, *gliA* and *gtmA*. GliT catalyzes disulfide formation during GT biosynthesis, whereas GliA is involved in GT efflux and both proteins provide self-protection against exogenous and endogenous GT [63–65]. The enzyme GtmA catalyzes the conversion of both the endogenous dithiol-GT (GT-[H_2S]) and the exogenous GT into bisdethiobis(metylthio)gliotoxin (BmGT), which is a negative modulator of GT biosynthesis, using S-adenosylmethionine (SAM) as a methyl donor [66]. Hence, the transcriptional profile of *gliZ*, *gliT* and *gliA* strongly suggests that either a much higher amount of GT is synthesized in zinc-limiting media than in zinc-replete conditions, or GT is far more noxious for fungal growth in zinc-limiting than in zinc-replete media. Besides, the GtmA-mediated bis-thiomethylation of GT is a SAM-dependent reaction that produces as a by-product S-adenosyl-homocysteine (SAH). SAH is then presumably hydrolyzed to homocysteine (Hcy) by the putative S-adenosyl-homocysteinase encoded by AFUA_1G10130/*sahA*, whose expression is also slightly up-regulated under zinc-limiting conditions (Table 2). It has been proposed that GliT, GliA and GtmA work in concert in *A. fumigatus* to resist the effect of exogenous GT in zinc-replete conditions [67], and that GliT and GtmA are up-synthesized in the presence of both GT and GT plus H_2O_2 under zinc-replete conditions [68]. In addition, GT inhibits H_2O_2-induced oxidative stress [68,69] because most likely GT is able to replace the function of 2-Cys peroxiredoxins as an electron acceptor in the thioredoxin-peroxiredoxin system [70], which is consistent with the lack of a Tsa1-like protein in *A. fumigatus*. Hence, it is very likely that the concerted action of the GliT, GliA, GtmA and SahA proteins has evolved in *A. fumigatus* as part of the adaptive response against oxidative stress caused by zinc starvation. However, the success of the GT-based strategy to reinforce the ROS detoxification capability of *A. fumigatus* relies on an efficient self-protection mechanism against the toxic effect of an excessive amount of GT. At the same time, a relatively high SAM:SAH ratio must be kept to prevent the competitive inhibition of specific methyltransferases by SAH.

The comparison of genes whose expression levels change in a wild-type strain in zinc-limiting versus zinc-replete conditions with those whose expression levels change in a Δ*zafA* mutant versus a wild-type strain when both are grown under in zinc-limiting conditions, produced a group of genes that was expected to be enriched in the most direct ZafA targets. Thus, we identified 153 putative ZafA target genes (35 down-regulated and 118 up-regulated) that represented about 1.56% of the 9824 predicted ORFs in *A. fumigatus*. Following a similar approach for the characterization of the Zap1 zinc-responsive regulon in *S. cerevisiae*, 111 genes were found to be putatively up-regulated by Zap1 [16], which represent about 1.82% of the 6091 biologically significant ORFs of *S. cerevisiae* [71]. In addition, by using a combination of in vitro and in silico approaches, it was determined that most of the 111 putative Zap1 target genes carried, at their promoter regions, at least one zinc response (ZR) consensus sequence 5′-ACCYYNAAGGT-3′ (or a degenerated version of it) to which Zap1 may bind [18,72]. Thus, it was concluded that a total of 81 genes in the yeast genome were direct targets of Zap1 [18]. Using a similar experimental approach, we have found 49 direct targets of ZafA, including 29 potential and 20 confirmed ZafA targets (Table 3). However, several DZR genes (*erg24A*, *gtmA*, *pyroA*, *azf1*, *gliT* and *frdA*) (Table 2), formally considered as direct targets of ZafA, lack obvious ZR motifs. This suggests that ZafA could be able to bind to ZR motifs with a relatively high degeneration degree. In this regard, it must be aware that, unlike Zap1 of *S. cerevisiae*, which binds to a 11-nucleotide sequence with a relatively low degeneration degree (5′-ACCYYNAAGGT-3′; with 16 [$2^2 \times 4$] different possible ZR sequences), the ZafA transcription factor of *A. fumigatus* binds to a 15-nucleotide zinc response sequence with a higher degeneration degree (5′-DYYVYCARGGTVYYY-3′; with 3456 [$3^3 \times 2^7$] different possible ZR sequences), even without considering that additional substitutions are possible out of the conserved core (5′-CARGGT-3′) of the ZR motif. Unlike this hexanucleotide sequence that is essential for ZafA to bind specifically to the ZR motifs, the high variability of both ends of the ZR motif could be intended to determine the affinity of ZafA binding to the ZRs. In either case, it appears that the diversity of ZR sequences to which ZafA can bind in *A. fumigatus* is noticeably higher than those recognized by Zap1 in *S. cerevisiae*. This fact complicates the identification of functionally relevant ZR motifs in many genes of *A. fumigatus*, including some of the most strongly expressed DZR genes, such as *gtmA* and *gliT*.

It is clear that ZafA plays a role in *A. fumigatus* similar to that of Zap1 in *S. cerevisiae* and in the pathogenic yeast *C. albicans* and *C. gattii*, although the only significant identity among these proteins is restricted to the C-terminal DNA binding domain. However, unlike ScZap1 that has four zinc-fingers for DNA binding (one of the CWCH2-type plus three of the C2H2-type), CgZap1 and CaZap1, similar to ZafA, have five (one of the CWCH2-type plus four of the C2H2-type) (Figure 1). Interestingly, given that a zinc-finger binds typically to a 3-nucleotide sequence [73], it may explain that ZafA binds to a 15-nucleotide ZR motif whereas ScZap1 binds to a 11-nucleotide ZR motif. It is interesting as well to note that the high hypersensitivity of the DNA fragments from the *zafA*, *zrfA*, *zrfB* and *zrfC* promoters to DNase I digestion, observed after performing the in vitro footprinting assays, could be an indication that binding of ZafA to the referred promoters causes DNA bending in vivo as part of the transcriptional regulatory mechanism mediated by ZafA, as reported for other regulators [74].

Finally, it is noticeable that most of the DZR genes that harbored ZR motifs in their promoters are up-regulated, which strongly suggests that ZafA mainly functions as an activator rather than as a repressor. Nevertheless, there are also some down-regulated genes that appear to be directly repressed by ZafA (e.g., *zrcA*, *srbA*, *alcC*, *sodA* and others without obvious ZR motifs in their promoters, such as *frdA* and *erg24A*) (Table 3). Similarly, Zap1 of *S. cerevisiae* appears to function nearly exclusively as a transcriptional activator since all 81 proposed Zap1 target genes appear to be induced by Zap1 [16,18], although it has been reported that Zap1 also functions paradoxically as a repressor of *ZRT2* in low zinc [75]. In addition, Zap1 under zinc deficiency represses the expression of the genes *ADH1* and *ADH3*, which encode zinc-dependent alcohol dehydrogenases, most likely as a mechanism to prevent their synthesis under zinc-limiting conditions [76]. Interestingly, a similar rationale could also be applied to explain the repression by ZafA of zinc-dependent enzymes of *A. fumigatus* such as *alcC* and *sodA*.

5. Conclusions

The analysis of the transcriptional profile of the ZafA regulon of *A. fumigatus*, under zinc-limiting conditions, confirmed that ZafA is the major regulator of the zinc homeostatic response to zinc starvation. It also indicated that ZafA, along with other regulators, was involved in a zinc/iron cross-homeostatic controlling network that allows the fungus to grow in media containing unbalanced Zn:Fe ratios. This study suggested as well that reduction of iron uptake and ergosterol biosynthesis might have co-evolved as part of the fungal adaptive response to iron excess under non-zinc-limiting conditions and to zinc starvation under non-iron-limiting conditions, even though this regulation appeared to be exerted only in part and indirectly by ZafA. In agreement with previous reports by other investigators, these results also suggested an increase in ROS production under zinc starvation that *A. fumigatus* counteracted by reducing the expression of genes encoding enzymes involved in ROS production and increasing the expression of genes encoding ROS-detoxifying enzymes and gliotoxin production, along with a self-protection mechanism against endogenous gliotoxin. Finally, it was shown that although ZafA appeared to function mainly as an inductor of gene expression under zinc-limiting conditions, it could also function as a repressor of a limited number of genes. Importantly, ZafA would exert its function as a transcriptional activator through binding to a well-defined zinc response consensus motif (5′-DYYVYCARGGTVYYY-3′) present in the promoters of its most direct target genes. However, ZafA could also bind to ZR motifs with a relatively high degeneration degree in nucleotides out of the conserved hexanucleotide core (5′-CARGGT-3′) and that could be present in the promoter regions of secondary target genes of ZafA.

Author Contributions: J.A.C. conceived and designed the experiments; R.V., J.A., L.M., and C.I.S. performed the experiments; J.A.C., R.V. and F.L. analyzed the data; J.A.C. wrote the paper.

Acknowledgments: R.V. was supported by a contract through grant SAF2013-48382-R to J.A.C.; C.I.S. was supported by a fellowship from the Universidad Industrial de Santander (Bucaramanga, Colombia) through resolution n° 2604 (18th December 2014).

References

1. Andreini, C.; Bertini, I.; Cavallaro, G.; Holliday, G.L.; Thornton, J.M. Metal ions in biological catalysis: From enzyme databases to general principles. *J. Biol. Inorg. Chem.* **2008**, *13*, 1205–1218. [CrossRef] [PubMed]
2. Auld, D.S. The ins and outs of biological zinc sites. *Biometals* **2009**, *22*, 141–148. [CrossRef] [PubMed]
3. Maret, W. Zinc and sulfur: a critical biological partnership. *Biochemistry* **2004**, *43*, 3301–3309. [CrossRef] [PubMed]
4. Eide, D.J. Zinc transporters and the cellular trafficking of zinc. *Biochim. Biophys. Acta* **2006**, *1763*, 711–722. [CrossRef] [PubMed]
5. Palmiter, R.D.; Findley, S.D. Cloning and functional characterization of a mammalian zinc transporter that confers resistance to zinc. *EMBO J.* **1995**, *14*, 639–649. [PubMed]
6. Maret, W. Zinc biochemistry: From a single zinc enzyme to a key element of life. *Adv. Nutr.* **2013**, *4*, 82–91. [CrossRef] [PubMed]
7. Simons, T.J. Intracellular free zinc and zinc buffering in human red blood cells. *J. Membr. Biol.* **1991**, *123*, 63–71. [CrossRef] [PubMed]
8. Bessman, J.D.; Johnson, R.K. Erythrocyte volume distribution in normal and abnormal subjects. *Blood* **1975**, *46*, 369–379. [PubMed]
9. Karthaus, M.; Buchheidt, D. Invasive aspergillosis: New insights into disease, diagnostic and treatment. *Curr. Pharm. Des.* **2013**, *19*, 3569–3594. [CrossRef] [PubMed]
10. Amich, J.; Calera, J.A. Zinc acquisition: A key aspect in *Aspergillus fumigatus* virulence. *Mycopathologia* **2014**, *178*, 379–385. [CrossRef] [PubMed]
11. Amich, J.; Vicentefranqueira, R.; Leal, F.; Calera, J.A. *Aspergillus fumigatus* survival in alkaline and extreme zinc-limiting environments relies on the induction of a zinc homeostasis system encoded by the *zrfC* and *aspf2* genes. *Eukaryot. Cell* **2010**, *9*, 424–437. [CrossRef] [PubMed]
12. Vicentefranqueira, R.; Moreno, M.A.; Leal, F.; Calera, J.A. The *zrfA* and *zrfB* genes of *Aspergillus fumigatus* encode the zinc transporter proteins of a zinc uptake system induced in an acid, zinc-depleted environment. *Eukaryot. Cell* **2005**, *4*, 837–848. [CrossRef] [PubMed]
13. Amich, J.; Vicentefranqueira, R.; Mellado, E.; Ruiz-Carmuega, A.; Leal, F.; Calera, J.A. The ZrfC alkaline zinc transporter is required for *Aspergillus fumigatus* virulence and its growth in the presence of the Zn/Mn-chelating protein calprotectin. *Cell Microbiol.* **2014**, *16*, 548–564. [CrossRef] [PubMed]
14. Moreno, M.A.; Ibrahim-Granet, O.; Vicentefranqueira, R.; Amich, J.; Ave, P.; Leal, F.; Latge, J.P.; Calera, J.A. The regulation of zinc homeostasis by the ZafA transcriptional activator is essential for *Aspergillus fumigatus* virulence. *Mol. Microbiol.* **2007**, *64*, 1182–1197. [CrossRef] [PubMed]
15. Eide, D.J. Homeostatic and adaptive responses to zinc deficiency in *Saccharomyces cerevisiae*. *J. Biol. Chem.* **2009**, *284*, 18565–18569. [CrossRef] [PubMed]
16. Lyons, T.J.; Gasch, A.P.; Gaither, L.A.; Botstein, D.; Brown, P.O.; Eide, D.J. Genome-wide characterization of the Zap1p zinc-responsive regulon in yeast. *Proc. Natl. Acad. Sci. USA* **2000**, *97*, 7957–7962. [CrossRef] [PubMed]
17. North, M.; Steffen, J.; Loguinov, A.V.; Zimmerman, G.R.; Vulpe, C.D.; Eide, D.J. Genome-wide functional profiling identifies genes and processes important for zinc-limited growth of *Saccharomyces cerevisiae*. *PLoS Genet.* **2012**, *8*, e1002699. [CrossRef] [PubMed]
18. Wu, C.Y.; Bird, A.J.; Chung, L.M.; Newton, M.A.; Winge, D.R.; Eide, D.J. Differential control of Zap1-regulated genes in response to zinc deficiency in *Saccharomyces cerevisiae*. *BMC Genom.* **2008**, *9*, 370. [CrossRef] [PubMed]
19. Nobile, C.J.; Nett, J.E.; Hernday, A.D.; Homann, O.R.; Deneault, J.S.; Nantel, A.; Andes, D.R.; Johnson, A.D.; Mitchell, A.P. Biofilm matrix regulation by *Candida albicans* Zap1. *PLoS Biol.* **2009**, *7*, e1000133. [CrossRef] [PubMed]
20. Schneider, R.O.; Fogaca, N.S.; Kmetzsch, L.; Schrank, A.; Vainstein, M.H.; Staats, C.C. Zap1 regulates zinc homeostasis and modulates virulence in *Cryptococcus gattii*. *PLoS ONE* **2012**, *7*, e43773. [CrossRef] [PubMed]
21. Hatayama, M.; Aruga, J. Gli protein nuclear localization signal. *Vitam. Horm.* **2012**, *88*, 73–89. [PubMed]
22. Espeso, E.A.; Tilburn, J.; Sanchez-Pulido, L.; Brown, C.V.; Valencia, A.; Arst, H.N., Jr.; Peñalva, M.A. Specific DNA recognition by the *Aspergillus nidulans* three zinc finger transcription factor PacC. *J. Mol. Biol.* **1997**, *274*, 466–480. [CrossRef] [PubMed]

23. Evans-Galea, M.V.; Blankman, E.; Myszka, D.G.; Bird, A.J.; Eide, D.J.; Winge, D.R. Two of the five zinc fingers in the Zap1 transcription factor DNA binding domain dominate site-specific DNA binding. *Biochemistry* **2003**, *42*, 1053–1061. [CrossRef] [PubMed]
24. Pavletich, N.P.; Pabo, C.O. Crystal structure of a five-finger GLI-DNA complex: New perspectives on zinc fingers. *Science* **1993**, *261*, 1701–1707. [CrossRef] [PubMed]
25. Calera, J.A.; Ovejero, M.C.; López-Medrano, R.; Segurado, M.; Puente, P.; Leal, F. Characterization of the *Aspergillus nidulans aspnd1* gene demonstrates that the ASPND1 antigen, which it encodes, and several *Aspergillus fumigatus* immunodominant antigens belong to the same family. *Infect. Immun.* **1997**, *65*, 1335–1344. [PubMed]
26. Priebe, S.; Kreisel, C.; Horn, F.; Guthke, R.; Linde, J. FungiFun2: A comprehensive online resource for systematic analysis of gene lists from fungal species. *Bioinformatics* **2015**, *31*, 445–446. [CrossRef] [PubMed]
27. Bailey, T.L.; Boden, M.; Buske, F.A.; Frith, M.; Grant, C.E.; Clementi, L.; Ren, J.; Li, W.W.; Noble, W.S. MEME SUITE: Tools for motif discovery and searching. *Nucleic Acids Res.* **2009**, *37*, W202–W208. [CrossRef] [PubMed]
28. Medina-Rivera, A.; Defrance, M.; Sand, O.; Herrmann, C.; Castro-Mondragon, J.A.; Delerce, J.; Jaeger, S.; Blanchet, C.; Vincens, P.; Caron, C.; et al. RSAT 2015: Regulatory Sequence Analysis Tools. *Nucleic Acids Res.* **2015**, *43*, W50–W56. [CrossRef] [PubMed]
29. Zianni, M.; Tessanne, K.; Merighi, M.; Laguna, R.; Tabita, F.R. Identification of the DNA bases of a DNase I footprint by the use of dye primer sequencing on an automated capillary DNA analysis instrument. *J. Biomol. Tech.* **2006**, *17*, 103–113. [PubMed]
30. Nierman, W.C.; Pain, A.; Anderson, M.J.; Wortman, J.R.; Kim, H.S.; Arroyo, J.; Berriman, M.; Abe, K.; Archer, D.B.; Bermejo, C.; et al. Genomic sequence of the pathogenic and allergenic filamentous fungus *Aspergillus fumigatus*. *Nature* **2005**, *438*, 1151–1156. [CrossRef] [PubMed]
31. Zhao, H.; Eide, D.J. Zap1p, a metalloregulatory protein involved in zinc-responsive transcriptional regulation in *Saccharomyces cerevisiae*. *Mol. Cell Biol.* **1997**, *17*, 5044–5052. [CrossRef] [PubMed]
32. Do, E.; Hu, G.; Caza, M.; Kronstad, J.W.; Jung, W.H. The ZIP family zinc transporters support the virulence of *Cryptococcus neoformans*. *Med. Mycol.* **2016**, *54*, 605–615. [CrossRef] [PubMed]
33. Schneider Rde, O.; Diehl, C.; dos Santos, F.M.; Piffer, A.C.; Garcia, A.W.; Kulmann, M.I.; Schrank, A.; Kmetzsch, L.; Vainstein, M.H.; Staats, C.C. Effects of zinc transporters on *Cryptococcus gattii* virulence. *Sci. Rep.* **2015**, *5*, 10104. [CrossRef] [PubMed]
34. Xu, W.; Solis, N.V.; Ehrlich, R.L.; Woolford, C.A.; Filler, S.G.; Mitchell, A.P. Activation and alliance of regulatory pathways in *C. albicans* during mammalian infection. *PLoS Biol.* **2015**, *13*, e1002076. [CrossRef] [PubMed]
35. Bottcher, B.; Palige, K.; Jacobsen, I.D.; Hube, B.; Brunke, S. Csr1/Zap1 maintains zinc homeostasis and influences virulence in *Candida dubliniensis* but is not coupled to morphogenesis. *Eukaryot. Cell* **2015**, *14*, 661–670. [CrossRef] [PubMed]
36. Kujoth, G.C.; Sullivan, T.D.; Merkhofer, R.; Lee, T.J.; Wang, H.; Brandhorst, T.; Wuthrich, M.; Klein, B.S. CRISPR/Cas9-mediated gene disruption reveals the importance of zinc metabolism for fitness of the dimorphic fungal pathogen *Blastomyces dermatitidis*. *MBio* **2018**, *9*, e00412-18. [CrossRef] [PubMed]
37. Wu, C.Y.; Bird, A.J.; Winge, D.R.; Eide, D.J. Regulation of the yeast TSA1 peroxiredoxin by ZAP1 is an adaptive response to the oxidative stress of zinc deficiency. *J. Biol. Chem.* **2007**, *282*, 2184–2195. [CrossRef] [PubMed]
38. Wu, C.Y.; Roje, S.; Sandoval, F.J.; Bird, A.J.; Winge, D.R.; Eide, D.J. Repression of sulfate assimilation is an adaptive response of yeast to the oxidative stress of zinc deficiency. *J. Biol. Chem.* **2009**, *284*, 27544–27556. [CrossRef] [PubMed]
39. Amich, J.; Schafferer, L.; Haas, H.; Krappmann, S. Regulation of sulphur assimilation is essential for virulence and affects iron homeostasis of the human-pathogenic mould *Aspergillus fumigatus*. *PLoS Pathog.* **2013**, *9*, e1003573. [CrossRef] [PubMed]
40. Haas, H. Fungal siderophore metabolism with a focus on *Aspergillus fumigatus*. *Nat. Prod. Rep.* **2014**, *31*, 1266–1276. [CrossRef] [PubMed]
41. Dix, D.R.; Bridgham, J.T.; Broderius, M.A.; Byersdorfer, C.A.; Eide, D.J. The *FET4* gene encodes the low affinity Fe(II) transport protein of *Saccharomyces cerevisiae*. *J. Biol. Chem.* **1994**, *269*, 26092–26099. [PubMed]

42. Schrettl, M.; Kim, H.S.; Eisendle, M.; Kragl, C.; Nierman, W.C.; Heinekamp, T.; Werner, E.R.; Jacobsen, I.; Illmer, P.; Yi, H.; et al. SreA-mediated iron regulation in *Aspergillus fumigatus*. *Mol. Microbiol.* **2008**, *70*, 27–43. [CrossRef] [PubMed]
43. Yasmin, S.; Abt, B.; Schrettl, M.; Moussa, T.A.; Werner, E.R.; Haas, H. The interplay between iron and zinc metabolism in *Aspergillus fumigatus*. *Fungal. Genet. Biol.* **2009**, *46*, 707–713. [CrossRef] [PubMed]
44. Schrettl, M.; Beckmann, N.; Varga, J.; Heinekamp, T.; Jacobsen, I.D.; Jochl, C.; Moussa, T.A.; Wang, S.; Gsaller, F.; Blatzer, M.; et al. HapX-mediated adaption to iron starvation is crucial for virulence of *Aspergillus fumigatus*. *PLoS Pathog.* **2010**, *6*, e1001124. [CrossRef] [PubMed]
45. Gsaller, F.; Hortschansky, P.; Beattie, S.R.; Klammer, V.; Tuppatsch, K.; Lechner, B.E.; Rietzschel, N.; Werner, E.R.; Vogan, A.A.; Chung, D.; et al. The Janus transcription factor HapX controls fungal adaptation to both iron starvation and iron excess. *EMBO J.* **2014**, *33*, 2261–2276. [CrossRef] [PubMed]
46. MacDiarmid, C.W.; Milanick, M.A.; Eide, D.J. Induction of the ZRC1 metal tolerance gene in zinc-limited yeast confers resistance to zinc shock. *J. Biol. Chem.* **2003**, *278*, 15065–15072. [CrossRef] [PubMed]
47. Miyabe, S.; Izawa, S.; Inoue, Y. Expression of *ZRC1* coding for suppressor of zinc toxicity is induced by zinc-starvation stress in Zap1-dependent fashion in *Saccharomyces cerevisiae*. *Biochem. Biophys. Res. Commun.* **2000**, *276*, 879–884. [CrossRef] [PubMed]
48. Blatzer, M.; Barker, B.M.; Willger, S.D.; Beckmann, N.; Blosser, S.J.; Cornish, E.J.; Mazurie, A.; Grahl, N.; Haas, H.; Cramer, R.A. SREBP coordinates iron and ergosterol homeostasis to mediate triazole drug and hypoxia responses in the human fungal pathogen *Aspergillus fumigatus*. *PLoS Genet.* **2011**, *7*, e1002374. [CrossRef] [PubMed]
49. Chung, D.; Barker, B.M.; Carey, C.C.; Merriman, B.; Werner, E.R.; Lechner, B.E.; Dhingra, S.; Cheng, C.; Xu, W.; Blosser, S.J.; et al. ChIP-seq and in vivo transcriptome analyses of the *Aspergillus fumigatus* SREBP SrbA reveals a new regulator of the fungal hypoxia response and virulence. *PLoS Pathog.* **2014**, *10*, e1004487. [CrossRef] [PubMed]
50. Vödisch, M.; Scherlach, K.; Winkler, R.; Hertweck, C.; Braun, H.P.; Roth, M.; Haas, H.; Werner, E.R.; Brakhage, A.A.; Kniemeyer, O. Analysis of the *Aspergillus fumigatus* proteome reveals metabolic changes and the activation of the pseurotin A biosynthesis gene cluster in response to hypoxia. *J. Proteome Res.* **2011**, *10*, 2508–2524. [CrossRef] [PubMed]
51. Maguire, S.L.; Wang, C.; Holland, L.M.; Brunel, F.; Neuveglise, C.; Nicaud, J.M.; Zavrel, M.; White, T.C.; Wolfe, K.H.; Butler, G. Zinc finger transcription factors displaced SREBP proteins as the major Sterol regulators during Saccharomycotina evolution. *PLoS Genet.* **2014**, *10*, e1004076. [CrossRef] [PubMed]
52. Baumann, K.; Dato, L.; Graf, A.B.; Frascotti, G.; Dragosits, M.; Porro, D.; Mattanovich, D.; Ferrer, P.; Branduardi, P. The impact of oxygen on the transcriptome of recombinant *S. cerevisiae* and *P. pastoris*—A comparative analysis. *BMC Genom.* **2012**, *12*, 218. [CrossRef] [PubMed]
53. Synnott, J.M.; Guida, A.; Mulhern-Haughey, S.; Higgins, D.G.; Butler, G. Regulation of the hypoxic response in *Candida albicans*. *Eukaryot. Cell* **2010**, *9*, 1734–1746. [CrossRef] [PubMed]
54. Kroll, K.; Pahtz, V.; Hillmann, F.; Vaknin, Y.; Schmidt-Heck, W.; Roth, M.; Jacobsen, I.D.; Osherov, N.; Brakhage, A.A.; Kniemeyer, O. Identification of hypoxia-inducible target genes of *Aspergillus fumigatus* by transcriptome analysis reveals cellular respiration as an important contributor to hypoxic survival. *Eukaryot. Cell* **2014**, *13*, 1241–1253. [CrossRef] [PubMed]
55. Camarasa, C.; Faucet, V.; Dequin, S. Role in anaerobiosis of the isoenzymes for *Saccharomyces cerevisiae* fumarate reductase encoded by OSM1 and FRDS1. *Yeast* **2007**, *24*, 391–401. [CrossRef] [PubMed]
56. Holmstrom, K.M.; Finkel, T. Cellular mechanisms and physiological consequences of redox-dependent signalling. *Nat. Rev. Mol. Cell Biol.* **2014**, *15*, 411–421. [CrossRef] [PubMed]
57. Messner, K.R.; Imlay, J.A. Mechanism of superoxide and hydrogen peroxide formation by fumarate reductase, succinate dehydrogenase, and aspartate oxidase. *J. Biol. Chem.* **2002**, *277*, 42563–42571. [CrossRef] [PubMed]
58. Chaiyen, P.; Fraaije, M.W.; Mattevi, A. The enigmatic reaction of flavins with oxygen. *Trends Biochem. Sci.* **2012**, *37*, 373–380. [CrossRef] [PubMed]
59. Korshunov, S.; Imlay, J.A. Two sources of endogenous hydrogen peroxide in *Escherichia coli*. *Mol. Microbiol.* **2010**, *75*, 1389–1401. [CrossRef] [PubMed]
60. Wu, C.Y.; Steffen, J.; Eide, D.J. Cytosolic superoxide dismutase (SOD1) is critical for tolerating the oxidative stress of zinc deficiency in yeast. *PLoS ONE* **2009**, *4*, e7061. [CrossRef] [PubMed]

61. MacDiarmid, C.W.; Taggart, J.; Kerdsomboon, K.; Kubisiak, M.; Panascharoen, S.; Schelble, K.; Eide, D.J. Peroxiredoxin chaperone activity is critical for protein homeostasis in zinc-deficient yeast. *J. Biol. Chem.* **2013**, *288*, 31313–31327. [CrossRef] [PubMed]
62. Bignell, E.; Cairns, T.C.; Throckmorton, K.; Nierman, W.C.; Keller, N.P. Secondary metabolite arsenal of an opportunistic pathogenic fungus. *Philos. Trans. R Soc. Lond. B Biol. Sci.* **2016**, *371*, 20160023. [CrossRef] [PubMed]
63. Scharf, D.H.; Remme, N.; Heinekamp, T.; Hortschansky, P.; Brakhage, A.A.; Hertweck, C. Transannular disulfide formation in gliotoxin biosynthesis and its role in self-resistance of the human pathogen *Aspergillus fumigatus*. *J. Am. Chem. Soc.* **2010**, *132*, 10136–10141. [CrossRef] [PubMed]
64. Schrettl, M.; Carberry, S.; Kavanagh, K.; Haas, H.; Jones, G.W.; O'Brien, J.; Nolan, A.; Stephens, J.; Fenelon, O.; Doyle, S. Self-protection against gliotoxin—A component of the gliotoxin biosynthetic cluster, GliT, completely protects *Aspergillus fumigatus* against exogenous gliotoxin. *PLoS Pathog.* **2010**, *6*, e1000952. [CrossRef] [PubMed]
65. Wang, D.N.; Toyotome, T.; Muraosa, Y.; Watanabe, A.; Wuren, T.; Bunsupa, S.; Aoyagi, K.; Yamazaki, M.; Takino, M.; Kamei, K. GliA in *Aspergillus fumigatus* is required for its tolerance to gliotoxin and affects the amount of extracellular and intracellular gliotoxin. *Med. Mycol.* **2014**, *52*, 506–518. [CrossRef] [PubMed]
66. Dolan, S.K.; Owens, R.A.; O'Keeffe, G.; Hammel, S.; Fitzpatrick, D.A.; Jones, G.W.; Doyle, S. Regulation of nonribosomal peptide synthesis: Bis-thiomethylation attenuates gliotoxin biosynthesis in *Aspergillus fumigatus*. *Chem. Biol.* **2014**, *21*, 999–1012. [CrossRef] [PubMed]
67. Owens, R.A.; O'Keeffe, G.; Smith, E.B.; Dolan, S.K.; Hammel, S.; Sheridan, K.J.; Fitzpatrick, D.A.; Keane, T.M.; Jones, G.W.; Doyle, S. Interplay between gliotoxin resistance, secretion, and the methyl/methionine cycle in *Aspergillus fumigatus*. *Eukaryot. Cell* **2015**, *14*, 941–957. [CrossRef] [PubMed]
68. Owens, R.A.; Hammel, S.; Sheridan, K.J.; Jones, G.W.; Doyle, S. A proteomic approach to investigating gene cluster expression and secondary metabolite functionality in *Aspergillus fumigatus*. *PLoS ONE* **2014**, *9*, e106942. [CrossRef] [PubMed]
69. Gallagher, L.; Owens, R.A.; Dolan, S.K.; O'Keeffe, G.; Schrettl, M.; Kavanagh, K.; Jones, G.W.; Doyle, S. The *Aspergillus fumigatus* protein GliK protects against oxidative stress and is essential for gliotoxin biosynthesis. *Eukaryot. Cell* **2012**, *11*, 1226–1238. [CrossRef] [PubMed]
70. Choi, H.S.; Shim, J.S.; Kim, J.A.; Kang, S.W.; Kwon, H.J. Discovery of gliotoxin as a new small molecule targeting thioredoxin redox system. *Biochem. Biophys. Res. Commun.* **2007**, *359*, 523–528. [CrossRef] [PubMed]
71. Lin, D.; Yin, X.; Wang, X.; Zhou, P.; Guo, F.B. Re-annotation of protein-coding genes in the genome of *Saccharomyces cerevisiae* based on support vector machines. *PLoS ONE* **2013**, *8*, e64477. [CrossRef] [PubMed]
72. Zhao, H.; Butler, E.; Rodgers, J.; Spizzo, T.; Duesterhoeft, S.; Eide, D. Regulation of zinc homeostasis in yeast by binding of the *ZAP1* transcriptional activator to zinc-responsive promoter elements. *J. Biol. Chem.* **1998**, *273*, 28713–28720. [CrossRef] [PubMed]
73. Pavletich, N.P.; Pabo, C.O. Zinc finger-DNA recognition: Crystal structure of a Zif268-DNA complex at 2.1 A. *Science* **1991**, *252*, 809–817. [CrossRef] [PubMed]
74. Nagaich, A.K.; Appella, E.; Harrington, R.E. DNA bending is essential for the site-specific recognition of DNA response elements by the DNA binding domain of the tumor suppressor protein p53. *J. Biol. Chem.* **1997**, *272*, 14842–14849. [CrossRef] [PubMed]
75. Bird, A.J.; Blankman, E.; Stillman, D.J.; Eide, D.J.; Winge, D.R. The Zap1 transcriptional activator also acts as a repressor by binding downstream of the TATA box in ZRT2. *EMBO J.* **2004**, *23*, 1123–1132. [CrossRef] [PubMed]
76. Bird, A.J.; Gordon, M.; Eide, D.J.; Winge, D.R. Repression of *ADH1* and *ADH3* during zinc deficiency by Zap1-induced intergenic RNA transcripts. *EMBO J.* **2006**, *25*, 5726–5734. [CrossRef] [PubMed]

11

New Concepts in Diagnostics for Invasive Mycoses: Non-Culture-Based Methodologies

Thomas F. Patterson * and J. Peter Donnelly

Division of Infectious Diseases, San Antonio Center for Medical Mycology, The University of Texas Health Science Center at San Antonio and the South Texas Veterans Health Care System, 7703 Floyd Curl Drive-MSC 7881, San Antonio, TX 78229-3900, USA; p.donnelly@usa.net

* Correspondence: patterson@uthscsa.edu

Abstract: Non-culture-based diagnostics have been developed to help establish an early diagnosis of invasive fungal infection. Studies have shown that these tests can significantly impact the diagnosis of infection in high risk patients. *Aspergillus* galactomannan EIA testing is well-recognized as an important adjunct to the diagnosis of invasive aspergillosis and can be detected in serum, bronchoalveolar lavage and other fluids. Galactomannan testing used along with PCR testing has been shown to be effective when integrated into care paths for high risk patients for both diagnoses and as a surrogate marker for outcome when used in serial testing. Beta-D-glucan assays are non-specific for several fungal genera including *Aspergillus* and *Candida* and in high risk patients have been an important tool to augment the diagnosis. Lateral flow technology using monoclonal antibodies to *Aspergillus* are available that allow rapid testing of clinical samples. While standard PCR for *Candida* remains investigational, T2 magnetic resonance allows for the rapid diagnosis of *Candida* species from blood cultures. *Aspergillus* PCR has been extensively validated with standardized approaches established for these methods and will be included in the diagnostic criteria in the revised European Organization for Research and Treatment of Cancer/Mycoses Study Group (EORTC-MSG) definitions. Finally, these non-culture-based tests can be used in combination to significantly increase the detection of invasive mycoses with the ultimate aim of establishing an early diagnosis of infection.

Keywords: invasive fungal infection; non-culture-based diagnostics; aspergillosis; candidiasis; *Aspergillus* PCR; galactomannan; lateral flow; beta-D-glucan; T2 *Candida*

---

1. Introduction

Invasive fungal infections remain a significant cause of morbidity and mortality in immunocompromised patients. The diagnosis of these infections is delayed due to lack of positive cultures from blood or from tissues, which require invasive procedures to obtain and are often difficult to perform in these critically ill patients. Non-culture-based diagnostics have been developed to help establish an early diagnosis of infection with the aim of allowing prompt initiation of antifungal therapy and improving patient outcomes.

Non-culture-based diagnostics have been developed for both *Aspergillus* and *Candida* along with other opportunistic fungal pathogens [1]. These assays have been largely focused on *Aspergillus* due to its prominence as the most common mold in immunocompromised hosts and for *Candida*, to augment diagnosis in the setting of negative or delayed positive blood cultures [2]. Assays are being developed for opportunistic pathogens including mucorales but are less widely available in clinical settings [3,4]. Additionally, for endemic fungi including *Coccidioides, Histoplasma,* and *Blastomyces* as well as *Cryptococcus*, non-culture-based methods for diagnosis are available but beyond the scope of this review.

Non-culture-based tests include galactomannan, which can be used in serum, bronchoalveolar lavage fluid and other samples; beta-D-glucan, a non-specific assay for *Aspergillus*, *Candida*, and other mycoses; lateral flow technology using an *Aspergillus* monoclonal antibody; and others including *Candida* PCR and T2 magnetic resonance. *Aspergillus* PCR has been extensively validated for standardized methodologies and is now included in the recent EORTC/MSG definition updates. In this review, the data supporting the use of clinically available non-culture-based methods for *Aspergillus* and *Candida* will be discussed and their utility alone and in combination will be summarized.

2. Risk Factors and Impact of Diagnostics

When approaching the use of these assays in the clinical setting, it is important to recognize the risk factors associated with invasive fungal infection, in order to improve the utility of their performance. The risk factors for invasive fungal infections have been extensively evaluated, as they significantly impact the incidence of invasive fungal infections and thus the performance of diagnostic assays. Herbrecht and colleagues outlined host factors for 'high risk patients', including those with allogeneic stem cell transplants, acute myelogenous leukemia/myelodysplastic syndrome, chronic granulomatous disease and others; those at 'intermediate' risk, including solid organ transplant recipients, other haematological malignancies, uncontrolled HIV infection, and others; while 'low risk' includes patients with autologous stem cell transplants, kidney transplant, solid tumors and others [5]. Additional risk factors influence the host condition, including innate immune defects; underlying conditions (neutropenia, graft vs. host disease, corticosteroid use, other biological agents, chemotherapy, etc); environmental factors and exposures; and other co-morbidities (diabetes, respiratory diseases and others) [5].

Fleming and colleagues established a risk stratification for patients with hematological malignancies. High risk patients are those with >10% incidence of invasive fungal disease, that is, patients with prolonged neutropenia ($<0.1 \times 10^9$/L for > 3 weeks or $<0.5 \times 10^9$/L for >5 weeks), unrelated, mismatched or cord blood donor SCT, graft vs. host disease (GVHD), high doses of corticosteroids, certain chemotherapeutic agents (high-dose cytarabine, fludarabine, alemtuzumab, and others), and certain hematological malignancies (acute myelogenous leukemia (AML) and acute lymphocytic leukemia (ALL)) [6]. An intermediate risk group with an incidence of invasive fungal disease of around 10% includes those with less profound neutropenia ($0.1–0.5 \times 10^9$/L for 3–5 weeks or $0.1–0.5 \times 10^9$/L for <3 weeks with lymphopenia), while low risk patients (~2% incidence of invasive fungal disease) would include autologous SCT and lymphoma [6]. Clearly, these patients with hematological malignancies have significant differences in risk for fungal infection and it becomes critically important to consider these differences when interpreting the clinical utility of these non-culture-based diagnostic tests, based on the prior probability of disease.

It is also critical to recognize the impact that diagnostic tests can have on underestimates of infection and the impact that diagnosis has on outcomes. Ceesay and colleagues evaluated a series of 203 patients with hematological malignancies using a strict diagnostic algorithm including a pre-treatment computed tomography of the chest, twice weekly serum galactomannan, and beta-D-glucan with suspicion of infection and tissue for diagnosis [7]. The series showed that the incidence of established infection rose from 10.5% with galactomannan alone to almost 20% with a combination of galactomannan and beta-D-glucan, and was 21.1% when all tests were combined. Furthermore, at 45%, the survival of those with proven/probable infection was significantly lower than those with possible disease, at 66%. The survival rate was 87% for those without infection ($p < 0.001$), supporting the importance of using these tools to establish a diagnosis of invasive fungal disease.

3. Galactomannan

The detection of galactomannan by EIA is a well-established and extensively studied method for the diagnosis of invasive aspergillosis [2,8,9]. Monoclonal antibody EB-A2 is used in a double sandwich ELISA to detect an antigenic side chain of β-1,5-galactofuronosyl with a linear core of mannan with α1,2 and α1,6 linkages [10]. Early studies by Maertens and others prior to the availability of anti-mold prophylaxis showed a sensitivity and specificity of 89% and 98%, respectively [11]. Subsequently, other studies showed more limited sensitivity (43–70%) but with specificity of 70–93% and studies confirmed the validation of a galactomannan index (GMI) of 0.5 as the threshold for positivity [12,13]. It was also appreciated that there were several sources for false-positive results including weakly positive samples, cross-reactivity with other fungi and antibiotics (such as pipercillin-tazobactam, which has now been resolved) [14]. Other sources of false-positives such as dietary reactivity, laboratory contamination or fluids for bronchoalveolar lavage (such as plasmalyte which also appears to have resolved) may continue [14–19]. A number of other factors may affect the performance of the galactomannan assay, including biological factors (such as site of infection, *Aspergillus* species, prior use of antifungals, renal clearance, hepatic metabolism, underlying condition, storage of the samples, and others) and epidemiological factors (such as the prevalence of disease, sampling strategies and definitions for positive results) [17]. An important study by Duarte and colleagues showed the dramatic impact of antifungal prophylaxis on the strategy of serial sampling [20]. In this study the positive predictive value dropped to 11.8%, but was still useful with a positive predictive value of 89.6% when used for the diagnosis of invasive fungal disease on suspicion of disease [20].

Galactomannan testing in bronchoalveolar (BAL) lavage fluid is very useful for establishing a diagnosis of infection. This method is more sensitive than cytology, culture, transbronchial biopsy or serum galactomannan testing [21]. Galactomannan detection increased the sensitivity from serum from 47% to 85% from BAL, with a positive predictive value approaching 100% and with a BAL GMI of <0.5, indicating that it is useful to exclude the diagnosis in high risk patients with hematological malignancies [22,23]. On the other hand, in solid organ transplant patients, false positive results were more likely in lung transplant patients and in those colonized with *Aspergillus* [24]. The utility of galactomannan has been shown to improve in combination with PCR. Reinwald and colleagues showed that positivity from BAL of both galactomannan (at a GMI of >0.5) with positive PCR results highly supported the diagnosis [25]. Notably, the consensus regarding the cutoff value for a positive BAL galactomannan is still lacking, as performance will also vary in different patient settings (i.e., hematological malignancy, solid organ transplantation, intensive care units, etc.) so that a higher cutoff threshold (GMI > 1.0) may correlate with better diagnostic utility [26,27].

Galactomannan along with PCR was evaluated in a diagnostic vs. empirical therapy approach by Morrissey and colleagues [28]. In this study, empirical antifungal therapy was reduced from 32% in the standard diagnosis group to 15% in the biomarker diagnosis group, even though the rate of proven/probable disease was increased from 1% to 15% [28]. Mortality was 15% in the standard diagnosis group and 10% in the biomarker group [28]. In this study, 10/39 (26%) of the patients receiving empirical antifungal therapy would have been diagnosed with invasive aspergillosis a median of 4 days earlier and 5/6 (83%) of those who died from invasive aspergillosis would have been diagnosed a median of 7 days earlier.

Finally, serial galactomannan measurements can also be used for the assessment of outcomes. Chai and colleagues showed that a GMI reduction of >35% between baseline and week 1 predicted a satisfactory response in patients enrolled in the Global Voriconazole Aspergillosis trial [29]. Poorer responses occurred with increasing GMI after 2 weeks. Similarly, outcomes are better in patients who become GMI negative during their course of treatment [9,30].

4. Beta-D-Glucan

Testing with (1-3)-β-D-glucan activates *Limulus* amebocyte lysate through factor G initiation of the complement cascade [31]. The output can be measured using a chromogenic substrate (Fungitell (Associates of Cape Cod, Falmouth, MA) and others or by turbidity after gel clot (Wako Pure Chemical Industries, Osaka, Japan) [31]. These assays detect a number of important fungal genera including *Aspergillus, Candida, Trichosporon, Fusarium,* and *Exerohilum* but not mucorales or cryptococcosis [32]. Early studies showed the value of the assay in candidemia and in invasive fungal disease in patients with acute leukemia, which allowed regulatory clearance as well as inclusion in the European Organization for Research and Treatment of Cancer/Mycoses Study Group (EORTC-MSG) definitions for fungal infection [33,34].

More recent studies in invasive candidiasis have evaluated the role of beta-D-glucan with *Candida*, real-time PCR and blood cultures [35]. In this study, both PCR and beta-D-glucan were more sensitive for deep seated *Candida* infection: 88% and 62%, respectively, vs. 17% for blood cultures. Beta-D-glucan was shown to anticipate the diagnosis of blood culture-negative intraabdominal candidiasis and may be an important adjunct to that diagnosis [36].

Beta-D-glucan testing has also shown utility in specific clinical settings. In pneumocystis pneumonia, beta-D-glucan levels are frequently extremely elevated (>500 pg/mL) so that in a likely clinical setting more invasive testing might be obviated [37]. In addition, during an outbreak of fungal meningitis due to contaminated steroids, it was recognized that *Exserohilum* spp. (the etiological cause of the outbreak) produces high levels of beta-D-glucan [38]. It was subsequently shown that beta-D-glucan is highly sensitive for the diagnosis and is correlated with response to therapy [38].

5. Lateral Flow Technology in Invasive Aspergillosis

Lateral flow assays for invasive aspergillosis offer the potential for a rapid diagnosis, ease of performance and point of care use. A murine monoclonal antibody, JF4, binds to an extracellular glycoprotein antigen secreted during the growth of *Aspergillus* and distinguishes between hyphae and conidia [39]. Earlier and more consistent detection compared to beta-D-glucan or galactomannan was seen in pre-clinical models [39–41]. A prototype lateral flow device (LFD) was evaluated in high risk hematological malignancy patients and was shown to improve the diagnostic yield, especially when combined with galactomannan and PCR [42–44]. In BAL samples this assay had an overall sensitivity of 73% and a specificity of 90% [45,46]. A recent European conformity (CE)-marked LFD (OLM Diagnostics, Newcastle-on-Tyne, UK) showed similar sensitivity to the prototype device of 71%, but with an improved sensitivity of 100% [46]. Another lateral flow assay for *Aspergillus* (IMMY, Norman, OK, USA) was compared in a small study to the LFD in BAL fluid and showed similar sensitivity and specificities of 89% and 88% [47].

6. T2 Magnetic Resonance

While real-time PCR for *Candida* remains investigational, the use of T2 magnetic resonance using nanoparticles has been cleared for clinical use (T2 *Candida*, T2 Biosystems, Lexington, MA, USA) [48–50]. The assay requires a dedicated instrument and detects *Candida* species directly from blood samples, but unlike blood cultures it does not require viable organisms [51]. The assay detects five major *Candida* species that are grouped based on typical susceptibility patterns. Using spiked blood samples, it was shown that this method could detect *C. albicans/C. tropicalis, C. parapsilosis*, and *C. krusei/C. glabrata* at a sensitivity of 91.1% with a time to positivity of 4.4 hrs and a limit of detection of 1–3 CFU/mL [52]. In a follow-up study of patients with candidemia, follow-up blood cultures were compared with the T2 *Candida* assay and showed T2 *Candida* positivity in 45% of the follow-up blood cultures compared to 24% with standard culture techniques. These results suggest that this method could be used to detect candidemia in patients who are receiving empirical antifungal therapy and could be very useful in allowing empirical therapy to be discontinued in patients with negative results [51]. In addition, T2 shortened the time to positivity to <3 h and identified a bloodstream infection not detected by blood cultures, while retaining sensitivity during antifungal therapy.

7. *Aspergillus* PCR Development and Standardization

PCR for *Aspergillus* species has been evaluated for more than 25 years to fulfil the mycological criteria for the diagnosis of invasive fungal disease [53]. The EORTC/MSG clinical definitions were published in 2002 and revised in 2008 and provided important guidelines for criteria of proven, probable and possible invasive fungal disease, in order to facilitate clinical research including drug trials, epidemiology, and diagnostic tests [54,55]. These were not intended as a guide to clinical practice, but the elements of the definitions have been widely used as an adjunct to clinical management. The 2008 definitions defined proven disease when fungi are detected in specimens from a sterile body site or in a biopsy. In contrast, possible and probable disease both require a host factor and a clinical feature. Possible disease is assigned in the absence of any mycological criteria. Probable disease is assigned when the mycological criteria are met by direct mycology–cytology, direct microscopy or culture, or indirectly, by the detection of galactomannan and beta-D-glucan, but not PCR, due to the lack of standardization and validation [55]. Subsequently, the European *Aspergillus* PCR Initiative (EAPCRI) was established to develop a standard for *Aspergillus* PCR methodology so that PCR could be incorporated into future consensus definitions for invasive fungal disease [56].

Initial efforts included a systemic review published in 2009 of more than 10,000 blood, serum or plasma samples from 1618 patients at risk for *Aspergillus* and concluded at that time that two positive tests were required to confirm the diagnosis due to the specificity of these tests and a single PCR-negative result was sufficient to exclude a diagnosis of invasive aspergillosis [57]. However, it was also noted that there was a lack of homogeneity of the PCR methods so that subsequent collaboration aimed at a formal validation of that process.

Aspergillus standardization was evaluated through a collaboration of 21 European medical centers [56]. While specific protocols were not developed, *compliant* and *non-compliant* centers were noted. Twelve centers used 10 different DNA extraction protocols and nine different PCR amplification procedures that were compliant. Nine centers used seven extraction protocols and seven different PCR amplification procedures that were noncompliant. The sensitivity, specificity, and diagnostic odds ratio (DOR) of compliant centers were 88.7%, 91.6%, and 119.9, respectively, for non-compliant centers these were and 57.7%, 77.2%, and 8.9, respectively. These results were highly statistically significant for sensitivity ($p = 0.008$) and DOR ($p = 0.006$). The factors with the most influence on PCR included compliance with the extraction method, bead beating of the sample, and use of an internal control PCR. This led to recommendations for the whole blood PCR of >3 mL of blood, bead-beating to lyse fungal cells, a real time PCR platform with multi-copy targets with specific probes, internal control PCR and others [56]. Subsequent work showed that most of the *Aspergillus* protocols used to test serum generated satisfactory analytical performance and that the testing serum required less standardization [58]. Additional evaluation evaluated plasma vs. serum and showed improved sensitivity with plasma with PCR positivity occurring earlier, while maintaining methodological simplicity [59].

An extensive Cochrane study was performed for the diagnosis of invasive aspergillosis in immunocompromised people [60]. The studies included were those that compared the results of blood PCR tests with reference to the EORTC/MSG standard and included false positive, true positive, false negative and true negative results and that evaluated the test(s) prospectively in cohorts from patients at high risk for invasive aspergillosis. Overall, 1672 records were identified and 155 were screened to eventually include 18 studies for the meta-analysis [60]. For one single PCR specimen a sensitivity of 80.5% and a specificity of 78.5 were reported in 17 studies. For two or more PCR specimens the sensitivity decreased to 57.9% and the specificity increased to 96.2%. The authors concluded that PCR shows moderate diagnostic accuracy when used for screening and has a high negative predictive value (NPV) that allows the diagnosis of invasive aspergillosis to be ruled out. A poor positive predictive value (PPV) when the prevalence of disease is low, limits the ability to rule in a diagnosis. Since other non-culture-based methods (such as galactomannan) detect different aspects of the disease, combinations of both together are likely to be more useful. PCR used in combination with galactomannan has been shown to improve the detection of invasive aspergillosis before detection by CT findings in high risk hematological patients [61] and to improve the sensitivity and specificity of testing [62]. In a randomized controlled trial, a combined monitoring strategy based on serum galactomannan and *Aspergillus* PCR was associated with an earlier diagnosis of invasive aspergillosis [63]. Robust recommendations for plasma and serum are available that establish a 'standard for PCR' but not a 'standard method for PCR' so that *Aspergillus* PCR will be included in the revised EORTC/MSG consensus definitions [64].

7. Clinical Utility and Summary

The importance of assessing risk and using non-culture-based diagnostics for invasive fungal disease is clear. Several methods have been evaluated and validated for clinical use including galactomannan, beta-D-glucan, lateral flow technology, T2 magnetic resonance, PCR and others. Non-culture-based biomarkers provide more reliable negative than positive predictive values. When the prevalence of disease is higher than 15%, negative test results exclude the diagnosis, while positive test results include the diagnosis. Clinicians and laboratories need to consider when a test is being requested for screening (when a patient is at risk for invasive fungal disease) as opposed to diagnosis (in which there is a high clinical suspicion of an invasive fungal disease), which will have a substantially higher pre-test probability. Finally, combinations of these tests may provide the greatest benefit in establishing a diagnosis of invasive fungal disease.

Author Contributions: Conceptualization, writing—review and editing, T.F.P and J.P.D.

References

1. Mikulska, M.; Furfaro, E.; Viscoli, C. Non-cultural methods for the diagnosis of invasive fungal disease. *Expert Rev. Anti Infect. Ther.* **2015**, *13*, 103–117. [CrossRef] [PubMed]
2. Hope, W.W.; Walsh, T.J.; Denning, D.W. Laboratory diagnosis of invasive aspergillosis. *Lancet Infect. Dis.* **2005**, *5*, 609–622. [CrossRef]
3. Baldin, C.; Soliman, S.S.M.; Jeon, H.H.; Alkhazraji, S.; Gebremariam, T.; Gu, Y.; Bruno, V.M.; Cornely, O.A.; Leather, H.L.; Sugrue, M.W.; et al. Pcr-based approach targeting mucorales-specific gene family for diagnosis of mucormycosis. *J. Clin. Microbiol.* **2018**, *56*. [CrossRef] [PubMed]
4. Scherer, E.; Iriart, X.; Bellanger, A.P.; Dupont, D.; Guitard, J.; Gabriel, F.; Cassaing, S.; Charpentier, E.; Guenounou, S.; Cornet, M.; et al. Quantitative pcr (qpcr) detection of mucorales DNA in bronchoalveolar lavage fluid to diagnose pulmonary mucormycosis. *J. Clin. Microbiol.* **2018**, *56*. [CrossRef] [PubMed]
5. Herbrecht, R.; Bories, P.; Moulin, J.C.; Ledoux, M.P.; Letscher-Bru, V. Risk stratification for invasive aspergillosis in immunocompromised patients. *Ann. N. Y. Acad. Sci.* **2012**, *1272*, 23–30. [CrossRef]
6. Fleming, S.; Yannakou, C.K.; Haeusler, G.M.; Clark, J.; Grigg, A.; Heath, C.H.; Bajel, A.; van Hal, S.J.; Chen, S.C.; Milliken, S.T.; et al. Consensus guidelines for antifungal prophylaxis in haematological malignancy and haemopoietic stem cell transplantation, 2014. *Intern. Med. J.* **2014**, *44*, 1283–1297. [CrossRef] [PubMed]
7. Ceesay, M.M.; Desai, S.R.; Berry, L.; Cleverley, J.; Kibbler, C.C.; Pomplun, S.; Nicholson, A.G.; Douiri, A.; Wade, J.; Smith, M.; et al. A comprehensive diagnostic approach using galactomannan, targeted beta-d-glucan, baseline computerized tomography and biopsy yields a significant burden of invasive fungal disease in at risk haematology patients. *Br. J. Haematol.* **2015**, *168*, 219–229. [CrossRef] [PubMed]
8. Miceli, M.H.; Maertens, J. Role of non-culture-based tests, with an emphasis on galactomannan testing for the diagnosis of invasive aspergillosis. *Semin. Respir. Crit. Care Med.* **2015**, *36*, 650–661.
9. Mercier, T.; Guldentops, E.; Lagrou, K.; Maertens, J. Galactomannan, a surrogate marker for outcome in invasive aspergillosis: Finally coming of age. *Front. Microbiol.* **2018**, *9*, 661. [CrossRef]
10. Stynen, D.; Goris, A.; Sarfati, J.; Latge, J.P. A new sensitive sandwich enzyme-linked immunosorbent assay to detect galactofuran in patients with invasive aspergillosis. *J. Clin. Microbiol.* **1995**, *33*, 497–500.
11. Maertens, J.; Verhaegen, J.; Lagrou, K.; Van Eldere, J.; Boogaerts, M. Screening for circulating galactomannan as a noninvasive diagnostic tool for invasive aspergillosis in prolonged neutropenic patients and stem cell transplantation recipients: A prospective validation. *Blood* **2001**, *97*, 1604–1610. [CrossRef] [PubMed]

12. Marr, K.A.; Balajee, S.A.; McLaughlin, L.; Tabouret, M.; Bentsen, C.; Walsh, T.J. Detection of galactomannan antigenemia by enzyme immunoassay for the diagnosis of invasive aspergillosis: Variables that affect performance. *J. Infect. Dis.* **2004**, *190*, 641–649. [CrossRef] [PubMed]
13. Herbrecht, R.; Letscher-Bru, V.; Oprea, C.; Lioure, B.; Waller, J.; Campos, F.; Villard, O.; Liu, K.L.; Natarajan-Ame, S.; Lutz, P.; et al. Aspergillus galactomannan detection in the diagnosis of invasive aspergillosis in cancer patients. *J. Clin. Oncol.* **2002**, *20*, 1898–1906. [CrossRef] [PubMed]
14. Mikulska, M.; Furfaro, E.; Del Bono, V.; Raiola, A.M.; Ratto, S.; Bacigalupo, A.; Viscoli, C. Piperacillin/tazobactam (tazocin) seems to be no longer responsible for false-positive results of the galactomannan assay. *J. Antimicrob. Chemother.* **2012**, *67*, 1746–1748. [CrossRef] [PubMed]
15. Machetti, M.; Majabo, M.J.; Furfaro, E.; Solari, N.; Novelli, A.; Cafiero, F.; Viscoli, C. Kinetics of galactomannan in surgical patients receiving perioperative piperacillin/tazobactam prophylaxis. *J. Antimicrob. Chemother.* **2006**, *58*, 806–810. [CrossRef] [PubMed]
16. Maertens, J.; Theunissen, K.; Verhoef, G.; Van Eldere, J. False-positive aspergillus galactomannan antigen test results. *Clin. Infect. Dis.* **2004**, *39*, 289–290. [CrossRef]
17. Mennink-Kersten, M.A.; Donnelly, J.P.; Verweij, P.E. Detection of circulating galactomannan for the diagnosis and management of invasive aspergillosis. *Lancet Infect. Dis.* **2004**, *4*, 349–357. [CrossRef]
18. Spriet, I.; Lagrou, K.; Maertens, J.; Willems, L.; Wilmer, A.; Wauters, J. Plasmalyte: No longer a culprit in causing false-positive galactomannan test results. *J. Clin. Microbiol.* **2016**, *54*, 795–797. [CrossRef]
19. Viscoli, C.; Machetti, M.; Cappellano, P.; Bucci, B.; Bruzzi, P.; Van Lint, M.T.; Bacigalupo, A. False-positive galactomannan platelia aspergillus test results for patients receiving piperacillin-tazobactam. *Clin. Infect. Dis.* **2004**, *38*, 913–916. [CrossRef]
20. Duarte, R.F.; Sanchez-Ortega, I.; Cuesta, I.; Arnan, M.; Patino, B.; Fernandez de Sevilla, A.; Gudiol, C.; Ayats, J.; Cuenca-Estrella, M. Serum galactomannan-based early detection of invasive aspergillosis in hematology patients receiving effective antimold prophylaxis. *Clin. Infect. Dis.* **2014**, *59*, 1696–1702. [CrossRef]
21. Nguyen, M.H.; Leather, H.; Clancy, C.J.; Cline, C.; Jantz, M.A.; Kulkarni, V.; Wheat, L.J.; Wingard, J.R. Galactomannan testing in bronchoalveolar lavage fluid facilitates the diagnosis of invasive pulmonary aspergillosis in patients with hematologic malignancies and stem cell transplant recipients. *Biol. Blood Marrow Transplant.* **2011**, *17*, 1043–1050. [CrossRef] [PubMed]
22. Becker, M.J.; Lugtenburg, E.J.; Cornelissen, J.J.; Van Der Schee, C.; Hoogsteden, H.C.; De Marie, S. Galactomannan detection in computerized tomography-based broncho-alveolar lavage fluid and serum in haematological patients at risk for invasive pulmonary aspergillosis. *Br. J. Haematol.* **2003**, *121*, 448–457. [CrossRef] [PubMed]
23. D'Haese, J.; Theunissen, K.; Vermeulen, E.; Schoemans, H.; De Vlieger, G.; Lammertijn, L.; Meersseman, P.; Meersseman, W.; Lagrou, K.; Maertens, J. Detection of galactomannan in bronchoalveolar lavage fluid samples of patients at risk for invasive pulmonary aspergillosis: Analytical and clinical validity. *J. Clin. Microbiol.* **2012**, *50*, 1258–1263. [CrossRef] [PubMed]
24. Husain, S.; Paterson, D.L.; Studer, S.M.; Crespo, M.; Pilewski, J.; Durkin, M.; Wheat, J.L.; Johnson, B.; McLaughlin, L.; Bentsen, C.; et al. Aspergillus galactomannan antigen in the bronchoalveolar lavage fluid for the diagnosis of invasive aspergillosis in lung transplant recipients. *Transplantation* **2007**, *83*, 1330–1336. [CrossRef] [PubMed]
25. Reinwald, M.; Spiess, B.; Heinz, W.J.; Vehreschild, J.J.; Lass-Florl, C.; Kiehl, M.; Schultheis, B.; Krause, S.W.; Wolf, H.H.; Bertz, H.; et al. Diagnosing pulmonary aspergillosis in patients with hematological malignancies: A multicenter prospective evaluation of an aspergillus pcr assay and a galactomannan elisa in bronchoalveolar lavage samples. *Eur. J. Haematol.* **2012**, *89*, 120–127. [CrossRef] [PubMed]
26. Maertens, J.; Maertens, V.; Theunissen, K.; Meersseman, W.; Meersseman, P.; Meers, S.; Verbeken, E.; Verhoef, G.; Van Eldere, J.; Lagrou, K. Bronchoalveolar lavage fluid galactomannan for the diagnosis of invasive pulmonary aspergillosis in patients with hematologic diseases. *Clin. Infect. Dis.* **2009**, *49*, 1688–1693. [CrossRef] [PubMed]
27. Clancy, C.J.; Jaber, R.A.; Leather, H.L.; Wingard, J.R.; Staley, B.; Wheat, L.J.; Cline, C.L.; Rand, K.H.; Schain, D.; Baz, M.; et al. Bronchoalveolar lavage galactomannan in diagnosis of invasive pulmonary aspergillosis among solid-organ transplant recipients. *J. Clin. Microbiol.* **2007**, *45*, 1759–1765. [CrossRef]

28. Morrissey, C.O.; Chen, S.C.; Sorrell, T.C.; Milliken, S.; Bardy, P.G.; Bradstock, K.F.; Szer, J.; Halliday, C.L.; Gilroy, N.M.; Moore, J.; et al. Galactomannan and pcr versus culture and histology for directing use of antifungal treatment for invasive aspergillosis in high-risk haematology patients: A randomised controlled trial. *Lancet Infect. Dis.* **2013**, *13*, 519–528. [CrossRef]
29. Chai, L.Y.; Kullberg, B.J.; Johnson, E.M.; Teerenstra, S.; Khin, L.W.; Vonk, A.G.; Maertens, J.; Lortholary, O.; Donnelly, P.J.; Schlamm, H.T.; et al. Early serum galactomannan trend as a predictor of outcome of invasive aspergillosis. *J. Clin. Microbiol.* **2012**, *50*, 2330–2336. [CrossRef]
30. Maertens, J.; Buve, K.; Theunissen, K.; Meersseman, W.; Verbeken, E.; Verhoef, G.; Van Eldere, J.; Lagrou, K. Galactomannan serves as a surrogate endpoint for outcome of pulmonary invasive aspergillosis in neutropenic hematology patients. *Cancer* **2009**, *115*, 355–362. [CrossRef]
31. Obayashi, T.; Negishi, K.; Suzuki, T.; Funata, N. Reappraisal of the serum (1–>3)-beta-d-glucan assay for the diagnosis of invasive fungal infections–a study based on autopsy cases from 6 years. *Clin. Infect. Dis.* **2008**, *46*, 1864–1870. [CrossRef] [PubMed]
32. Odabasi, Z.; Paetznick, V.L.; Rodriguez, J.R.; Chen, E.; McGinnis, M.R.; Ostrosky-Zeichner, L. Differences in beta-glucan levels in culture supernatants of a variety of fungi. *Med. Mycol.* **2006**, *44*, 267–272. [CrossRef] [PubMed]
33. Odabasi, Z.; Mattiuzzi, G.; Estey, E.; Kantarjian, H.; Saeki, F.; Ridge, R.J.; Ketchum, P.A.; Finkelman, M.A.; Rex, J.H.; Ostrosky-Zeichner, L. Beta-d-glucan as a diagnostic adjunct for invasive fungal infections: Validation, cutoff development, and performance in patients with acute myelogenous leukemia and myelodysplastic syndrome. *Clin. Infect. Dis.* **2004**, *39*, 199–205. [CrossRef]
34. Ostrosky-Zeichner, L.; Alexander, B.D.; Kett, D.H.; Vazquez, J.; Pappas, P.G.; Saeki, F.; Ketchum, P.A.; Wingard, J.; Schiff, R.; Tamura, H.; et al. Multicenter clinical evaluation of the (1–>3) beta-d-glucan assay as an aid to diagnosis of fungal infections in humans. *Clin. Infect. Dis.* **2005**, *41*, 654–659. [CrossRef]
35. Nguyen, M.H.; Wissel, M.C.; Shields, R.K.; Salomoni, M.A.; Hao, B.; Press, E.G.; Shields, R.M.; Cheng, S.; Mitsani, D.; Vadnerkar, A.; et al. Performance of candida real-time polymerase chain reaction, beta-d-glucan assay, and blood cultures in the diagnosis of invasive candidiasis. *Clin. Infect. Dis.* **2012**, *54*, 1240–1248. [CrossRef] [PubMed]
36. Tissot, F.; Lamoth, F.; Hauser, P.M.; Orasch, C.; Fluckiger, U.; Siegemund, M.; Zimmerli, S.; Calandra, T.; Bille, J.; Eggimann, P.; et al. Beta-glucan antigenemia anticipates diagnosis of blood culture-negative intraabdominal candidiasis. *Am. J. Respir. Crit. Care Med.* **2013**, *188*, 1100–1109. [CrossRef] [PubMed]
37. Koo, S.; Baden, L.R.; Marty, F.M. Post-diagnostic kinetics of the (1 –> 3)-beta-d-glucan assay in invasive aspergillosis, invasive candidiasis and pneumocystis jirovecii pneumonia. *Clin. Microbiol. Infect.* **2012**, *18*, E122–E127. [CrossRef]
38. Litvintseva, A.P.; Lindsley, M.D.; Gade, L.; Smith, R.; Chiller, T.; Lyons, J.L.; Thakur, K.T.; Zhang, S.X.; Grgurich, D.E.; Kerkering, T.M.; et al. Utility of (1-3)-beta-d-glucan testing for diagnostics and monitoring response to treatment during the multistate outbreak of fungal meningitis and other infections. *Clin. Infect. Dis.* **2014**, *58*, 622–630. [CrossRef]
39. Thornton, C.R. Development of an immunochromatographic lateral-flow device for rapid serodiagnosis of invasive aspergillosis. *Clin. Vaccine Immunol.* **2008**, *15*, 1095–1105. [CrossRef]
40. Thornton, C.R. Breaking the mould—novel diagnostic and therapeutic strategies for invasive pulmonary aspergillosis in the immune deficient patient. *Expert Rev. Clin. Immunol.* **2014**, *10*, 771–780. [CrossRef]
41. Wiederhold, N.P.; Thornton, C.R.; Najvar, L.K.; Kirkpatrick, W.R.; Bocanegra, R.; Patterson, T.F. Comparison of lateral flow technology and galactomannan and (1->3)-beta-d-glucan assays for detection of invasive pulmonary aspergillosis. *Clin. Vaccine Immunol.* **2009**, *16*, 1844–1846. [CrossRef] [PubMed]
42. Eigl, S.; Prattes, J.; Lackner, M.; Willinger, B.; Spiess, B.; Reinwald, M.; Selitsch, B.; Meilinger, M.; Neumeister, P.; Reischies, F.; et al. Multicenter evaluation of a lateral-flow device test for diagnosing invasive pulmonary aspergillosis in icu patients. *Crit. Care* **2015**, *19*, 178. [CrossRef] [PubMed]
43. Hoenigl, M.; Prattes, J.; Spiess, B.; Wagner, J.; Prueller, F.; Raggam, R.B.; Posch, V.; Duettmann, W.; Hoenigl, K.; Wolfler, A.; et al. Performance of galactomannan, beta-D-glucan, aspergillus lateral-flow device, conventional culture, and pcr tests with bronchoalveolar lavage fluid for diagnosis of invasive pulmonary aspergillosis. *J. Clin. Microbiol.* **2014**, *52*, 2039–2045. [CrossRef] [PubMed]

44. White, P.L.; Parr, C.; Thornton, C.; Barnes, R.A. Evaluation of real-time pcr, galactomannan enzyme-linked immunosorbent assay (elisa), and a novel lateral-flow device for diagnosis of invasive aspergillosis. *J. Clin. Microbiol.* **2013**, *51*, 1510–1516. [CrossRef] [PubMed]
45. Willinger, B.; Lackner, M.; Lass-Florl, C.; Prattes, J.; Posch, V.; Selitsch, B.; Eschertzhuber, S.; Honigl, K.; Koidl, C.; Sereinigg, M.; et al. Bronchoalveolar lavage lateral-flow device test for invasive pulmonary aspergillosis in solid organ transplant patients: A semiprospective multicenter study. *Transplantation* **2014**, *98*, 898–902. [CrossRef] [PubMed]
46. Hoenigl, M.; Eigl, S.; Heldt, S.; Duettmann, W.; Thornton, C.; Prattes, J. Clinical evaluation of the newly formatted lateral-flow device for invasive pulmonary aspergillosis. *Mycoses* **2018**, *61*, 40–43. [CrossRef]
47. Jenks, J.D.; Mehta, S.R.; Taplitz, R.; Aslam, S.; Reed, S.L.; Hoenigl, M. Point-of care diagnosis of invasive aspergillosis in in non-neutropenic patients: Aspergillus galactomannan lateral flow assay versus aspergillus-specific lateral flow device test in bronchoalveolar lavage. *Mycoses* **2018**. [CrossRef]
48. Clancy, C.J.; Nguyen, M.H. T2 magnetic resonance for the diagnosis of bloodstream infections: Charting a path forward. *J. Antimicrob. Chemother.* **2018**, *73*, iv2–iv5. [CrossRef]
49. Clancy, C.J.; Nguyen, M.H. Non-culture diagnostics for invasive candidiasis: Promise and unintended consequences. *J. Fungi (Basel)* **2018**, *4*, 27. [CrossRef]
50. Zacharioudakis, I.M.; Zervou, F.N.; Mylonakis, E. T2 magnetic resonance assay: Overview of available data and clinical implications. *J. Fungi (Basel)* **2018**, *4*, 45. [CrossRef]
51. Clancy, C.J.; Pappas, P.G.; Vazquez, J.; Judson, M.A.; Kontoyiannis, D.P.; Thompson, G.R., 3rd; Garey, K.W.; Reboli, A.; Greenberg, R.N.; Apewokin, S.; et al. Detecting infections rapidly and easily for candidemia trial, part 2 (direct2): A prospective, multicenter study of the t2candida panel. *Clin. Infect. Dis.* **2018**, *66*, 1678–1686. [CrossRef]
52. Mylonakis, E.; Clancy, C.J.; Ostrosky-Zeichner, L.; Garey, K.W.; Alangaden, G.J.; Vazquez, J.A.; Groeger, J.S.; Judson, M.A.; Vinagre, Y.M.; Heard, S.O.; et al. T2 magnetic resonance assay for the rapid diagnosis of candidemia in whole blood: A clinical trial. *Clin. Infect. Dis.* **2015**, *60*, 892–899. [CrossRef] [PubMed]
53. Spreadbury, C.; Holden, D.; Aufauvre-Brown, A.; Bainbridge, B.; Cohen, J. Detection of aspergillus fumigatus by polymerase chain reaction. *J. Clin. Microbiol.* **1993**, *31*, 615–621. [PubMed]
54. Ascioglu, S.; Rex, J.H.; de Pauw, B.; Bennett, J.E.; Bille, J.; Crokaert, F.; Denning, D.W.; Donnelly, J.P.; Edwards, J.E.; Erjavec, Z.; et al. Defining opportunistic invasive fungal infections in immunocompromised patients with cancer and hematopoietic stem cell transplants: An international consensus. *Clin. Infect. Dis.* **2002**, *34*, 7–14. [CrossRef] [PubMed]
55. De Pauw, B.; Walsh, T.J.; Donnelly, J.P.; Stevens, D.A.; Edwards, J.E.; Calandra, T.; Pappas, P.G.; Maertens, J.; Lortholary, O.; Kauffman, C.A.; et al. Revised definitions of invasive fungal disease from the european organization for research and treatment of cancer/invasive fungal infections cooperative group and the national institute of allergy and infectious diseases mycoses study group (eortc/msg) consensus group. *Clin. Infect. Dis.* **2008**, *46*, 1813–1821.
56. White, P.L.; Bretagne, S.; Klingspor, L.; Melchers, W.J.; McCulloch, E.; Schulz, B.; Finnstrom, N.; Mengoli, C.; Barnes, R.A.; Donnelly, J.P.; et al. Aspergillus pcr: One step closer to standardization. *J. Clin. Microbiol.* **2010**, *48*, 1231–1240. [CrossRef]
57. Mengoli, C.; Cruciani, M.; Barnes, R.A.; Loeffler, J.; Donnelly, J.P. Use of pcr for diagnosis of invasive aspergillosis: Systematic review and meta-analysis. *Lancet Infect. Dis.* **2009**, *9*, 89–96. [CrossRef]
58. White, P.L.; Mengoli, C.; Bretagne, S.; Cuenca-Estrella, M.; Finnstrom, N.; Klingspor, L.; Melchers, W.J.; McCulloch, E.; Barnes, R.A.; Donnelly, J.P.; et al. Evaluation of aspergillus pcr protocols for testing serum specimens. *J. Clin. Microbiol.* **2011**, *49*, 3842–3848. [CrossRef]
59. White, P.L.; Barnes, R.A.; Springer, J.; Klingspor, L.; Cuenca-Estrella, M.; Morton, C.O.; Lagrou, K.; Bretagne, S.; Melchers, W.J.; Mengoli, C.; et al. Clinical performance of aspergillus pcr for testing serum and plasma: A study by the european aspergillus pcr initiative. *J. Clin. Microbiol.* **2015**, *53*, 2832–2837. [CrossRef]
60. Cruciani, M.; Mengoli, C.; Loeffler, J.; Donnelly, P.; Barnes, R.; Jones, B.L.; Klingspor, L.; Morton, O.; Maertens, J. Polymerase chain reaction blood tests for the diagnosis of invasive aspergillosis in immunocompromised people. *Cochrane Database Syst. Rev.* **2015**, CD009551. [CrossRef]
61. Rogers, T.R.; Morton, C.O.; Springer, J.; Conneally, E.; Heinz, W.; Kenny, C.; Frost, S.; Einsele, H.; Loeffler, J. Combined real-time pcr and galactomannan surveillance improves diagnosis of invasive aspergillosis in high risk patients with haematological malignancies. *Br. J. Haematol.* **2013**, *161*, 517–524. [CrossRef] [PubMed]

62. Arvanitis, M.; Anagnostou, T.; Mylonakis, E. Galactomannan and polymerase chain reaction-based screening for invasive aspergillosis among high-risk hematology patients: A diagnostic meta-analysis. *Clin. Infect. Dis.* **2015**, *61*, 1263–1272. [CrossRef] [PubMed]
63. Aguado, J.M.; Vazquez, L.; Fernandez-Ruiz, M.; Villaescusa, T.; Ruiz-Camps, I.; Barba, P.; Silva, J.T.; Batlle, M.; Solano, C.; Gallardo, D.; et al. Serum galactomannan versus a combination of galactomannan and polymerase chain reaction-based aspergillus DNA detection for early therapy of invasive aspergillosis in high-risk hematological patients: A randomized controlled trial. *Clin. Infect. Dis.* **2015**, *60*, 405–414. [CrossRef] [PubMed]
64. Barnes, R.A.; White, P.L.; Morton, C.O.; Rogers, T.R.; Cruciani, M.; Loeffler, J.; Donnelly, J.P. Diagnosis of aspergillosis by pcr: Clinical considerations and technical tips. *Med. Mycol.* **2018**, *56*, 60–72. [CrossRef] [PubMed]

12

Transcriptomic and Genomic Approaches for Unravelling *Candida albicans* Biofilm Formation and Drug Resistance

Pei Pei Chong [1,*], Voon Kin Chin [1], Won Fen Wong [2,*], Priya Madhavan [3], Voon Chen Yong [1] and Chung Yeng Looi [1]

1 School of Biosciences, Faculty of Health and Medical Sciences, Taylor's University Malaysia, Subang Jaya, 47500 Selangor, Malaysia; VoonKin.Chin@taylors.edu.my (V.K.C.); PhelimVoonChen.Yong@taylors.edu.my (V.C.Y.); ChungYeng.Looi@taylors.edu.my (C.Y.L.)
2 Department of Medical Microbiology, Faculty of Medicine, University Malaya, 50603 Kuala Lumpur, Malaysia
3 School of Medicine, Faculty of Health and Medical Sciences, Taylor's University Malaysia, Subang Jaya, 47500 Selangor, Malaysia; Priya.Madhavan@taylors.edu.my
* Correspondence: PeiPei.Chong@taylors.edu.my (P.P.C.); wonfen@um.edu.my (W.F.W.)

Abstract: *Candida albicans* is an opportunistic fungal pathogen, which causes a plethora of superficial, as well as invasive, infections in humans. The ability of this fungus in switching from commensalism to active infection is attributed to its many virulence traits. Biofilm formation is a key process, which allows the fungus to adhere to and proliferate on medically implanted devices as well as host tissue and cause serious life-threatening infections. Biofilms are complex communities of filamentous and yeast cells surrounded by an extracellular matrix that confers an enhanced degree of resistance to antifungal drugs. Moreover, the extensive plasticity of the *C. albicans* genome has given this versatile fungus the added advantage of microevolution and adaptation to thrive within the unique environmental niches within the host. To combat these challenges in dealing with *C. albicans* infections, it is imperative that we target specifically the molecular pathways involved in biofilm formation as well as drug resistance. With the advent of the -omics era and whole genome sequencing platforms, novel pathways and genes involved in the pathogenesis of the fungus have been unraveled. Researchers have used a myriad of strategies including transcriptome analysis for *C. albicans* cells grown in different environments, whole genome sequencing of different strains, functional genomics approaches to identify critical regulatory genes, as well as comparative genomics analysis between *C. albicans* and its closely related, much less virulent relative, *C. dubliniensis*, in the quest to increase our understanding of the mechanisms underlying the success of *C. albicans* as a major fungal pathogen. This review attempts to summarize the most recent advancements in the field of biofilm and antifungal resistance research and offers suggestions for future directions in therapeutics development.

Keywords: *Candida albicans*; biofilm; antifungal resistance; transcriptomics

1. Introduction

Candida albicans is the leading etiological agent for fungemia and disseminated candidiasis, which are associated with high mortality rates. According to statistics provided by the Centre for Disease Control, *C. albicans* is the third most commonly isolated microbe from bloodstream infections among hospitalized patients in the US [1]. The success of this eukaryotic microbe in causing a myriad range of human infections from superficial skin and nail infections, oral and vaginal candidiasis, to the more serious invasive candidemia and deep organ infections, is in part due to its arsenal of virulence factors and its morphology switching capability. Unlike most other fungi, *C. albicans* is able to exist in yeast, pseudohyphal as well as hyphal forms depending on the in vivo surrounding environment or in vitro culture conditions.

This versatile fungus is able to grow in biofilms on medical devices such as intravenous catheters, urinary catheters, heart pacers and other equipment that is in contact with biological fluids or organs. A huge problem encountered by clinicians treating invasive candidiasis is the enhanced antifungal drug resistance displayed by *Candida* sp. biofilms. Indeed, *C. albicans* biofilm cells have been reported in multiple studies to display up to 1000-fold greater drug resistance than planktonic, non-biofilm cells [2–4]. Globally, the impact of medical device-related candidiasis is undeniably serious considering the high mortality and morbidity rates ascribed to these infections that are often recalcitrant to routine antifungal therapies.

In this review, we summarize the switch from commensalism to colonization and active infection for *C. albicans* in host cells and discuss the various stages, biochemical processes and molecular changes that are essential for biofilm development and pathogenesis. The intricate transcription regulatory networks that play a critical part in biofilm formation are discussed. Next, drug resistance associated with biofilm growth of *C. albicans* will be dissected. A section will be dedicated to the chief genomic differences observed between *C. albicans* and its relatively less virulent close relative, *C. dubliniensis*. This is in line with our efforts to understand the inherent genetic factors that contribute to the success of *C. albicans* as a human pathogen. Recent studies, which report the transcriptomic analysis of genes and metagenomic profiling of antifungal drug resistance related to biofilms, are also highlighted. The final section of this review focuses on the strategies for future research on targeted therapeutics that could combat *C. albicans* biofilm formation.

2. Morphology Switching and Pathogenesis of Biofilm Formation

Owing to its dimorphic switching property, *C. albicans* is able to switch from a yeast to a hyphal form thereby exiting the "harmless" commensal stage to become a pathogen. In addition, the fungus possesses the trait of biofilm development; another major contributor to its pathogenesis. Normally, in healthy hosts, *C. albicans* is a commensal microbe that inhabits mucosal surfaces especially in the intestines and is almost ubiquitous in the human microbiome. Factors such as the normal microbial flora, innate immunity and also epithelial barriers prevent *C. albicans* from overgrowing or invading the deeper layers of skin or penetrating the intestinal barrier. Constant interaction between the fungus and the host immune system is believed to take place during this commensal stage [5].

During the transition from commensalism to pathogenesis, three distinct yet dynamic stages are seen, namely (i) adhesion, (ii) invasion, and (iii) damage [6]. Wächtler and colleagues were the first to show that the three stages are mediated by distinct factors. In the adhesion stage, factors that play a crucial role include the adhesins from the Als family and the cell wall components Hwp1 and Als3 [6]. The adhesion factor Eap1 was separately shown by another study to be involved in adhesion [7]. Several of these adhesins are linked to the cell membrane whereas others are linked to the cell wall via glycosylphosphatidylinositol moieties. In a study by Wächtler, a *C. albicans* microarray from Eurogentec (Belgium) was used for transcriptional profiling of genes during the adhesion, invasion and damage stages in interactions with oral epithelial cells. Many hyphal associated genes including *ALS3*, *HWP1*, *ECE1*, *SOD5*, *PHR1*, *PRA1*, and *RBT1* were found to be upregulated when in contact with the oral epithelial cells [6].

The Hwp1 and also the Als3 proteins are produced predominantly during hypha formation, to allow for the adhesion of the fungal cells either to the host cells or to a substrate surface [8]. In the invasion stage, a different set of genes are expressed; although the common involvement of Als3, a multifunctional adhesin and invasin protein, is also present. The proteases such as secreted aspartyl proteinases (Saps) and phospholipases have long been known to be crucial players in the hyphal invasion of host cells. On the other hand, the onset of host cell damage is a key feature of pathogenesis. Tissue damage occurs when *C. albicans* hyphae penetrate deep into or through the epithelial layer (interepithelial layer), a process facilitated by secreted hydrolases [9]. A previous study by Wächtler [6] suggested that Icl1, Sod5 and Yhb1 are involved in the active infection of epithelial cells in particular during epithelial damage. In a recent study, Allert and coworkers screened libraries of *C. albicans* deletion mutants in a quest to delineate genes involved in host epithelial damage and translocation through the intestine barrier. They found that candidalysin, a peptide toxin of *C. albicans*, is crucial for this process [10].

Biofilms are complex three-dimensional structures that are composed of a core microbial cell community (either a single species or a mixed species) attached to host tissue or abiotic surfaces surrounded by an extracellular matrix (ECM) of polysaccharides that provide a shield or scaffold for the microbes beneath [11,12]. Not surprisingly, a biofilm provides protection against antimicrobials for the microbes associated with it, and thus biofilm-associated infections are notoriously difficult to treat. Among the clinical isolates of *Candida* species and even across different species, there is great heterogeneity in terms of the biofilm forming capability. The ability of clinical *Candida* isolates to form a biofilm has been shown by many studies to correlate with a higher virulence and hence an increased mortality [13–15].

In *C. albicans* biofilm formation, several stages are distinguishable: (i) adhesion, (ii) initiation, (iii) maturation, (iv) dispersal; which typically progress in sequence over a period of 24–48 h [16,17]. In the adhesion step, single *C. albicans* yeast cells adhere to the substrate to form a basal layer of yeast cells. The cell proliferation phase ensues followed by filamentation whereby the yeast cells begin to elongate and develop into filamentous hyphae. This is the initiation step whereby the cells change their morphology and invade either the host mucosal site or plastic or other polymer surfaces in inert medical devices. An arsenal of hydrolytic enzymes such as proteinases, haemolysins, and phospholipase are secreted by *C. albicans*, which enables the fungus to invade host tissue or other solid substrates. The secreted aspartyl proteinases (Saps), comprising a family of ten genes (*SAP1–10*), are the most well studied among the many secreted enzymes [16,17].

In the maturation step, the production of hyphae is a key feature accompanied by the secretion of ECM of polysaccharides. The biofilm ECM of *C. albicans* is complex, where the major polysaccharides include α-mannan, β-1,6 glucan and β-1,3 glucan [18]. Among these, although β-1,3 glucan is a minor constituent, it is the chief matrix polysaccharide linked to biofilm resistance to antifungals as it could block drug diffusion [19]. The hyphal invasion into tissues is driven by physical hydrostatic forces (turgor), which drive the cytoplasmic forces. The cells could communicate with other cells through quorum sensing mechanisms and one of the most studied quorum sensing molecules that could regulate biofilm formation is farnesol [20].

Finally, in the dispersal stage, lateral yeast cells are released from the matured biofilm and are then able to disseminate to distant sites to initiate a new cycle of biofilm formation. The dispersal stage of biofilm is of immense clinical relevance, as the newly released cells from the mature biofilm located in either indwelling catheter or an infectious nidus are able to not only initiate new rounds of biofilm formation but also enter into the bloodstream to establish a distant focus of infection. This is the reason why biofilm formation is closely associated with candidemia and disseminated invasive candidiasis clinically [21]. Importantly, a previous study had shown that the dispersed cells are predominantly yeast cells, with associated enhanced adherence, filamentation capacity, biofilm formation, increased resistance to azole drugs, and are more pathogenic than their planktonic counterparts [22]. Interestingly, in the latest study by Uppuluri and colleagues, they demonstrated that a portion (~33%) of dispersed yeast cells express the hypha-specific hyphal wall protein *HWP1* gene, whereas the yeast wall protein *YWP1* gene was expressed in ~64% of the dispersal yeast cells [23]. It is intriguing that up to a third of the lateral yeast cells express *HWP1* and although the underlying cause is still yet unknown, we postulate that this may be a clever strategy for the fungus so that these *HWP1*-expressing cells are "primed" and ready to colonize and invade the host cells as soon as they land on another site. The same authors also found that *PES1*, which is essential for yeast cell growth, had upregulated expression in dispersal yeast cells compared to biofilm, presumably as an inducer for generating more lateral yeast cells for dispersal [23].

In previous studies, differential expression analysis of the genes involved in various stages of biofilm production in *C. albicans* was mostly assessed via qualitative reverse transcription PCR (RT-PCR) or sometimes quantitative real-time RT-PCR systems. More recent transcriptomic and genomic approaches for studying regulatory networks involved in biofilm formation and the associated antifungal drug mechanisms are discussed in a later section in this review.

3. Transcription Regulatory Network of Biofilm Formation

As discussed in the above section, there are still many unanswered questions pertaining to biofilm formation by *C. albicans* in terms of the pathogenesis and the virulence mechanism. In this section, we will further dissect *C. albicans* biofilm formation in the context of the transcriptional regulatory network involved in this phenomenon.

Based on earlier literature, a master transcriptional regulatory network that consists of six major transcription regulators Efg1, Bcr1, Brg1, Ndt80, Tec1 and Rob1 are involved in controlling the normal process of biofilm formation. These regulators were discovered via screening a mutant library and in vivo studies in animal models [24,25]. Efg1 and Tec1 are involved in cell morphology regulation while Ndt80 is involved in biofilm formation. Meanwhile, Brg1 and Rob1 are present only in a species closely linked with *C. albicans* whereas, for Bcr1, its functions are yet to be fully characterized. Nobile et al deduced that transcription regulators form a complex and interconnected network with more than one thousand genes in controlling biofilm formation [25], where most of the target genes were bound by at least two or more transcriptional regulators. The same authors also surmised that the complexity in the biofilm network could be due to a number of factors including environmental influences and formation of cell memory to coordinate the cooperation between cells in order to maintain the dynamism and stability of the biofilm over generations. The authors also postulate that the complexity in the architecture of regulatory network helps to control the gene expression more precisely. On the other hand, evolutionary analysis suggests that transcriptional circuitry for the biofilm network in *C. albicans* has just evolved recently, where broad changes in the cis-regulatory sequence and regulators such as Brg1 and Rob1 are necessary for this modernized biofilm circuit [25].

A few years later, by screening the expanded library for biofilm formation at four different time points (immediately after adherence, at 8, 24 and 48 h), Fox and his coworkers [26] have identified three new transcriptional regulators involved in the biofilm circuit. These new regulators include Rfx2, Gal4 and Flo8, which are imperative and have specific roles in the development of the biofilm over time. The authors suggest that Flo8 is the most critical regulator identified in addition to the six master regulators identified earlier by Nobile [25], as double deletion mutants of Flo8 had severe disruption of biofilm formation at all time-points and the biofilm formed was similar to those formed by strains that resulted from deletions of any one of the previously discovered master regulators. Additionally, Flo8 is speculated to be a biofilm-specific regulator, as the upregulation of its expression was not affected by the form of reference cells (either yeast or filamentous form). Meanwhile, the authors reported that Rfx2 and Gal4 are involved in the biofilms formed at intermediate time points. Additionally, the authors hypothesized that Rfx2 and Gal4 are negative regulators for biofilms, where the enhancement of biofilm formation was observed in both rfx2Δ/Δ and gal4Δ/Δ mutant strains. Furthermore, through chromatin immunoprecipitation studies, the authors reported that *FLO8* is bound by Efg1, Brg1 and Ndt80 while *RFX2* and *GAL4* are bound by Ndt80. These findings further prove that Rfx2, Gal4 and Flo8 are well integrated into the existing *C. albicans* transcriptional biofilm regulatory network [26].

The pathogenesis of a biofilm often begins with adherence and colonization of *C. albicans* on the cell surface. Thus, analyzing the regulatory processes that occur during *C. albicans* adherence could provide a new paradigm to further understand the initial stage of biofilm formation. Finkel et al first reported that adherence of *C. albicans* on a silicone surface is under the control of 29 transcription factors [27]. Amongst these transcription factors, only mutants for Ace2p, Arg81p, Bcr1p, and Snf5p exhibit the anti-adherence properties in vitro. Meanwhile, the deletion of Zcf28p, Zfu2p and Crz2p is only able to disrupt biofilm formation on catheters in animal models [27]. Lee et al adopted a functional genomic analysis approach to screen for a library consisting of 1481 double barcoded doxycycline-repressible conditional gene expression strains which encompass approximately 25% of the *C. albicans* genome [28]. The authors have identified five important adherence regulators namely *ARC18, PMT1, MNN9, SPT7,* and *orf19.831* where transcriptional repression of these genes impaired the adherence of *C. albicans*. Of all, transcriptional repression of *ARC18* results in the strongest adherence defect and cell wall physiology changes in *C. albicans*. Arc18 is one of the putative members of the Arp2/3 complex. The authors demonstrated that perturbation of the Arp2/3 complex reduces biofilm formation, impairs the adherence process, and increases the cell surface hydrophobicity. Additionally, the disruption of the Arp2/3 complex also leads to hyperactivation of small G-protein Rho1-mediated cell wall related stress pathways, where extensive fungal cell wall remodeling is taking place. Taken together, in this study, the authors have identified a novel molecular mechanism between Arp2/3 complex and Rho1 in regulating *C. albicans* adhesion and biofilm formation [28].

Previous findings from Nobile [25], which used genome-wide approaches, have revealed that the transcription regulatory network of biofilm formation is highly integrated. Nevertheless, the functional consequences of this integration and the interactions between transcriptional regulators in this transcriptional circuitry remain obscure. Additionally, the study by Nobile and other studies on transcriptional circuitry for biofilm formation usually employed double homozygous deletion mutants of particular transcriptional regulator genes to study its effect on biofilm formation [24–26]. This genetic analysis approach will eventually limit the potential to discover novel genes that contribute towards alterations in biofilm formation, particularly for a single homozygous strain. To address this limitation, Glazier and his workers [29] have adopted a simple haploinsufficiency genetic analysis approach to analyze the transcription regulatory network of biofilm formation. The authors generated and analyzed the interaction between all possible double heterozygous mutants of the transcriptional regulators (Efg1, Bcr1, Brg1, Ndt80, Tec 1 and Rob1). From the study, the authors reported that the biofilm network is remarkably susceptible to genetic perturbation where all of the six transcriptional regulator mutants showed changes in biofilm formation. Additionally, the double heterozygous mutants showed a comparable or more severe disruption in biofilm development than the double homozygous mutants. In this study, the authors also shed light on the functions and involvement of individual transcriptional regulators. The authors revealed that *TEC1* expression is highly sensitive to small disruptions by other transcriptional regulators while *NDT80* expression is under the influence of *TEC1*. Meanwhile, *ROB1* expression was found to be dependent on the cooperative interaction among transcriptional regulators and auto-regulation mechanism [29]. Figure 1 summarizes and highlights the involvement of different transcription factors, master regulators and effectors in the complex biofilm regulatory circuitry according to the distinct stages of biofilm development in *C. albicans*.

4. Drug Resistance in *Candida albicans* Biofilm

The five major groups of antifungal agents that are used in the treatment of *C. albicans* infections are azoles, allylamines, echinocandins, polyenes and nucleoside analogues. The azoles and allylamines inhibit the ergosterol synthesis by blocking different enzymes respectively, whereas echinocandins disrupt the cell wall integrity by inhibiting the enzyme β-1,3-glucan synthase. Polyenes bind to sterols and cause intracellular leakage, whereas nucleoside analogues perturb DNA/RNA synthesis thus inhibiting cell growth [30].

Treatment of *Candida* biofilm was shown to be effective with amphotericin B and echinochandins in some previous studies [31–37]. However, antifungal drug resistance in biofilms of *C. albicans* has been reported in the past few years. Furthermore, the pyrimidine analogs, allylamines and classic formulations of polyenes are not effective against biofilms of *C. albicans* [3,38–40]. Factors contributing to antifungal resistance in *C. albicans* have been described. One of the more prominent factors is the ability of this species to effectively pump out drugs via its efflux pumps mechanism [41]. Besides the drug efflux pumps mechanism, the biofilm architecture, which is a thick layer of matrix and its constituents such as the polysaccharide β-1,3-glucan, has the ability to bind to the antifungal agents, preventing them from reaching their targets, which eventually increases the resistance of *C. albicans* towards these drugs [41,42].

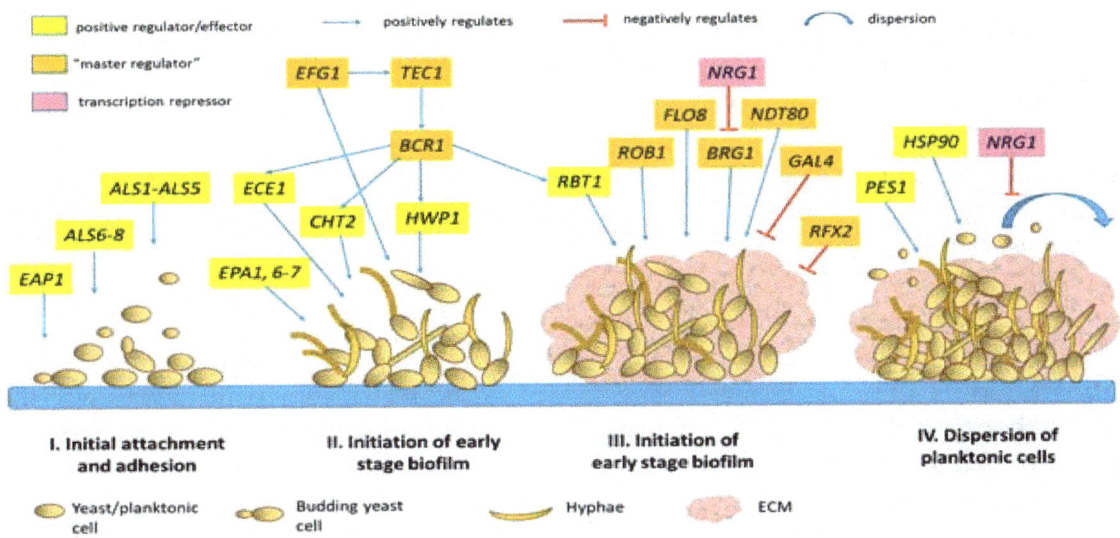

Figure 1. Schematic diagram depicting the stages of biofilm formation in *Candida albicans* and the transcription regulatory network involved in the process. The information on the "master regulators" originated from Nobile [25], Fox [26] and Glazier [29].

Persister cells that exist within the biofilms as metabolically inactive cells are also known to be resistant to many antifungal drugs such as amphotericin B [16,40]. Due to the dormancy of these persister cells, it is difficult for antifungal drugs to evoke an effect as these drugs normally target actively metabolizing cells. In this case, where persister cells exist within the biofilm matrix, much higher minimum inhibitory concentrations (MICs) of the drugs may be required to achieve the intended therapeutic goal. The acquisition of drug resistance in *C. albicans* has been studied using transcriptomes. The RNAseq analyses have been shown to be more accurate and sensitive when compared to microarray and, thus, provide a better platform to unravel the complexity of drug resistance genes in *C. albicans* [43,44]. Using RNA seq, more than 50 genes were found to be overexpressed in drug-resistant *C. albicans* [45]. The transcriptional factor encoded by the *CZF1* gene that is associated with hyphal transition and white/opaque switching was upregulated along with the *CDR1* and *CDR2* genes. This gene is also known to negatively control the expression of one of the three genes which encode β-1,3-glucan synthase, i.e., *GSL1*. Besides these genes, several other genes regulating adherence (*ALS1*), carbon metabolism (*CIT1, HGT10, GAL7, GUT1, FUM12* and *GDH3*), cell wall maintenance (*MNN4* and *CHR11*), drug transport (*YOR1*) and morphogenesis (*WHI1, ADAEC, SFL2, SCH9, CZF1, ECE1, DLD1, GPR1* and *SRR1*) of *C. albicans* were overexpressed. The study also revealed a few other genes that were repressed such as gene regulating adherence (*ALS2*), carbon metabolism (*HGT12, MAL2* and *MAE1*), copper and iron homeostasis (*HEM13, CRP1* and *SMF3*), drug transport (*CDR4* and *MFS*), extracellular proteins (*PLB1, ALS2* and *MAL2*), morphogenesis (*NAT4* and *PHHB*) and steroid binding (*EBP1* and *CBP1*). A new transcribed region was identified upstream of the *TAC1* gene, which encodes the major *CDR* transcriptional regulator, which is yet to be characterized [45].

5. Comparative Studies on *C. albicans* vs. "Avirulent" *C. dubliniensis*

C. albicans is the most commonly found opportunistic yeast that can exist as a normal microflora in healthy individuals or as an etiological agent in human candidiasis. *C. dubliniensis*, first identified in 1995, is a pathogenic species that is phylogenetically close to *C. albicans* [46,47]. Similar to *C. albicans*,

C. dubliniensis is able to form a chlamydospore and germ tube and to cause oral candidiasis, particularly in human immunodeficiency virus (HIV)-infected patients [48]. Despite the phylogenetic similarities between *C. dubliniensis* and *C. albicans*, the former exhibits a poorer virulence and lower prevalence rate due to the reduced capability to colonize the host and to form filaments [48–50]. Previous studies have focused on elucidating the phenotypical differences between these two closely related species to understand the fungal virulence mechanism. Some of the prominent findings from these studies indicate that *C. dubliniensis* exhibits impaired growth kinetics at 42 °C [51], has no β-glucosidase activity [52] and fails to produce true hyphae under *N*-acetylglucosamine stimulation or a nutrient-rich environment [46,53]. However, it shows a higher extracellular proteinase expression, adheres more strongly to buccal epithelial cells and is less susceptible to 5-flucytosine compared to *C. albicans* [54].

Using an in vivo animal infection model, Vilela demonstrated that mice intravenously infected with *C. dubliniensis* show higher survival rates than those infected with *C. albicans* and this is likely due to a more effective host inflammatory immune response to *C. dubliniensis* [48]. This is supported by in vitro culture experiment whereby *C. dubliniensis* had a lower survival rate in the presence of human polymorphonuclear leukocytes [55]. Furthermore, in an immunosuppressed mouse model, Stoke demonstrated that *C. dubliniensis* poses a weaker degree of expansion and dissemination to internal organs than *C. albicans* [50]. When co-cultured with oral reconstituted human epithelial cells, *C. dubliniensis* appears predominantly in yeast form that renders minimal effect to the cells; whereas *C. albicans* forms abundant hyphae that damage the epithelial cells in vitro [50].

Given that *C. albicans* and *C. dubliniensis* share a close phylogenetic relationship, the puzzle remains as to how these two species are varied in terms of virulence. Studies have used genomics and transcriptomics approaches to gain further insights into the different morphogenesis pathways in both species [53,55–57]. Moran has a utilized comparative genomic hybridization (CGH) method by co-hybridizing *C. albicans* microarrays with fluorescently labelled *C. albicans* and *C. dubliniensis* genomic DNA to assess the cross species genomic homology [55]. The outcome from this experiment shows a high genome similarity between the two species. Up to 95.6% of *C. dubliniensis* genomic DNA is homologous to, and hybridizes with, nucleotides from the *C. albicans* genome; while only a small proportion (4.4%, 247 genes) shows sequence divergence. The divergent genes include those encoding the hypha-specific human transglutaminase substrate *HWP1P*, which are important for hyphae formation. It is also noted that two of the *C. albicans* virulence factors implicated in invasion, the secreted aspartyl proteinase-encoding genes (*SAP5*, and either one of the *SAP4* or *SAP6*), are missing in the *C. dubliniensis* genome. Further, Jackson and coworkers sequenced the 14.6-megabase genome of *C. dubliniensis* and compared it to that of *C. albicans* using whole-genome shotgun sequencing at 11-fold average coverage [56]. Similar to results from Moran [55], that utilize the CGH method, a highly conserved sequence and synteny are shown throughout the genome of both species and only a total of 168 species-specific genes are identified. The absence of *SAP4* and *SAP5* genes in *C. dubliniensis* genome is reconfirmed in this study. Other genes reported in this study include the proposed invasin *ALS3* and a group of 115 pseudogenes that are orthologs of filamentous growth regulator (*FGR*) genes with predicted functions in fungal pathogenesis. A study by Butler compared eight *Candida* species (without *C. dubliniensis*) and shows some genes involved in mating and meiosis pathways are missing throughout evolution in certain species [58]. This suggests that distinct *Candida* species may have modified their genomes during evolutionary adaptation, which may contribute to the different virulence levels of each species. Figure 2 provides a summary of the differences between *C. albicans* and *C. dubliniensis* in different aspects, which contribute to the differences in virulence.

Compared to the genomic data, transcriptomic analysis provides more vital information of transactive genes under different stimuli or conditions. Transcriptomic analysis has been used to analyze the cross species gene expression between *Candida* versus other fungal species [57,59–61]. In 2013, Grumaz [57] used RNA-sequencing (RNA-Seq) on the Illumina (San Diego, CA, USA) next generation sequencing platform to compare the transcriptional landscapes between *C. dubliniensis* and *C. albicans* in both hyphal and yeast stages. A comparison of the differentially expressed orthologs was quantitatively determined. Recently, an RNA-Seq approach has also been used to compare the transcriptome of *C. albicans* versus *C. africana*, a biovariant with a low degree of virulence and inability to produce chlamydospores; which unveiled two novel transcriptionally active regions in both species [61]. A recent study by Caplice [53] uses a microarray meta-analysis to compare the transcriptional response of *C. dubliniensis* and *C. albicans* to different stimuli such as pH and temperature [53]. Interestingly, *C. dubliniensis* displays no or minimal expression of several Efg1-regulated, hypha-induced genes, such as the extent of cell elongation 1 (*ECE1*) and *HWP1* in response to 37 °C incubation. Other genes that are induced in *C. albicans* but not *C. dubliniensis* include those involved in the cell cycle, cytoskeleton organization, and the maintenance of hyphal growth and DNA replication. Hence, -omics approaches to compare between a less virulent and less versatile pathogen *C. dubliniensis* (or *C. africana*) to the highly virulent *C. albicans* provide important clues for the intricate gene regulatory network of the virulence process.

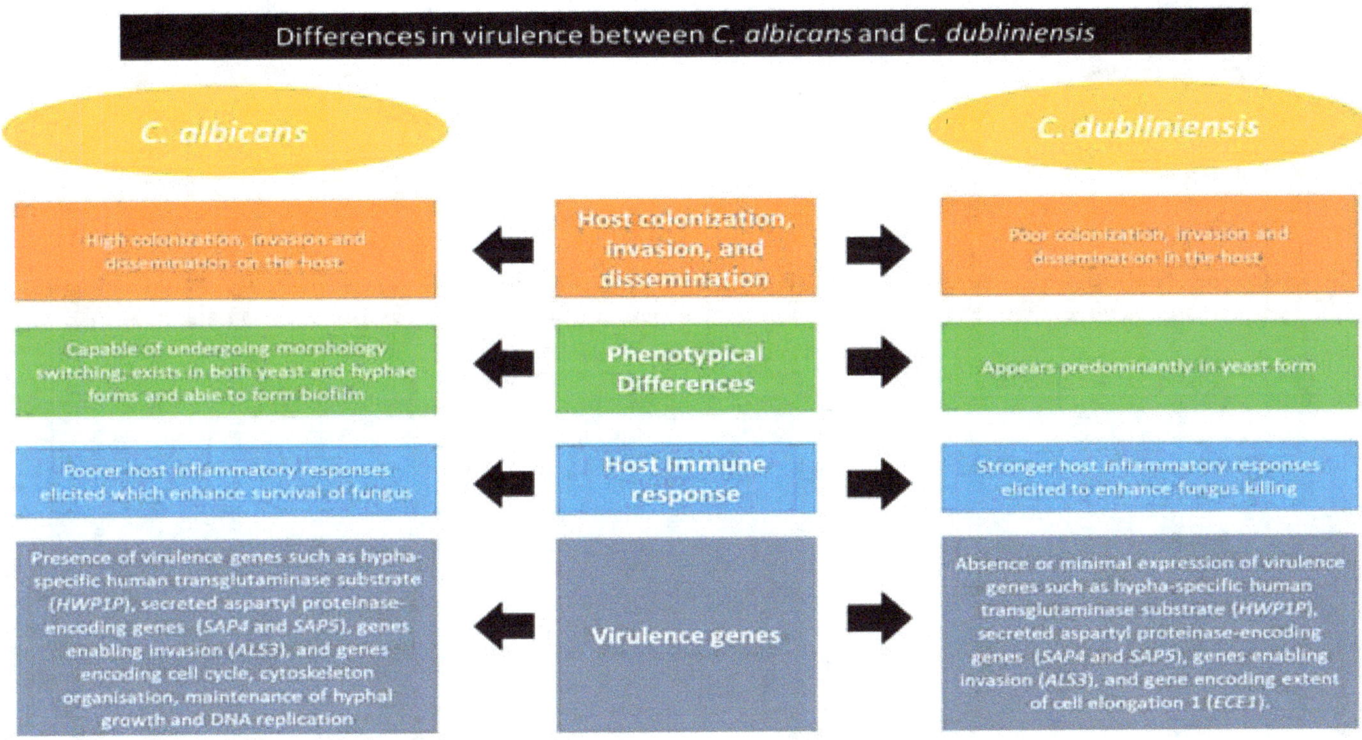

Figure 2. Comparative differences in the virulence determinants between *C. albicans* and *C. dubliniensis*. Differences in (i) host colonization, invasion, and dissemination; (ii) morphology; (iii) host immune response; and (iv) virulence genes are highlighted.

6. Exploitation of Transcriptomic and Genomic Technologies for Dissecting *C. albicans* Biofilm Formation and Drug Resistance

The *C. albicans* genome was sequenced and annotated via the efforts of the Stanford Genome Technology Centre as well as the European Galar Fungail network. The CandidaDB genome database for *C. albicans* pathogenomics was first launched in January 2002. Later, the release of CandidaDB launched in June 2004 represented an up-to-date annotation of Assembly 19 of the *C.albicans* genome sequence [62]. The genome database provided a strong impetus for and an indispensable base, which spurred numerous whole-genome related transcriptomics and proteomic studies. Table 1 below is a summary of the key publications within the last decade, which helped to advance our knowledge in *C. albicans* biofilm formation and drug resistance, particularly through those that describe the use of new -omics platforms. The list is in no way exhaustive but merely a snapshot of the studies that have contributed to this field.

Table 1. Gene expression studies on *C. albicans* biofilm and drug resistance.

Methodology/Platform	Biological Issue Studied	Major Findings	Reference
Microarrays with probes for *C. albicans* genes/Eurogentec (Seraing, Belgium)	Transcription profiles of biofilm cells vs. planktonic cells under different conditions of flow, oxygenation, and glucose concentration	Gcn4p, a regulator of amino acid metabolism, is required for biofilm growth	[63]
Microarrays/Eurogentec SA (Ivoz-Ramet, Belgium) in collaboration with European Galar Fungail Consortium (www.pasteur.fr)	Genome-wide expression profile of *C. albicans* to polyene, pyrimidine, azole, and echinocandin antifungal agents	Different expression profile signatures obtained in exposure to different classes of antifungals with various genes overexpressed	[64]
Oligonucleotide microarray (Agilent Technologies, Santa Clara, CA, USA) with *C. albicans* Assembly 21 genome (http://www.candidagenome.org/), Full Genome Chromatin Immunoprecipitation Tiling Microarray (ChIP-chip), RNA Sequencing (RNA-seq)	Comparative transcriptional analysis of *C. albicans* biofilm and planktonic cells, with *C. albicans* transcription regulator (TR) deletion mutants that are deficient in biofilm formation	Six master regulators Bcr1, Tec1, Efg1, Ndt80, Rob1, and Brg1 are essential for biofilm formation.	[25]
NanoString expression profiling and nCounter platform (NanoString Technologies, Inc., Seattle, US) with ~150 probes from cell wall-related genes, ~50 host-pathogen interaction genes, ~100 genes highly regulated during hypha development or biofilm formation, oxidative or osmotic stress	Expression profiling of genes involved in *C. albicans* adherence to substrate (silicone), an early step in medical device-related infections	Biofilm regulators Bcr1 and Ace2 have a role in adherence. A large regulatory network of 11 adherence regulators, the zinc-response regulator Zap1, and approximately 25% of the predicted cell surface protein genes known as Cell Surface Targets of Adherence Regulators (CSTARs) are involved in adherence.	[27]
RNA-sequencing (mRNA-Seq 8, Illumina) and Genome Analyzer (Illumina Inc.)	Transcriptome analysis of a *Candida* Drug Resistance (*CDR*) strain against its isogenic drug susceptible counterpart	Identified ∼50 genes overexpressed in *CDR* strain: *CZF1* which is involved in transcription regulation of white/opaque switching and hypha formation is upregulated with *CDR1* and *CDR2*, 5′UTR region of TAC1	[45]
Gene expression microarrays (Agilent Technologies), Chromatin immunoprecipitation quantitative real-time PCR (ChIP-qPCR)	Genome-wide expression analysis of biofilm formation at different intervals, immediately after adherence, at 8, 24 and 48 h	Identified Flo8, Gal4, and Rfx2 to be involved in different time points of biofilm formation	[26]
High-throughput next-generation sequencing/Hi-Seq 2500 platform (Illumina)	Use pooled Gene Replacement and Conditional Expression (GRACE) library conditional expression strains to identify novel regulators of cell-to-surface adherence	Novel functional relationship between the Arp2/3 complex and Rho1 important for modulating actin cytoskeleton, endocytosis and cell wall remodeling,	[28]
RNA-seq with TruSeq RNA v2 kit/HiSeq2500 platform (Illumina)	Transcriptomic profiling of 124 mutant *C. albicans* strains in 10 in vitro conditions for filamentation ability	Genes encoding cell wall/membrane proteins, adhesins, alcohol dehydrogenases, and iron uptake and utilization genes were common genes upregulated across different conditions	[65]
Candida genome microarray (CapitalBio Corp., Beijing, China) with *C. albicans* genome database (http://www.candidagenome.org/)/CapitalBio BioMixer II hybridization station	Gene expression profiling of fluconazole-resistant *C. albicans* strain treated with osthole (a natural coumarin) in synergy with fluconazole	Genes in oxidation-reduction process (e.g., catalase encoded by *CAT1* and mitochondrial glycosylase encoded by *OGG1*); *CTN1* (carnitine acetyltransferase) and *ICL1* (isocitrate lyase) were upregulated	[66]
RNA-seq with BIOO Scientific NEXTflex Directional RNA-seq kit/HiSeq2000 platform (Illumina)	To decipher transcriptional gene expression patterns of dispersal cells versus core biofilm cells and planktonic cells	Transcription pattern of dispersal cells mostly similar to parent biofilm, *YWP1* expression ~2-fold higher in dispersal > biofilm > planktonic cells; ~33% of dispersal yeast cells express *HWP1*	[23]

7. Future Directions of Research on New Antifungal Drugs Targeted at *Candida* Biofilm

Undoubtedly, biofilm formation by *C. albicans* is a complicated process leading to life-threatening infections, which are difficult to eradicate. Additionally, current antifungal therapies have minimal effects on biofilm formation and there is no effective solution to solve this problem. Moreover, the development of resistance and toxicity further hindered the efficacy of antifungal drugs. Nonetheless, there are some promising strategies that could be carried out to tackle biofilm formation. These strategies include lock therapies for an infected catheter, catheter coatings, natural products and synthetic products screening, photodynamic inactivation, and targeting of the molecular pathways related to *C. albicans* biofilm formation.

The "lock therapy" is where high concentrations of antifungal drugs are directly administered into the catheter lumen for a period of time, such as several hours to days, prior to contact with patients. This approach allows the antifungal agent to eliminate biofilm formation in the catheter and also to avoid undesirable systemic toxicity build-up in patients as the high dosage of the antifungal agent only acts in the catheter [67]. This therapy has been tested on silicone catheters infected with different *C. glabrata* and *C. albicans* strains, using caspofungin, micafungin and posaconazole as antifungal agents. The outcomes were positive where all antifungal agents used in the study have successfully reduced biofilm formation, with micafungin showing the most promising result [68]. Meanwhile, another lock therapy using amphotericin B lipid formulation (L-AMB) was not effective to eradicate *Candida* biofilms [69]. There are several concerns when considering lock therapy in catheter-related candidemia including (1) the higher failure rate for biofilm infection on the outer surface or on the catheter tip; (2) the possibility of the development of antifungal drug resistance and (3) concomitant systemic antifungal treatment may need to be considered for disseminated infection. To counter these concerns, the choice of non-antifungal agents or antiseptics such as ethanol, EDTA or a high dose of minocycline are more preferable in the lock therapy against *C. albicans* and non-*albicans* biofilms [70].

Another alternative to counter *C. albicans* biofilm formation is through the modification of the catheter coating. A study has shown that the modification of the catheter coating with chlorhexidine, minocycline-rifampin or silver sulfadiazine could reduce the incidence of bloodstream infections caused by central venous catheters in the intensive care unit [71]. Meanwhile, a novel silane system coated on the implant surfaces of titanium and zirconia has been shown to inhibit *C. albicans* biofilm formation [72]. On the other hand, Karlsson fabricated and coated antifungal β-peptide-containing multilayered polymer films onto surfaces and demonstrated a profound inhibition of the antifungal-containing polymer films on the growth and proliferation of *C. albicans*. The authors suggest that this approach could be used to suppress the biofilm formation caused by *C. albicans* on film-coated surfaces, which could be further applied onto the surface of medical devices to inhibit *C. albicans* biofilm in clinical settings [73]. Hoque also demonstrated that by coating the surface of medical devices with water-insoluble and organo-soluble polymeric materials inhibition on the growth and proliferation for a number of bacteria and fungi including *C. albicans* was remarkable [74].

Exploiting the efficacy and synergistic effect of combinations of antifungal therapies with other drug classes could be another strategy for new antifungal development against *C. albicans* biofilm formation. For example, synergistic effects between cyclosporine A with fluconazole, caspofungin, voriconazole, nystatin and amphotericin B against *C. albicans* biofilm formation were observed [75]. Additionally, our previous work also demonstrated that allicin, a pure compound from garlic extract, when combined with fluconazole reduced the *C. albicans* biofilm formation and altered the expression of biofilm-related genes in vitro [76]. Besides that, the combination of Hsp90 inhibitors and the non-steroidal anti-inflammatory drugs (NSAIDs) with antifungal drugs also showed a promising synergistic activity against *C. albicans* biofilm formation [77,78]. The additive effects of different drugs such as that between fluconazole and doxycycline were also effective against *C. albicans* biofilms [79]. Nevertheless, the possibility of the development of cell toxicity has to be considered when adopting such an approach.

On the other hand, formulation of new drugs based on existing antifungal drugs could be another approach against *C. albicans* biofilm formation. Hitherto, several new formulated drugs, including an amphotericin B lipid complex and liposomal amphotericin B, showed efficacy against *C. albicans* biofilm in a bioprosthetic model [32]. Caspofungin, echinocandin, and micafungin also showed similar effects against *C. parapsilosis* and *C. albicans* biofilms in the same model [32]. Recent studies also documented the efficacy of amphotericin B lipid and echinocandin against *Candida* biofilm formation both in vitro (34) and in vivo (35,37). Meanwhile, aspirin was shown to inhibit *C. albicans* filamentation and biofilm formed by *C. albicans*, *C. parapsilosis* and *C. glabrata* [80]. Taken together, future work on the discovery of new antifungal drugs through in silico modeling or structural modification of existing antifungal drugs can help us in reducing the emergence of antifungal drug resistance.

Targeting the biofilm-related pathways in *C. albicans* could serve as a promising strategy in combating *C. albicans* biofilm formation. One instance is targeting the quorum-sensing pathway. Farnesol is a quorum-sensing molecule involved in facilitating the communication between *Candida* cells during cell proliferation. Previous studies have shown that farnesol is able to inhibit *C. albicans* biofilm formation and augment the efficacy of azoles [22,81–83]. Further evaluation of the efficacy of farnesol in vivo and the discovery of more quorum sensing molecules could shed light on the possibility of targeting the quorum-sensing pathway for *C. albicans* biofilm treatment. Meanwhile, targeting the biofilm ECM of *C. albicans*, such as β-1,3 glucan and extracellular DNA (eDNA) could be another potential approach for anti-biofilm therapy. As such, studies have shown fluconazole activity is enhanced upon digestion of β-1,3 glucan while amphotericin B activity is enhanced by the degradation of eDNA [11,42,84]. More studies identifying potential inhibitors for targeting the biofilm matrix and pathways could help us in designing better antifungal drugs for anti-biofilm therapy.

On-going and intense research has explored natural products or synthetic peptides against *C. albicans* biofilm formation. Compounds under investigation include terpenoids, polyphenols and phenylpropanoids from plant and tea extracts [85,86] and also phenazines produced by *P. aeruginosa* [87]. These compounds can suppress *C. albicans* biofilm formation and inhibit yeast-to-hyphal transition. Additionally, some synthetic peptides, such as KSL-W have significant effects on biofilm formation, growth and yeast-to-hypha transition of *C. albicans* [88]. On the other hand, several high-throughput screenings aimed at identifying small-molecule inhibitors against *C. albicans* filamentation and biofilm formation have been conducted. Siles screened for 1200 off-patent drugs approved by the Food and Drug Administration within the Prestwick Chemical Library and identified 38 bioactive compounds with ability in suppressing *C. albicans* biofilm [89]. Subsequently, Wong screened for 50,240 small molecules from a library and identified SM21 as a potent inhibitor for *C. albicans* yeast-to-hypha transition [90]. Pierce identified a series of diazaspiro-decane structural analogs which inhibit the filamentation and biofilm formation of *C. albicans* from a chemical library (NOVACore™) of 20,000 small molecules [91]. Meanwhile, Romo screened for 30,000 small-molecules within ChemBridge's DIVERSet chemical library and identified *N*-[3-(allyloxy)-phenyl]-4-methoxybenzamide as the leading compound for preventing *C. albicans* filamentation and biofilm formation [92].

Another potential approach to eliminate *C. albicans* biofilm is through photodynamic inactivation. This technique adopts the use of a nontoxic dye (photosensitizer) and visible light to produce reactive oxygen species, which are able to destroy the DNA, cell membrane or proteins of microbial cells and subsequently kill them. Several photosensitizers have been tested on *Candida* biofilm formation including methylene blue and toluidine blue [93,94]. A study has shown that toluidine blue (0.1 mg/mL) is able to reduce *C. albicans* biofilm at up to 60% [93]. In addition to that, when combined with chitosan, a greater reducing effect on *C albicans* biofilm formation was observed [95]. This non-toxic and yet cost-effective technique will definitely serve as a future expansion field in reducing biofilm formation of *Candida* spp.

In recent years, nanoparticles with antifungal properties have been described. There is rife interest on the anti-biofilm properties of silver (Ag) nanoparticles, which have been shown to damage the cell wall and membrane of *C. albicans* biofilm cells and inhibit filamentation [96]. A recent study also showed that Ag nanoparticles have altered multiple cellular targets including ergosterol content, fatty acid composition, cell membrane integrity and ultrastructure [97]. Another biopolymer with promising anti-biofilm property is chitosan nanoparticles, which were demonstrated by a recent study to be effective in *C. albicans* biofilm inhibition on a resin denture surface [98]. Moreover, the efficacy of other nanoparticles namely gold nanoparticles [99], silica nanoparticles [100] and selenium nanoparticles either alone or as a carrier for antifungal drugs has also been explored [101].

Vaccination is another potential strategy in preventing invasive fungal infections, particularly on high-risk groups with identifiable risk factors [102,103]. The key protection lies in the ability of vaccines to boost host immunity, including pro-inflammatory, cell-mediated, Th1 or Th17 responses to enhance phagocytic killing of the fungus [103]. Dedicated studies have been conducted by researchers in recent years to develop safe and effective fungal vaccines [104,105]. Though no specific vaccine has been developed to prevent *Candida* biofilms, however, two promising fungal vaccines against invasive candidiasis have been developed and they are currently under clinical trials. The first *Candida* vaccine containing the rAls3p-N antigen is presently under a phase IIa clinical trial whereby the results indicated that this vaccine hinders fungal adhesion and invasion in immunized subjects [105,106]. The second *Candida* vaccine is a virosome-based vaccine comprising of Sap2 antigen/truncated recombinant Sap2 antigen, which confers protection for both systemic and mucosal candidiasis [107]. Concerted efforts should be given to unravel new compounds and molecules that can be applied in the prophylaxis and treatment of *Candida* infections.

In conclusion, the majority of the data generated on *C. albicans* biofilms has mainly relied on in vitro models, which pose limitations in translating the findings from bench to bedside. Each in vitro biofilm model could be limited by the species/strains used, the specific environmental conditions and the choices of biotic interphase. It is important to take into consideration the clinical relevance of the adopted model as well. The lack of in vivo studies also warrants the development of reliable and novel in vitro biofilm models that resemble the conditions in vivo, which can be utilized for long-term anti-biofilm and antimicrobial activity prediction. On the other hand, from the accumulated data derived from transcriptome expression profiles of *C. albicans* biofilm, various key regulators of biofilm development have been identified. Dispersal cells, in particular, should be targeted as they are programmed to survive in nutrient-starved niches and to infect new sites in the host. Using the latest molecular docking and in silico modeling software to screen libraries of small molecules and peptides for candidates that could bind to and inactivate selected CSTARs targets and key regulators such as *PES1*, *YWP1*, *HWP1* and the Arp2/3 complex, we might be able to identify potential anti-*C. albicans* molecules that could become the next marketed antifungal drugs.

Acknowledgments: PPC's research was funded by the University Putra Malaysia Research University Grants Scheme (RUGS). WFW was funded by Institut Mérieux Young Investigator Award Grant to University of Malaya (UM.0000107/HIF.IF; IF039-2017).

References

1. Wisplinghoff, H.; Bischoff, T.; Tallent, S.M.; Seifert, H.; Wenzel, R.P.; Edmond, M.B. Nosocomial bloodstream infections in U.S. hospitals: Analysis of 24,179 cases from a prospective nationwide surveillance study. *Clin. Infect. Dis.* **2004**, *39*, 309–317. [CrossRef] [PubMed]
2. Baillie, G.S.; Douglas, L.J. Role of dimorphism in the development of *Candida albicans* biofilms. *J. Med. Microbiol.* **1999**, *48*, 671–679. [CrossRef] [PubMed]
3. Mukherjee, P.K.; Chandra, J.; Kuhn, D.M.; Ghannoum, M.A. Mechanism of fluconazole resistance in *Candida albicans* biofilms: Phase-specific role of efflux pumps and membrane sterols. *Infect. Immun.* **2003**, *71*, 4333–4340. [CrossRef] [PubMed]

4. LaFleur, M.D.; Kumamoto, C.A.; Lewis, K. *Candida albicans* biofilms produce antifungal-tolerant persister cells. *Antimicrob. Agents Chemother.* **2006**, *50*, 3839–3846. [CrossRef] [PubMed]
5. Mochon, A.B.; Ye, J.; Kayala, M.A.; Wingard, J.R.; Clancy, C.J.; Nguyen, M.H.; Felgner, P.; Baldi, P.; Liu, H. Serological profiling of a *Candida albicans* protein microarray reveals permanent host-pathogen interplay and stage-specific responses during candidemia. *PLoS Pathog.* **2010**, *6*, e1000827. [CrossRef]
6. Wächtler, B.; Wilson, D.; Haedicke, K.; Dalle, F.; Hube, B. From attachment to damage: Defined genes of *Candida albicans* mediate adhesion, invasion and damage during interaction with oral epithelial cells. *PLoS ONE* **2011**, *6*, e17046. [CrossRef] [PubMed]
7. Zordan, R.; Cormack, B. Adhesins in Opportunistic Fungal Pathogens. In *Candida and Candidiasis*, 2nd ed.; Calderone, R.A., Clancy, C.J., Eds.; ASM Press: Washington, DC, USA, 2012; pp. 243–259.
8. Liu, Y.; Filler, S.G. *Candida albicans* Als3, a multifunctional adhesin and invasin. *Eukaryot. Cell* **2011**, *10*, 168–173. [CrossRef] [PubMed]
9. Dalle, F.; Wächtler, B.; L'Ollivier, C.; Holland, G.; Bannert, N.; Wilson, D.; Labruere, C.; Bonnin, A.; Hube, B. Cellular interactions of *Candida albicans* with human oral epithelial cells and enterocytes. *Cell. Microbiol.* **2010**, *12*, 248–271. [CrossRef] [PubMed]
10. Allert, S.; Förster, T.M.; Svensson, C.M.; Richardson, J.P.; Pawlik, T.; Hebecker, B.; Rudolphi, S.; Juraschitz, M.; Schaller, M.; Blagojevic, M.; et al. *Candida albicans*-induced epithelial damage mediates translocation through intestinal barriers. *MBio* **2018**, *9*, e00915-18. [CrossRef] [PubMed]
11. Al-Fattani, M.A.; Douglas, L.J. Biofilm matrix of *Candida albicans* and *Candida tropicalis*: Chemical composition and role in drug resistance. *J. Med. Microbiol.* **2006**, *55*, 999–1008. [CrossRef] [PubMed]
12. Ghannoum, M.A.; Roilides, E.; Katragkou, A.; Petraitis, V.; Walsh, T.J. The role of echinocandins in *Candida* biofilm-related vascular catheter infections: In vitro and in vivo model systems. *Clin. Infect. Dis.* **2015**, *61*, S618–S621. [CrossRef] [PubMed]
13. Tumbarello, M.; Fiori, B.; Trecarichi, E.M.; Posteraro, P.; Losito, A.R.; De Luca, A.; Sanguinetti, M.; Fadda, G.; Cauda, R.; Posteraro, B. Risk factors and outcomes of candidemia caused by biofilm-forming isolates in a tertiary care hospital. *PLoS ONE* **2012**, *7*, e33705. [CrossRef] [PubMed]
14. Sherry, L.; Nile, C.J.; Sherriff, A.; Johnson, E.M.; Hanson, M.F.; Williams, C.; Munro, C.A.; Jones, B.J.; Ramage, G. Biofilm formation is a risk factor for mortality in patients with *Candida albicans* bloodstream infection-Scotland, 2012–2013. *Clin. Microbiol. Infect.* **2016**, *22*, 87–93.
15. Soldini, S.; Posteraro, B.; Vella, A.; De Carolis, E.; Borghi, E.; Falleni, M.; Losito, A.R.; Maiuro, G.; Trecarichi, E.M.; Sanguinetti, M.; et al. Microbiological and clinical characteristics of biofilm-forming *Candida parapsilosis* isolates associated with fungaemia and their impact on mortality. *Clin. Microbiol. Infect.* **2018**, *24*, 771–777. [CrossRef] [PubMed]
16. Mathé, L.; Van Dijck, P. Recent insights into *Candida albicans* biofilm resistance mechanisms. *Curr. Genet.* **2013**, *59*, 251–264. [CrossRef] [PubMed]
17. Tsui, C.; Kong, E.F.; Jabra-Rizk, M.A. Pathogenesis of *Candida albicans* biofilm. *Pathog. Dis.* **2016**, *74*, ftw018. [CrossRef] [PubMed]
18. Mitchell, K.F.; Zarnowski, R.; Andes, D.R. Fungal super glue: The biofilm matrix and its composition, assembly, and functions. *PLoS Pathog.* **2016**, *12*, e1005828. [CrossRef] [PubMed]
19. Taff, H.T.; Mitchell, K.F.; Edward, J.A.; Andes, D.R. Mechanisms of *Candida* biofilm drug resistance. *Future Microbiol.* **2013**, *8*, 1325–1337. [CrossRef] [PubMed]
20. Polke, M.; Leonhardt, I.; Kurzai, O.; Jacobsen, I.D. Farnesol signalling in *Candida albicans*—More than just communication. *Crit. Rev. Microbiol.* **2018**, *44*, 230–243. [CrossRef] [PubMed]
21. Tournu, H.; Van Dijck, P. *Candida* biofilms and the host: Models and new concepts for eradication. *Int. J. Microbiol.* **2012**, *2012*, 845352. [CrossRef] [PubMed]
22. Uppuluri, P.; Chaturvedi, A.K.; Srinivasan, A.; Banerjee, M.; Ramasubramaniam, A.K.; Köhler, J.R.; Kadosh, D.; Lopez-Ribot, J.L. Dispersion as an important step in the *Candida albicans* biofilm developmental cycle. *PLoS Pathog.* **2010**, *6*, e1000828. [CrossRef] [PubMed]
23. Uppuluri, P.; Zaldívar, M.A.; Anderson, M.Z.; Dunn, M.J.; Berman, J.; Ribot, J.L.L.; Köhler, J.R. *Candida albicans* dispersed cells are developmentally distinct from biofilm and planktonic cells. *mBio* **2018**, *9*, e01338-18. [CrossRef] [PubMed]

24. Fox, E.P.; Nobile, C.J. A sticky situation: Untangling the transcriptional network controlling biofilm development in *Candida albicans*. *Transcription* **2012**, *3*, 315–322. [CrossRef] [PubMed]
25. Nobile, C.J.; Fox, E.P.; Nett, J.E.; Sorrells, T.R.; Mitrovich, Q.M.; Hernday, A.D.; Tuch, B.B.; Andes, D.R.; Johnson, A.D. A recently evolved transcriptional network controls biofilm development in *Candida albicans*. *Cell* **2012**, *148*, 126e38. [CrossRef] [PubMed]
26. Fox, E.P.; Bui, C.K.; Nett, J.E.; Hartooni, N.; Mui, M.C.; Andes, D.R.; Nobile, C.J.; Johnson, A.D. An expanded regulatory network temporally controls *Candida albicans* biofilm formation. *Mol. Microbiol.* **2015**, *96*, 1226–1239. [CrossRef] [PubMed]
27. Finkel, J.S.; Xu, W.; Huang, D.; Hill, E.M.; Desai, J.V.; Woolford, C.A.; Nett, J.E.; Taff, H.; Norice, C.T.; Andes, D.R.; et al. Portrait of *Candida albicans* adherence regulators. *PLoS Pathog.* **2012**, *8*, e1002525. [CrossRef] [PubMed]
28. Lee, J.A.; Robbins, N.; Xie, J.L.; Ketela, T.; Cowen, L.E. Functional genomic analysis of *Candida albicans* adherence reveals a key role for the arp2/3 complex in cell wall remodelling and biofilm formation. *PLoS Genet.* **2016**, *12*, e1006452. [CrossRef] [PubMed]
29. Glazier, V.E.; Murante, T.; Murante, D.; Koselny, K.; Liu, Y.; Kim, D.; Koo, H.; Krysan, D.J. Genetic analysis of the *Candida albicans* biofilm transcription factor network using simple and complex haploinsufficiency. *PLoS Genet.* **2017**, *8*, e1006948. [CrossRef] [PubMed]
30. Fox, E.P.; Singh-babak, S.D.; Hartooni, N.; Nobile, C.J. Biofilms and antifungal resistance. In *Antifungals from Genomics to Resistance and the Development of Novel Agents*; Coste, A.T., Vandeputte, P., Eds.; Caister Academic Press: Poole, UK, 2015; p. 71e90.
31. Bachmann, S.P.; VandeWalle, K.; Ramage, G.; Patterson, T.F.; Wickes, B.L.; Graybill, J.R.; López-Ribot, J.L. In vitro activity of echinocandins against *Candida albicans* biofilms. *Antimicrob. Agents Chemother.* **2002**, *46*, 3591–3596. [CrossRef] [PubMed]
32. Kuhn, D.M.; George, T.; Chandra, J.; Mukherjee, P.K.; Ghannoum, M.A. Antifungal susceptibility of *Candida* biofilms: Unique efficacy of amphotericin B lipid formulations and echinocandins. *Antimicrob. Agents Chemother.* **2002**, *46*, 1773–1780. [CrossRef] [PubMed]
33. Ramage, G.; VandeWalle, K.; Bachmann, S.P.; Wickes, B.L.; Lopez-Ribot, J.L. In vitro pharmacodynamic properties of three antifungal agents against preformed *Candida albicans* biofilms determined by time-kill studies. *Antimicrob. Agents Chemother.* **2002**, *46*, 3634–3636. [CrossRef] [PubMed]
34. Ramage, G.; Jose, A.; Sherry, L.; Lappin, D.F.; Jones, B.; Williams, C. Liposomal amphotericin B displays rapid dose-dependent activity against *Candida albicans* biofilms. *Antimicrob. Agents Chemother.* **2013**, *57*, 2369–2371. [CrossRef] [PubMed]
35. Mukherjee, P.K.; Long, L.A.; Kim, H.G.; Ghannoum, M.A. Amphotericin B lipid complex is efficacious in the treatment of *Candida albicans* biofilms using a model of catheter-associated *Candida* biofilms. *Int. J. Antimicrob. Agents* **2009**, *33*, 149–153. [CrossRef] [PubMed]
36. Kucharíková, S.; Tournu, H.; Holtappels, M.; Van Dijck, P.; Lagrou, K. In vivo efficacy of anidulafungin against *Candida albicans* mature biofilms in a novel rat model of catheter-associated candidiasis. *Antimicrob. Agents Chemother.* **2010**, *54*, 4474–4478. [CrossRef] [PubMed]
37. Kucharicová, S.; Sharma, N.; Spriet, I.; Maertens, J.; Van Dijck, P.; Lagrou, K. Activities of systematically administered echinocandins against in vivo mature *Candida albicans* biofilms developed in a rat subcutaneous model. *Antimicrob. Agents Chemother.* **2013**, *57*, 2365–2368. [CrossRef] [PubMed]
38. Ramage, G.; Bachmann, S.; Patterson, T.F.; Wickes, B.L.; Lopez-Ribot, J.L. Investigation of multidrug efflux pumps in relation to fluconazole resistance in *Candida albicans* biofilms. *J. Antimicrob. Chemother.* **2002**, *49*, 973e80. [CrossRef]
39. Anderson, J.B. Evolution of antifungal-drug resistance: Mechanisms and pathogen fitness. *Nat. Rev. Microbiol.* **2005**, *3*, 547e56. [CrossRef] [PubMed]
40. Nobile, C.J.; Johnson, A.D. *Candida albicans* biofilms and human disease. *Annu. Rev. Microbiol.* **2015**, *69*, 71e92. [CrossRef] [PubMed]
41. Nett, J.; Lincoln, L.; Marchillo, K.; Massey, R.; Holoyda, K.; Hoff, B.; VanHandel, M.; Andes, D. Putative role of β-1,3 glucans in *Candida albicans* biofilm resistance. *Antimicrob. Agents Chemother.* **2007**, *51*, 510e20. [CrossRef] [PubMed]

42. Vediyappan, G.; Rossignol, T.; d' Enfert, C. Interaction of *Candida albicans* biofilms with antifungals: Transcriptional response and binding of antifungals to β-glucans. *Antimicrob. Agents Chemother.* **2010**, *54*, 2096e111. [CrossRef] [PubMed]
43. Nagalakshmi, U.; Wang, Z.; Waern, K.; Shou, C.; Raha, D.; Gerstein, M.; Snyder, M. The transcriptional landscape of the yeast genome defined by RNA sequencing. *Science* **2008**, *320*, 1344–1349. [CrossRef] [PubMed]
44. Xiong, Y.; Chen, X.; Chen, Z.; Wang, X.; Shi, S.; Wang, X.; Zhang, J.; He, X. RNA sequencing shows no dosage compensation of the active X-chromosome. *Nat. Genet.* **2010**, *42*, 1043–1047. [CrossRef] [PubMed]
45. Dhamgaye, S.; Bernard, M.; Lelandais, G.; Sismeiro, O.; Lemoine, S.; Coppée, J.Y.; Le Crom, S.; Prasad, R.; Devaux, F. RNA sequencing revealed novel actors of the acquisition of drug resistance in *Candida albicans*. *BMC Genom.* **2012**, *13*, 396. [CrossRef] [PubMed]
46. Gilfillan, G.D.; Sullivan, D.J.; Haynes, K.; Parkinson, T.; Coleman, D.C.; Gow, N.A. *Candida dubliniensis*: Phylogeny and putative virulence factors. *Microbiology* **1998**, *144*, 829–838. [CrossRef] [PubMed]
47. Schorling, S.R.; Kortinga, H.C.; Froschb, M.; Muhlschlegel, F.A. The role of *Candida dubliniensis* in oral candidiasis in human immunodeficiency virus-infected individuals. *Crit. Rev. Microbiol.* **2000**, *26*, 59–68. [CrossRef] [PubMed]
48. Vilela, M.M.; Kamei, K.; Sano, A.; Tanaka, R.; Uno, J.; Takahashi, I.; Ito, J.; Yarita, K.; Miyaji, M. Pathogenicity and virulence of *Candida dubliniensis*: Comparison with *C. albicans*. *Med. Mycol.* **2002**, *40*, 249–257. [CrossRef] [PubMed]
49. Sullivan, D.J.; Moran, G.P.; Pinjon, E.; Al-Mosaid, A.; Stokes, C.; Vaughan, C.; Coleman, D.C. Comparison of the epidemiology, drug resistance mechanisms, and virulence of *Candida dubliniensis* and *Candida albicans*. *FEMS Yeast Res.* **2004**, *4*, 369–376. [CrossRef]
50. Stokes, C.; Moran, G.P.; Spiering, M.J.; Cole, G.T.; Coleman, D.C.; Sullivan, D.J. Lower filamentation rates of *Candida dubliniensis* contribute to its lower virulence in comparison with *Candida albicans*. *Fungal. Genet. Biol.* **2007**, *44*, 920–931. [CrossRef] [PubMed]
51. Sullivan, D.; Coleman, D. *Candida dubliniensis*: Characteristics and identification. *J. Clin. Microbiol.* **1998**, *36*, 329–334. [PubMed]
52. Schoofs, A.; Odds, F.C.; Colebunders, R.; Ieven, M.; Goossens, H. Use of specialised isolation media for recognition and identification of *Candida dubliniensis* isolates from HIV-infected patients. *Eur. J. Clin. Microbiol. Infect. Dis.* **1997**, *16*, 296–300. [CrossRef] [PubMed]
53. Caplice, N.; Moran, G.P. *Candida albicans* exhibits enhanced alkaline and temperature induction of Efg1-regulated transcripts relative to *Candida dubliniensis*. *Genom. Data* **2015**, *6*, 130–135. [CrossRef] [PubMed]
54. McCullough, M.; Ross, B.; Reade, P. Characterization of genetically distinct subgroup of *Candida albicans* strains isolated from oral cavities of patients infected with human immunodeficiency virus. *J. Clin. Microbiol.* **1995**, *33*, 696–700. [PubMed]
55. Moran, G.; Stokes, C.; Thewes, S.; Hube, B.; Coleman, D.C.; Sullivan, D. Comparative genomics using *Candida albicans* DNA microarrays reveals absence and divergence of virulence-associated genes in *Candida dubliniensis*. *Microbiology* **2004**, *150*, 3363–3382. [CrossRef] [PubMed]
56. Jackson, A.P.; Gamble, J.A.; Yeomans, T.; Moran, G.P.; Saunders, D.; Harris, D.; Aslett, M.; Barrell, J.F.; Butler, G.; Citiulo, F.; et al. Comparative genomics of the fungal pathogens *Candida dubliniensis* and *Candida albicans*. *Genom. Res.* **2009**, *19*, 2231–2244. [CrossRef] [PubMed]
57. Grumaz, C.; Lorenz, S.; Stevens, P.; Lindemann, E.; Schock, U.; Retey, J.; Rupp, S.; Sohn, K. Species and condition specific adaptation of the transcriptional landscapes in *Candida albicans* and *Candida dubliniensis*. *BMC Genom.* **2013**, *14*, 212. [CrossRef] [PubMed]
58. Butler, G.; Rasmussen, M.D.; Lin, M.F.; Santos, M.A.; Sakthikumar, S.; Munro, C.A.; Rheinbay, E.; Grabherr, M.; Forche, A.; Reedy, J.L.; et al. Evolution of pathogenicity and sexual reproduction in eight *Candida* genomes. *Nature* **2009**, *459*, 657–662. [CrossRef] [PubMed]
59. Bruno, V.M.; Wang, Z.; Marjani, S.L.; Euskirchen, G.M.; Martin, J.; Sherlock, G.; Snyder, M. Comprehensive annotation of the transcriptome of the human fungal pathogen *Candida albicans* using RNA-seq. *Genom. Res.* **2010**, *20*, 1451–1458. [CrossRef] [PubMed]
60. Movahed, E.; Munusamy, K.; Tan, G.M.; Looi, C.Y.; Tay, S.T.; Wong, W.F. Genome-wide transcription study of *Cryptococcus neoformans* H99 clinical strain versus environmental strains. *PLoS ONE* **2015**, *10*, e0137457. [CrossRef] [PubMed]

61. Giosa, D.; Felice, M.R.; Lawrence, T.J.; Gulati, M.; Scordino, F.; Giuffre, L.; Lo Passo, C.; D'Alessandro, E.; Criseo, G.; Ardell, D.H.; et al. Whole RNA-sequencing and transcriptome assembly of *Candida albicans* and *Candida africana* under chlamydospore-inducing conditions. *Genom. Biol. Evol.* **2017**, *9*, 1971–1977. [CrossRef] [PubMed]
62. d' Enfert, C.; Goyard, S.; Rodriguez-Arnaveilhe, S.; Frangeul, L.; Jones, L.; Tekaia, F.; Bader, O.; Albrecht, A.; Castillo, L.; Dominguez, A.; et al. CandidaDB: A genome database for *Candida albicans* pathogenomics. *Nucleic Acids Res.* **2005**, *33*, D353–D357. [CrossRef] [PubMed]
63. García-Sánchez, S.; Aubert, S.; Iraqui, I.; Janbon, G.; Ghigo, J.M.; d' Enfert, C. *Candida albicans* biofilms: A developmental state associated with specific and stable gene expression patterns. *Eukaryot. Cell* **2004**, *3*, 536–545. [CrossRef] [PubMed]
64. Liu, T.T.; Znaidi, S.; Barker, K.S.; Xu, L.; Homayouni, R.; Saidane, S.; Morschhäuser, J.; Nantel, A.; Raymond, M.; Rogers, P.D. Genome-wide expression and location analyses of the *Candida albicans* Tac1p regulon. *Eukaryot. Cell* **2007**, *6*, 2122–2238. [CrossRef] [PubMed]
65. Azadmanesh, J.; Gowen, A.M.; Creger, P.E.; Schafer, N.D.; Blankenship, J.R. Filamentation involves two overlapping, but distinct, programs of filamentation in the pathogenic fungus *Candida albicans*. *Genes Genom. Genet.* **2017**, *7*, 3797–3808. [CrossRef] [PubMed]
66. Li, D.D.; Chai, D.; Huang, X.W.; Guan, S.X.; Du, J.; Zhang, H.Y.; Sun, Y.; Jiang, Y.Y. Potent in vitro synergism of fluconazole and osthole against fluconazole-resistant *Candida albicans*. *Antimicrob. Agents Chemother.* **2017**, *61*, e00436-17. [CrossRef] [PubMed]
67. Carratalà, J. The antibiotic-lock technique for therapy of 'highly needed' infected catheters. *Clin. Microbiol. Infect.* **2002**, *8*, 282–289. [CrossRef] [PubMed]
68. Cateau, E.; Berjeaud, J.M.; Imbert, C. Possible role of azole and echinocandin lock solutions in the control of *Candida* biofilms associated with silicone. *Int. J. Antimicrob. Agents* **2011**, *37*, 380–384. [CrossRef] [PubMed]
69. Toulet, D.; Debarre, C.; Imbert, C. Could liposomal amphotericin B (L-AMB) lock solutions be useful to inhibit *Candida* spp. biofilms on silicone biomaterials? *J. Antimicrob. Chemother.* **2012**, *67*, 430–432. [CrossRef] [PubMed]
70. Raad, I.; Hanna, H.; Dvorak, T.; Chaiban, G.; Hachem, R. Optimal antimicrobial catheter lock solution, using different combinations of minocycline, EDTA, and 25-percent ethanol, rapidly eradicates organisms embedded in biofilm. *Antimicrob. Agents. Chemother.* **2007**, *51*, 78–83. [CrossRef] [PubMed]
71. Bonne, S.; Mazuski, J.E.; Sona, C.; Schallom, M.; Boyle, W.; Buchman, T.G.; Bochicchio, G.V.; Coopersmith, C.M.; Schuerer, D.J. Effectiveness of minocycline and rifampin vs chlorhexidine and silver sulfadiazine-impregnated central venous catheters in preventing central line-associated bloodstream infection in a high-volume academic intensive care unit: A before and after trial. *J. Am. Coll. Surg.* **2015**, *221*, 739–747. [CrossRef] [PubMed]
72. Villard, N.; Seneviratne, C.; Tsoi, J.K.H.; Heinonen, M.; Matinlinna, J. *Candida albicans* aspects of novel silane system-coated titanium and zirconia implant surfaces. *Clin. Oral Implants Res.* **2015**, *26*, 332–341. [CrossRef] [PubMed]
73. Karlsson, A.J.; Flessner, R.M.; Gellman, S.H.; Lynn, D.M.; Palecek, S.P. Polyelectrolyte multilayers fabricated from antifungal β-peptides: Design of surfaces that exhibit antifungal activity against *Candida albicans*. *Biomacromolecules* **2010**, *11*, 2321–2328. [CrossRef] [PubMed]
74. Hoque, J.; Akkapeddi, P.; Yadav, V.; Manjunath, G.B.; Uppu, D.S.; Konai, M.M.; Yarlagadda, V.; Sanyal, K.; Haldar, J. Broad spectrum antibacterial and antifungal polymeric paint materials: Synthesis, structure-activity relationship, and membrane-active mode of action. *ACS. Appl. Mater. Interfaces* **2015**, *7*, 1804–1815. [CrossRef] [PubMed]
75. Shinde, R.B.; Chauhan, N.M.; Raut, J.S.; Karuppayil, S.M. Sensitization of *Candida albicans* biofilms to various antifungal drugs by cyclosporine A. *Ann. Clin. Microbiol. Antimicrob.* **2012**, *11*, 27. [CrossRef] [PubMed]
76. Khodavandi, A.; Harmal, N.S.; Alizadeh, F.; Scully, O.J.; Sidik, S.M.; Othman, F.; Sekawi, Z.; Ng, K.P.; Chong, P.P. Comparison between allicin and fluconazole in *Candida albicans* biofilm inhibition and in suppression of *HWP1* gene expression. *Phytomedicine* **2011**, *19*, 56–63. [CrossRef] [PubMed]
77. Robbins, N.; Uppuluri, P.; Nett, J.; Rajendran, R.; Ramage, G.; Lopez-Ribot, J.L.; Andes, D.; Cowen, L.E. Hsp90 governs dispersion and drug resistance of fungal biofilms. *PLoS Pathog.* **2011**, *7*, e1002257. [CrossRef] [PubMed]

78. Bink, A.; Kucharíková, S.; Neirinck, B.; Vleugels, J.; Van Dijck, P.; Cammue, B.P.; Thevissen, K. The nonsteroidal antiinflammatory drug diclofenac potentiates the in vivo activity of caspofungin against *Candida albicans* biofilms. *J. Infect. Dis.* **2012**, *206*, 1790–1797. [CrossRef] [PubMed]
79. Gao, Y.; Zhang, C.; Lu, C.; Liu, P.; Li, Y.; Li, H.; Sun, S. Synergistic effect of doxycycline and fluconazole against *Candida albicans* biofilms and the impact of calcium channel blockers. *FEMS Yeast Res.* **2013**, *13*, 453–462. [CrossRef] [PubMed]
80. Stepanovic, S.; Vukovic, D.; Jesic, M.; Ranin, L. Influence of acetylsalicylic acid (aspirin) on biofilm production by *Candida* species. *J. Chemother.* **2004**, *16*, 134–138. [CrossRef] [PubMed]
81. Ramage, G.; Saville, S.P.; Wickes, B.L.; Lopez-Ribot, J.L. Inhibition of *Candida albicans* biofilm formation by farnesol, a quorum-sensing molecule. *Appl. Environ. Microbiol.* **2002**, *68*, 5459–5463. [CrossRef] [PubMed]
82. Sharma, M.; Prasad, R. The quorum-sensing molecule farnesol is a modulator of drug efflux mediated by ABC multidrug transporters and synergizes with drugs in *Candida albicans*. *Antimicrob. Agents Chemother.* **2011**, *55*, 4834–4843. [CrossRef] [PubMed]
83. Yu, L.H.; Wei, X.; Ma, M.; Chen, X.J.; Xu, S.B. Possible inhibitory molecular mechanism of farnesol on the development of fluconazole resistance in *Candida albicans* biofilm. *Antimicrob. Agents Chemother.* **2012**, *56*, 770–775. [CrossRef] [PubMed]
84. Martin, M.; Henriques, M.; Lopez-Ribot, J.L.; Oliveira, R. Addition of DNase improves the in vitro activity of antifungal drugs against *Candida albicans* biofilms. *Mycoses* **2012**, *55*, 80–85. [CrossRef] [PubMed]
85. Raut, J.S.; Shinde, R.B.; Chauhan, N.M.; Karuppayil, S.M. Phenylpropanoids of plant origin as inhibitors of biofilm formation by *Candida albicans*. *J. Microbiol. Biotechnol.* **2014**, *24*, 1216–1225. [CrossRef] [PubMed]
86. Raut, J.S.; Shinde, R.B.; Chauhan, N.M.; Mohan Karuppayil, S. Terpenoids of plant origin inhibit morphogenesis, adhesion, and biofilm formation by *Candida albicans*. *Biofouling* **2013**, *29*, 87–96. [CrossRef] [PubMed]
87. Morales, D.K.; Grahl, N.; Okegbe, C.; Dietrich, L.E.; Jacobs, N.J.; Hogan, D.A. Control of *Candida albicans* metabolism and biofilm formation by *Pseudomonas aeruginosa* phenazines. *MBio* **2013**, *4*, 1–9. [CrossRef] [PubMed]
88. Theberge, S.; Semlali, A.; Alamri, A.; Leung, K.P.; Rouabhia, M. *C. albicans* growth, transition, biofilm formation, and gene expression modulation by antimicrobial decapeptide KSL-W. *BMC Microbiol.* **2013**, *13*, 246. [CrossRef] [PubMed]
89. Siles, S.A.; Srinivasan, A.; Pierce, C.G.; Lopez-Ribot, J.L.; Ramasubramanian, A.K. High-throughput screening of a collection of known pharmacologically active small compounds for the identification of *Candida albicans* biofilm inhibitors. *Antimicrob. Agents Chemother.* **2013**, *57*, 3681–3687. [CrossRef] [PubMed]
90. Wong, S.S.; Kao, R.Y.; Yuen, K.Y.; Wang, Y.; Yang, D.; Samaranayake, L.P.; Seneviratne, C.J. In vitro and in vivo activity of a novel antifungal small molecule against *Candida* infections. *PLoS ONE* **2014**, *9*, e85836. [CrossRef] [PubMed]
91. Pierce, C.G.; Chaturvedi, A.K.; Lazzell, A.L.; Powell, A.T.; Saville, S.P.; McHardy, S.F.; Lopez-Ribot, J.L. A novel small molecule inhibitor of *Candida albicans* biofilm formation, filamentation and virulence with low potential for the development of resistance. *NPJ Biofilms Microb.* **2015**, *1*, 15012. [CrossRef] [PubMed]
92. Romo, J.A.; Pierce, C.G.; Chaturvedi, A.K.; Lazzell, A.L.; McHardy, S.F.; Saville, S.P.; Lopez-Ribot, J.L. Development of anti-virulence approaches for candidiasis via a novel series of small-molecule inhibitors of *Candida albicans* Filamentation. *mBio* **2017**, *8*, e01991-17. [CrossRef] [PubMed]
93. Rosseti, I.B.; Chagas, L.R.; Costa, M.S. Photodynamic antimicrobial chemotherapy (PACT) inhibits biofilm formation by *Candida albicans*, increasing both ROS production and membrane permeability. *Lasers Med. Sci.* **2014**, *29*, 1059–1064. [CrossRef] [PubMed]
94. Černáková, L.; Chupáčová, J.; Židlíková, K.; Bujdáková, H. Effectiveness of the photoactive dye methylene blue versus caspofungin on the *Candida parapsilosis* biofilm in vitro and ex vivo. *Photochem. Photobiol.* **2015**, *91*, 1181–1190. [CrossRef] [PubMed]
95. Chien, H.F.; Chen, C.P.; Chen, Y.C.; Chang, P.H.; Tsai, T.; Chen, C.T. The use of chitosan to enhance photodynamic inactivation against *Candida albicans* and its drug-resistant clinical isolates. *Int. J. Mol. Sci.* **2013**, *14*, 7445–7456. [CrossRef] [PubMed]
96. Lara, H.H.; Romero-Urbina, D.G.; Pierce, C.; Lopez-Ribot, J.L.; Arellano-Jiménez, M.J.; Jose-Yacaman, M. Effect of silver nanoparticles on *Candida albicans* biofilms: An ultrastructural study. *J. Nanobiotechnol.* **2015**, *13*, 91. [CrossRef] [PubMed]

97. Radhakrishnan, V.S.; Reddy Mudiam, M.K.; Kumar, M.; Dwivedi, S.P.; Singh, S.P.; Prasad, T. Silver nanoparticles induced alterations in multiple cellular targets, which are critical for drug susceptibilities and pathogenicity in fungal pathogen (*Candida albicans*). *Int. J. Nanomed.* **2018**, *13*, 2647–2663. [CrossRef] [PubMed]
98. Gondim, B.L.C.; Castellano, L.R.C.; de Castro, R.D.; Machado, G.; Carlo, H.L.; Valença, A.M.G.; de Carvalho, F.G. Effect of chitosan nanoparticles on the inhibition of *Candida* spp. biofilm on denture base surface. *Arch. Oral. Biol.* **2018**, *94*, 99–107. [CrossRef] [PubMed]
99. de Alteriis, E.; Maselli, V.; Falanga, A.; Galdiero, S.; Di Lella, F.M.; Gesuele, R.; Guida, M.; Galdiero, E. Efficiency of gold nanoparticles coated with the antimicrobial peptide indolicidin against biofilm formation and development of *Candida* spp. clinical isolates. *Infect. Drug Resist.* **2018**, *11*, 915–925. [CrossRef] [PubMed]
100. Baigorria, E.; Reynoso, E.; Alvarez, M.G.; Milanesio, M.E.; Durantini, E.N. Silica nanoparticles embedded with water insoluble phthalocyanines for the photoinactivation of microorganisms. *Photodiagn. Photodyn. Ther.* **2018**, *23*, 261–269. [CrossRef] [PubMed]
101. Mosallam, F.M.; El-Sayyad, G.S.; Fathy, R.M.; El-Batal, A.I. Biomolecules-mediated synthesis of selenium nanoparticles using *Aspergillus oryzae* fermented Lupin extract and gamma radiation for hindering the growth of some multidrug-resistant bacteria and pathogenic fungi. *Microb. Pathog.* **2018**, *122*, 108–116. [CrossRef] [PubMed]
102. Perlroth, J.; Choi, B.; Spellberg, B. Nosocomial fungal infections: Epidemiology, diagnosis, and treatment. *Med. Mycol.* **2007**, *45*, 321–346. [CrossRef] [PubMed]
103. Spellberg, B. Vaccines for invasive fungal infections. *F1000 Med. Rep.* **2011**, *3*, 13. [CrossRef] [PubMed]
104. Santos, E.; Levitz, S.M. Fungal vaccines and immunotherapeutics. *Cold Spring Harb. Perspect. Med.* **2014**, *4*, a019711. [CrossRef] [PubMed]
105. Shahid, S.K. Newer patents in antimycotic therapy. *Pharm. Pat Anal.* **2016**, *5*, 115–134. [CrossRef] [PubMed]
106. Edwards, J.E. Fungal cell wall vaccines: An update. *J. Med. Microbiol.* **2012**, *61*, 895–903. [CrossRef] [PubMed]
107. Vecchiarelli, A.; Pericolini, E.; Gabrielli, E.; Pietrella, D. New approaches in the development of a vaccine for mucosal candidiasis: Progress and challenges. *Front. Microbiol.* **2012**, *3*, 294. [CrossRef] [PubMed]

13

Immunomodulation as a Therapy for *Aspergillus* Infection: Current Status and Future Perspectives

Chris D. Lauruschkat, Hermann Einsele and Juergen Loeffler *

Department of Internal Medicine II, University Hospital Wuerzburg, WÜ4i, Building C11, 97080 Wuerzburg, Germany; Lauruschka_c@ukw.de (C.D.L.); Einsele_h@ukw.de (H.E.)

* Correspondence: Loeffler_j@ukw.de

Abstract: Invasive aspergillosis (IA) is the most serious life-threatening infectious complication of intensive remission induction chemotherapy and allogeneic stem cell transplantation in patients with a variety of hematological malignancies. *Aspergillus fumigatus* is the most commonly isolated species from cases of IA. Despite the various improvements that have been made with preventative strategies and the development of antifungal drugs, there is an urgent need for new therapeutic approaches that focus on strategies to boost the host's immune response, since immunological recovery is recognized as being the major determinant of the outcome of IA. Here, we aim to summarize current knowledge about a broad variety of immunotherapeutic approaches against IA, including therapies based on the transfer of distinct immune cell populations, and the administration of cytokines and antibodies.

Keywords: Immunotherapy; invasive aspergillosis; *Aspergillus fumigatus*; fungal infections; innate immunity; adaptive immunity; cell therapy; cytokine therapy

---

1. Introduction

Within the last decade, the filamentous fungus *Aspergillus fumigatus* (*A. fumigatus*) has underlined its role as one of the most clinically relevant fungal pathogens. Conidia of this saprobic fungus can be isolated ubiquitously. Because of this high abundance, hundreds of spores of *Aspergillus* are inhaled daily by each individual [1]. Mucociliary clearance and phagocytic cells in the lung prevent disease in immunocompetent individuals. This includes alveolar macrophages, the major resident cells in the lung alveoli, which most efficiently engulf conidia in the lung [2].

The most severe disease caused by *Aspergillus* is invasive aspergillosis (IA). Major risk factors include immunosuppression, neutropenia, lymphopenia, and depletion of T cells [3]. Thus, IA occurs almost exclusively in immunocompromised patients. The incidence in allogeneic stem cell transplantation (allo-SCT) patients ranges from 4%–10%. Although many *Aspergilli* cause IA, *A. fumigatus* is responsible for more than 90% of all systemic *Aspergillus* infections [4].

Innate immunity is of major importance for the defense against *A. fumigatus*. In contrast to most bacterial pathogens, *A. fumigatus* undergoes major morphological changes during the early phase of infection. In the alveoli, inert spores swell, germinate, and grow into lung tissue, becoming subsequently angioinvasive and lastly undergoing hematogenous dissemination [5]. Cells of the innate immunity recognize the different fungal morphologies by distinct pattern recognition receptors (e.g., TLR2, TLR4, and dectin-1), which induce cell-specific and general defense mechanisms [6]. Upon stimulation with *A. fumigatus* in vitro, polymorphonuclear neutrophils (PMNs) release reactive oxygen intermediates and form neutrophil extracellular traps. Dendritic cells (DCs) release inflammatory cytokines (e.g., TNF-α and IL-1) and chemokines (e.g., IL-8 and CXCL10), which attract and activate other innate immune cell populations and build a bridge between the innate and the adaptive immunity by processing fungal antigens and presenting them to T cells. Natural killer (NK) cells degranulate and secrete cytotoxic proteins (perforin, granzymes) in response to *A. fumigatus*, causing fungal damage, and produce Th1 cytokines and chemokines, again attracting and activating other innate immune cell populations [7–9].

Unfortunately, there is still a lack of reliable diagnostic and therapeutic tools, resulting in high mortality rates of up to 90%, depending on the patient cohort and the localization of the fungus [10]. Therapy of *Aspergillus* infection remains limited to only a handful of antifungal agents. Voriconazole is the drug of choice for primary therapy of IA, with isavuconazole and the liposomal formulation of amphotericin B serving as alternatives. Echinocandins (e.g., anidulafungin) and other mold-active azoles (e.g., itraconazole and posaconazole) remain for salvage therapy [11]. Recently, triazole-resistant *A. fumigatus* strains have increasingly been isolated from patients. These strains emerge most likely due to the extensive use of azole fungicidals in agriculture and massively hinder antifungal treatment [12].

The following pages describe how different options of immune modulation have or will become alternatives to treat *Aspergillus* infection. In the case of immunocompromised patients, this usually involves therapeutic enhancement of immunity, including cell therapy approaches such as the transfusion of cells of the innate (granulocytes, dendritic cells, natural killer cells) and adaptive immune systems (T cells) as well as the administration of different cytokines, chemokines, and antibodies (Figure 1).

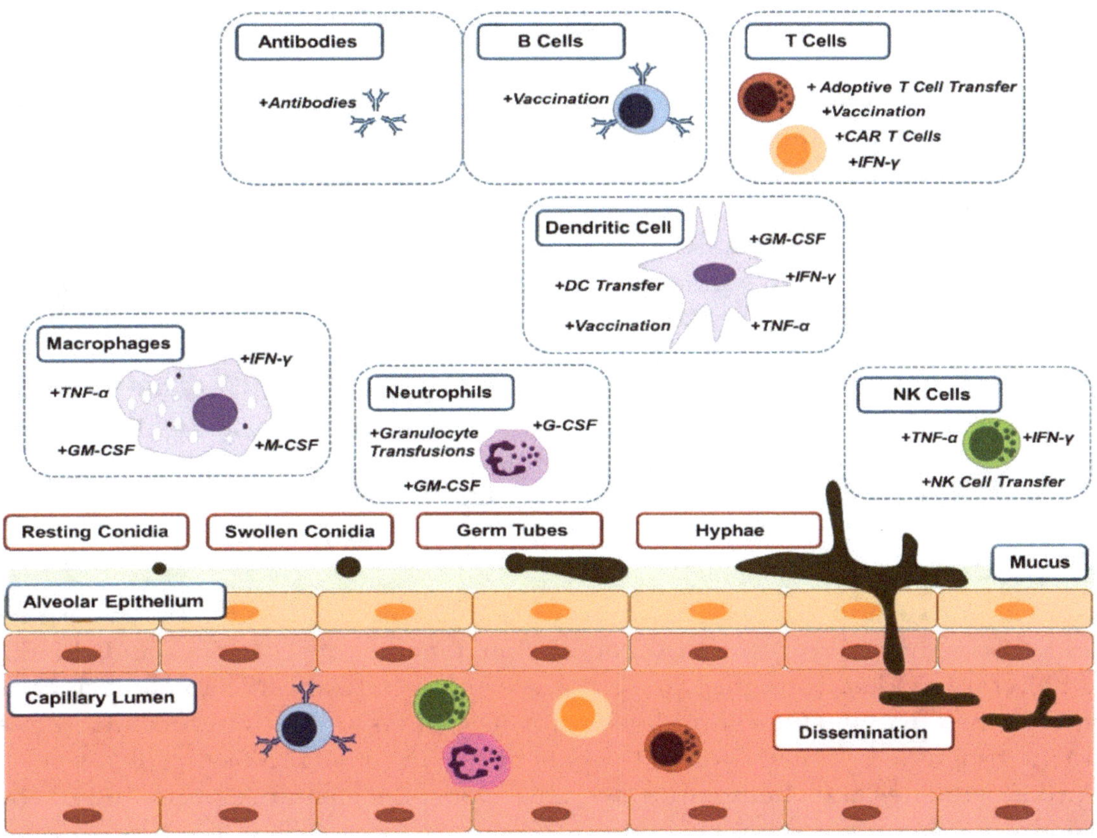

Figure 1. Cells of the innate and adaptive immune systems interact with different morphotypes of *Aspergillus fumigatus*. Macrophages clear resting and swollen conidia. Neutrophils attack all morphotypes of the fungus, while natural killer (NK) cells react to germ tubes and hyphae. Dendritic cells bridge the innate immune system to the adaptive immune system, which orchestrates fungal clearance of all morphotypes. Immunotherapeutic treatment options supporting these cells of the innate and adaptive immune systems are indicated next to the cell type they affect. Abbreviations: dendritic cell (DC); chimeric antigen receptor (CAR); granulocyte-macrophage colony stimulating factor (GM-CSF); granulocyte CSF (G-CSF); macrophage CSF (M-CSF); interferon (IFN) γ; tumor necrosis factor (TNF) α.

2. Cell Therapy

2.1. Granulocyte Transfusion

PMNs are able to engulf fungus, release antimicrobial peptides, and form extracellular traps [13,14]. After allo-SCT, especially during neutropenia, the ability of the immune system to effectively clear fungus is severely limited. Numerous studies have evaluated the transfusion of high numbers of neutrophils to patients during neutropenia in the past decades. Allogeneic granulocyte transfusions (GTs) dramatically increase neutrophil counts, which is speculated to reverse the increased susceptibility to infections in allo-SCT patients [15,16]. GTs have shown low toxicity in allo-SCT patients and are considered to be safe [16,17].

In a phase I/II clinical trial, allogeneic neutrophil transfusion in combination with dexamethasone and granulocyte colony stimulating factors (G-CSF) increased neutrophil counts and response; however, none of the five patients suffering from aspergillosis survived [16]. Mousset et al. reported that in hematological patients, who received either prophylactic or interventional GTs, *Aspergillus* infection could be controlled in 17 out of 22 cases. This result, however, was limited by the inclusion of possible IA cases into the study population and the trial's nonrandomized nature [18]. In contrast, in a randomized phase III clinical trial in which GTs were given to neutropenic patients, no difference in 100-day survival of fungal infections was found. The authors of the study did not discriminate between different fungal infections; nonetheless, 49 of the 55 cases were *Aspergillus* infections [17]. In a randomized multicenter controlled study, 58 neutropenic subjects were treated with GTs plus G-CSF and dexamethasone in addition to standard microbial treatment. This arm of the trial was compared to 56 neutropenic patients on standard microbial treatment alone. No difference in infections between the groups was found. Both the control and treatment groups included only three proven aspergillosis cases [19], which made it difficult to draw conclusions for *Aspergillus* infections. Moreover, to improve the limited life span of transfused granulocytes, granulocyte progenitors for transfusion could be used. Bitmansour et al. have shown protection of neutropenic mice from *A. fumigatus* infection by granulocyte/monocyte progenitors [20,21].

In summary, although GTs have a lot of potential and new trials should be performed to further clarify the effect of GTs, no recommendation of treating allo-SCT patients with GTs is currently given [22]. The limited success of GT transfusions up to date might be a result of the transfusion of too low granulocyte numbers in some patients [19] and points to the necessity of overcoming multifactorial dysfunctions of the immune system after allo-SCT in order to prevent and clear IA.

2.2. Dendritic Cells (DCs)

DCs connect innate and adaptive immunity. They recognize fungus by pattern recognition receptors and process fungal antigens. After activation, they secrete cytokines and chemokines and migrate to the lymph nodes. Here they present these antigens to specific T cells, which in turn are activated and primed. Ex vivo DCs stimulated with *Aspergillus* antigens induce protective immune responses to the fungus after transfusion to the patient due to activation of *Aspergillus*-specific T cells and secretion of cytokines and chemokines, which support the clearance of the fungus by both the innate and adaptive immune systems [23–25].

DC stimulation with unmethylated CpG oligodeoxynucleotides as an adjuvant in combination with one of the major *A. fumigatus* allergens, Asp f 16, induced a protective Th1 response in a hematopoietic stem cell transplantation (HSCT) mouse model of IA [26]. The same protective Th1 response was found when DCs were stimulated by *A. fumigatus* conidia and transfected with IL-12 in a similar murine model [27]. In addition, DCs that had been transduced with IL-12 and stimulated by *A. fumigatus* were administered to neutropenic mice in a model for IA. The treatment led to less mortality and decreased fungal burden due to a strong Th1 response [28]. Asp f 16-stimulated DCs were more effective in generating a cytotoxic T lymphocyte response against *Aspergillus* when antigen presentation of DCs was succeeded by a second antigen presentation using Epstein–Barr virus-transformed B lymphoblastoid cell lines. This method was described as more effective in generating Asp f 16-specific cytotoxic T lymphocytes (CTLs), and therefore would require less initial blood volume of the patient compared to DC stimulation alone [29].

In conclusion, an ex vivo stimulation of DCs and subsequent administration to the patient is cost inefficient, difficult to scale, and labor intensive. It shows, however, the therapeutic potential of fungal vaccination [30].

2.3. Natural Killer Cell Therapy

NK cells participate in the control of numerous pathogens, including viruses and fungi [31]. They have been shown to interact with *A. fumigatus*, *Cryptococcus neoformans*, *Candida albicans*, and Mucorales [32].

NK cells directly interact with *A. fumigatus* through the neural cell adhesion molecule (NCAM-1, CD56), and this interaction leads to the secretion of CC chemokine ligands CCL3, 4, and 5 [33]. After contact with *A. fumigatus*, NK cells become activated and release soluble factors such as perforin and granzyme, which mediate antifungal activity [34].

Higher reactive oxygen species (ROS) production and NK cell counts were associated with better control of IA in allo-SCT patients [35]. Referring to this study, Fernández-Ruiz et al. investigated NK cell counts of solid organ transplant recipients and correlated them to fungal infections. During the median follow-up period of 504.5 days, 10 out of 396 patients suffered from invasive fungal infection (IFI), and 4/10 IFI cases were classified as IA. Higher NK cell counts one month after transplantation decreased the incidence of fungal infections. In vivo, NK cells were the most significant contributor to IFN-γ secretion during the early stages of *Aspergillus* infection in the lungs of neutropenic mice. NK cell depletion resulted in higher mortality. In turn, fungal clearance was increased by transferring activated NK cells of wild-type mice to IFN-γ-deficient or wild-type neutropenic mice. The transfer of NK cells of IFN-γ-deficient mice into the same murine models, however, showed no effect [36]. Moreover, *Aspergillus niger* growth was partly inhibited due to increased NK cell activity in a murine model [37].

These results suggest that allogeneic NK cell transfer might be beneficial for the prevention of IA. Allogeneic NK cell transfer and transfer of the cell line NK92 after irradiation, which is already FDA-approved for clinical testing in certain types of cancer, were used in clinical studies and have a good safety profile in patients [38–42]. Nonetheless, they have to show their efficacy against IA in future studies.

2.4. Adoptive T Cell Transfer

The protective effect of *Aspergillus*-specific CD4$^+$ cells of the Th1 lineage has been shown throughout the literature [43]. After allo-SCT, the adaptive immune system reconstitutes much slower than the innate immune system. Only a few *Aspergillus*-specific T cells can be measured 9–12 months after allo-SCT [44]. Therefore, an artificial increase of these specific T cells might help to clear *Aspergillus* in immunocompromised patients. For adoptive T cell transfer, T cells are isolated from the patient and stimulated with defined antigens. Consequently, T cell populations that are specific for the antigens are activated and proliferate. In turn, high numbers of these specific T cells are injected into the patient, where they recognize their target and aid the immune system in its elimination [45]. While the benefits of adoptive T cell transfer were illustrated in viral infections after transplantation, the development of similar techniques for the transfer of fungus-specific T cells lags behind [45].

One major obstacle to successful specific T cell transfer for *Aspergillus* in allo-SCT patients is the generation of an adequate number of *Aspergillus*-specific T cells with sufficient purity, using Good Manufacturing Practice (GMP) guidelines. Because of the fast progression of IA, the enrichment process needs to be as fast as possible. Many groups have worked toward complying with these requirements [46–49]. Bacher et al. reported a GMP-compliant protocol, in which they were able to enrich *Aspergillus*-specific T cells 200-fold in the T cell population. After isolation, they depleted cytotoxic and regulatory T cells, stimulated the remaining T cells with a GMP-grade *A. fumigatus* lysate, and isolated *A. fumigatus*-specific T cells with the help of the T cell activation marker CD137. This protocol is being used in an ongoing clinical trial (EudraCT Nr.2013-002914-11) [50]. However, another group has demonstrated that immunosuppressants such as cyclosporine A, methylprednisolone, as well as mycophenolic acid, lowered the number and activation of *Aspergillus*-specific protective Th1 cells. These immunosuppressants are frequently used after allo-SCT, complicating the application of adoptive T cell transfer in allo-SCT patients [51].

Up to this point, to our knowledge, there is only one clinical trial testing the efficacy and safety of adoptive T cell transfer in invasive fungal diseases. In this study, 10 patients with IA were treated by adoptive T cell transfer, while 13 IA patients in the control group did not receive a cell transfusion. The IA clearance rate was 90% in the treatment group compared to 53% in the control group. Infused cells did not cause graft versus host disease (GvHD) and showed a high IFN-γ to IL-10 ratio, indicating Th1 priming in the first three weeks after infusion. In contrast, patients in the control group had only a few naturally occurring *Aspergillus*-specific T cells 9–12 months after transplantation, exhibiting a nonprotective Th2 profile. In addition, patients receiving adoptive T cell transfer showed significantly decreased galactomannan antigenemia in comparison to the levels in the control group [44]. In order to shorten the time in between diagnosis and the transfusion of the cell product, off-the-shelf T cells specific for certain viruses were developed. They were found to be safe and only rarely caused mild GvHD (grade 1) [52]. Production of off-the-shelf T cells for transfusing IA patients is desirable.

Current findings have indicated that not only $CD4^+$ T cell responses are important against *Aspergillus*, but cytotoxic $CD8^+$ T cells might play an important role as well [53,54]. CTLs stimulated with Asp f 16 were able to induce increased Th1 responses. The transfer of Asp f 16-specific CTLs resulted in higher survival in a murine model of IA [55]. In consequence, adoptive T cell transfer for IA might not only be limited to $CD4^+$ cells.

Adoptive T cell transfer is a promising tool for the fight against IA. GMP-compliant protocols for the production of sufficient numbers of *Aspergillus*-specific T cells are available, and off-the-shelf cell products against the infection might be developed soon. The results of the first clinical trial have been very promising, and there should be strong incentives for additional clinical trials.

2.5. Chimeric Antigen Receptors (CARs)

Chimeric antigen receptor (CAR) T cells are one of the most promising immunotherapeutic tools available and have shown their efficacy in primary clinical trials of B cell malignancies [56]. The FDA has already approved CAR T cell therapies for the treatment of acute lymphoblastic leukemia (ALL) and B cell lymphoma in appropriate patient groups [57]. CARs are artificially designed receptors that are introduced into T cells. MHC unrestricted antigen recognition and the capability to recognize glycoproteins and lipids are only two of the many advantages of this approach [58,59]. CARs consist of two extracellular, one transmembrane, and one intracellular element. The task of the extracellular targeting element is to recognize the target. The single chain variable fragment (scFv) region of a monoclonal antibody targeting the desired antigen is usually used, but other targeting elements such as extracellular parts of naturally occurring receptors are also tested. The targeting element is linked to a spacer or linker, which gives the targeting element the flexibility to bind to the intended target [60]. The most common transmembrane domain used in CARs is the transmembrane spanning region of CD28 [61]. The intracellular domain assures signal delivery, resulting in the activation of the cell. In first-generation CARs, CD3-ζ was used for signal transduction. In second-generation CARs, a costimulatory domain, most commonly CD28 and 4-1BB, was added to CD3-ζ, resulting in better persistence of CAR T cells [62] (Figure 2).

The success of CAR T cells in B cell malignancies led to the attempt to use CARs for infections like aspergillosis. The group of Cooper et al. swapped the CD19 targeting element of a second-generation CAR, which is currently being evaluated in a clinical trial, with the extracellular part of Dectin-1 [63,64]. Dectin-1 is a naturally occurring receptor of the innate immune system that is not expressed on T cells. Its ligand ß-glucan is a polysaccharide found on the surface of many fungi, including *Aspergillus*. In addition to the extracellular part of Dectin-1, the Dectin-1 CAR (D-CAR) consisted of an IgG4 spacer, a CD28 transmembrane domain, and an intracellular domain of CD28 and CD3-ζ. The authors demonstrated that the D-CAR was activated by ß-glucan and inhibited the growth of *A. fumigatus*. In addition, IFN-γ concentration increased after stimulation, and the perforin/granzyme pathway was likely activated [63]. Interestingly, steroid treatment did not inhibit the antifungal activity of the D-CAR.

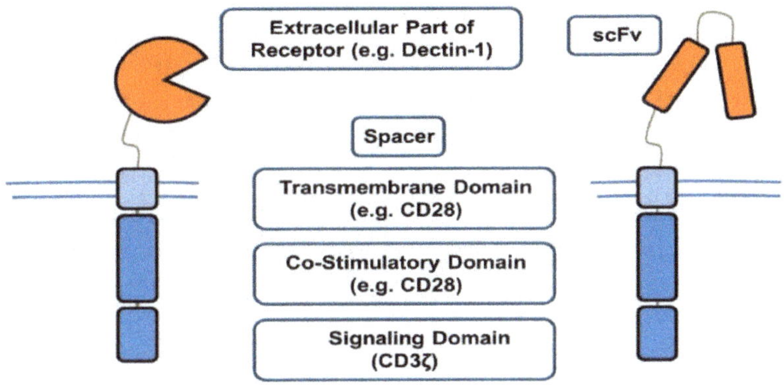

Figure 2. Second-generation chimeric antigen receptors (CARs) include a spacer, transmembrane domain, costimulatory domain, and signaling domain, as well as a targeting element. The two depicted CARs differ in their targeting element, which is usually the single chain variable fragment (scFv) of an antibody, but can also consist of the extracellular part of a receptor.

In light of this report, CAR T cells might not only be helpful for the treatment of B cell malignancies, but also for *Aspergillus* infections. However, there is only one report about the efficacy of CAR T cells against *Aspergillus* available, and more data needs to be generated. Additional CAR constructs containing alternative costimulatory domains and new targeting elements could be more efficient and should be evaluated. Moreover, the autologous generation of sufficient numbers of CAR T cells takes from just over one up to several weeks, which might lose critical time in an acute infection like IA [60].

3. Cytokine Therapy

One approach to fight aspergillosis after allo-SCT is to strengthen the immune system by administering cytokines. The most discussed cytokines are available as recombinant forms approved by the FDA, resulting in a more efficient evaluation on new patient cohorts. Cytokine therapies aimed at innate or both innate and adaptive immune systems have been assessed in several studies.

3.1. Colony Stimulating Factors

CSF treatment is aimed at increasing the capacity of the innate immune system to clear *Aspergillus*. This might be achieved by a faster reconstitution of innate immune cells mitigating risk factors such as neutropenia as well as increasing the activity of these cells against the fungus.

3.1.1. G-CSF

G-CSF increases neutrophil proliferation as well as maturation and is FDA-approved [65]. After stem cell transplantation, it is frequently administered during febrile episodes of neutropenia. Even though G-CSF does not decrease mortality caused by infections, it reduces time of neutropenia and febrile neutropenia-related hospitalization periods [66]. In an *A. fumigatus* mouse model, the addition of G-CSF to the antifungal caspofungin or caspofungin combined with amphotericin B-intralipid, resulted in higher survival rates of up to 78.9%, decreased fungal burden in organs, and reduced serum galactomannan [67]. It also increased neutrophil counts and led to a four-fold higher killing of *A. fumigatus* conidia by PMNs compared to untreated controls [68].

Research shows that G-CSF shortens neutropenia in patients, but more studies investigating the effects of G-CSF on the prevalence and outcomes of *Aspergillus* infections have to be conducted [69,70].

3.1.2. M-CSF

In contrast to G-CSF and granulocyte-macrophage CSF (GM-CSF), macrophage CSF (M-CSF) is not FDA-approved. Its main function is the stimulation of macrophage growth [71]. In a clinical phase I/II trial, the regular antifungal therapy of 46 bone marrow transplant patients was supplemented by recombinant human M-CSF. While the clinical outcome of patients infected with various *Candida* species improved compared to historical controls, no positive effect on patients suffering from aspergillosis was observed [72]. Treating transplanted mice with M-CSF before *A. fumigatus* challenge not only reduced fungal organ burden, but also increased survival rates from 10% in saline-treated animals to 60% [73]. Prophylactic administration of M-CSF to neutropenic rabbits in a model of pulmonary aspergillosis lowered pulmonary injury and increased survival, most likely due to increased macrophage numbers and phagocytosis activity [74].

Only a few experiments have been performed with M-CSF. M-CSF treatment has shown some promise in animal models for aspergillosis and should be evaluated further for the treatment of patients after allo-SCT.

3.1.3. GM-CSF

Like G-CSF, GM-CSF is FDA-approved, but has a broader effect on immune cells. It plays a role in the differentiation of dendritic cells, as well as macrophages, and stimulates the proliferation and activation of many cell types, including neutrophils, macrophages, eosinophils, and dendritic cells [75,76]. Therefore, GM-CSF treatment increases numbers of tissue macrophages, circulating monocytes, neutrophils, and platelets, as well as eosinophils [77,78].

After allo-SCT, GM-CSF administration is considered safe [79]. In a prospective multicenter randomized phase IV clinical trial, 206 allogeneic stem cell patients were prophylactically administered with either G-CSF or GM-CSF alone, or a combination of both. Although GM-CSF and GM-CSF + G-CSF decreased combined 600-day IFI-related mortality and yeast incidence, no benefit for IA incidence was found [78].

GM-CSF might partly mitigate the effect of certain immunosuppressive drugs but inhibit the ability of the immune system to clear *Aspergillus*. Brummer et al. illustrated that GM-CSF prevents the immunosuppressive effects of dexamethasone on murine bronchoalveolar macrophages, leading to increased killing of *A. fumigatus* conidia [80]. Supportively, GM-CSF exposure lowered the fungal burden in the lung among cyclophosphamide immunosuppressed mice in a model of pulmonary aspergillosis [81]. Macrophage suppression by the corticosteroid cortisone acetate was also inhibited by GM-CSF. This effect lasted for more than a week after treatment in a murine model. In addition, GM-CSF has been shown to counteract corticosteroid-induced downregulation of pro-inflammatory cytokines such as TNF-α, which are crucial to early defense mechanisms of the innate immune system against *Aspergillus* conidia [82].

Even though GM-CSF shortens the time of neutropenia, which is the major risk factor for IA, no benefit concerning incidence or course of IA in larger patient cohorts has been found to date. Again, this demonstrates that addressing one of the many dysfunctions of the immune system after allo-SCT might not be sufficient to prevent or clear IA. However, GM-CSF potential to partly reverse undesired immunosuppressive effects after allo-SCT, which hamper infection control, might be an additional advantage of GM-CSF administration.

3.2. IFN-γ

A strong Th1 response is essential to clear *Aspergillus* [83–85]. In order to increase the Th1 response of patients, FDA-approved forms of IFN-γ might be administered. In vivo, IFN-γ is secreted by T and NK cells. It has the capacity to induce protective responses of the innate and adaptive immune systems against *Aspergillus* [43]. Numerous clinical studies have investigated the benefit of supplementing antifungal therapy with IFN-γ.

Case reports describing the positive effect of adjunctive IFN-γ administration on aspergillosis have been published [86–89]. In a randomized prospective placebo-controlled double-blinded clinical study of 128 patients undergoing chronic granulomatous disease, decreased frequencies of infections were observed after frequent IFN-γ administration compared to controls. However, only one patient in the IFN-γ-treated group and four patients in the placebo group suffered from aspergillosis, which highly limited the predictive value of the study. The study was also limited by the short follow-up period of only 10 months [90]. A case series of IFIs on renal transplant patients included three patients suffering from disseminated IA. All three cases were cured after six weeks of combined amphotericin B and IFN-γ treatment [91]. In a prospective case series of eight patients, including three aspergillosis cases, Delsing et al. showed increased ability of peripheral blood mononuclear cells (PBMCs) to produce pro-inflammatory cytokines IL-1β and TNF-α, Th17-stimulating cytokines IL-17 and IL-22, and heightened HLA-DR expression after combined IFN-γ and antifungal treatment, all of which play an important role in protecting the host from IA. While lymphocyte and monocyte numbers were increased, granulocyte numbers were slightly decreased [92]. In order to reverse the drop in granulocyte numbers, the addition of IFN-γ with a granulocyte count-increasing cytokine such as GM-CSF might be beneficial. Combination therapy of IFN-γ and GM-CSF, supporting antifungal treatment in two HIV-negative and one HIV-positive patient suffering from progressive pulmonary aspergillosis, showed promising results. Peripheral leukocyte numbers increased and Th1 response was strengthened. This resulted in an improved control of the fungal infection [93]. In vitro, pre-incubation of human PMNs with IFN-γ and GM-CSF led to enhanced *Aspergillus flavus* hyphal damage and increased release of oxygen radicals by PMNs. This effect disappeared when pre-incubating PMNs with only either one of the cytokines [94]. Another report demonstrated that IFN-γ treatment of PMNs and PBMCs resulted in increased hyphal damage of *A. fumigatus* [95].

Even though adjunctive IFN-γ treatment has many potential advantages and is well tolerated in allo-SCT patients [96], the evidence supporting the use in patients is still weak [22]. More trials need to be conducted.

3.3. TNF-α

TNF-α is one of the most important cytokines in the defense against *Aspergillus* [97]. Comparable to IFN-γ, addition of TNF-α stimulates PMNs, which in turn increase oxygen radical release and cause enhanced hyphal damage against *A. fumigatus* in vitro. Although intracellular killing of *A. fumigatus* conidia by alveolar macrophages was not increased, phagocytosis was enhanced [98]. Administration of TNF-α to immunosuppressed mice in a model for pulmonary aspergillosis increased survival [99]. A time-dependent increase in TNF-α levels of the lung was correlated with higher migration of PMNs to the lung and increased survival of neutropenic and non-neutropenic mice after challenge with *A. fumigatus* conidia. In turn, blocking of TNF-α resulted in higher mortality and fungal lung burden in neutropenic mice. Prophylactic treatment of neutropenic mice with TNF-α increased their survival [100]. However, the major limitation of using TNF-α in the treatment of aspergillosis is its serious toxicity after systemic administration, including hepatotoxicity, nephrotoxicity, and neurotoxicity [101].

4. Other Immunotherapeutic Approaches

4.1. Vaccination

Successful vaccination elicits an adaptive immune response to a pathogen, leading to the generation of memory cells, which are able to fight subsequent infections with the same pathogen much more efficiently. There are different forms of vaccination available. First of all, inactivated whole-cell vaccines can be used; however, they have known limitations. They are complex and therefore difficult to standardize, and usually only elicit weak immune responses [102]. Live vaccines are more immunogenic, but are considered unsafe in immunocompromised patients, as they can potentially cause disease [103]. Subunit vaccines, which consist of purified elements, in combination with an adjuvant, could be the best method available in order to vaccinate immunocompromised patients, as they are easy to standardize and also considered safe in this cohort [53].

Subcutaneous vaccination using a hyphal sonicate protected immunocompromised mice in a model of IA [104]. The vaccination of mice with heat-killed *S. cerevisiae* before *A. fumigatus* challenge increased survival and decreased fungal organ burden. The major limitation of this study was the usage of immunocompetent mice without any immunosuppression. The usefulness of this approach in an immunocompromised setting cannot be predicted [105]. In another study, mice were vaccinated by intranasal inhalation of either filtrates of viable *A. fumigatus*, viable *A. fumigatus*, or heat-inactivated *A. fumigatus*. Thereafter, mice were immunosuppressed and challenged with the fungus. The filtrate and the live fungus vaccination were able to prolong survival and induced a protective Th1 response. In contrast, no prolonged protection was found in mice vaccinated with heat-inactivated fungus, which provoked a Th2 response [106]. Furthermore, vaccination with recombinant *Aspergillus* antigens Asp f 3, Asp f 9, Asp f 16 (all major allergens), Gel1 (a protein associated with cell wall morphogenesis), and Pep1 (an extracellular endopeptidase) resulted in protective effects in murine models of aspergillosis [107,108]. These antigens could potentially be used as the basis of subunit vaccines. The same is true for mannans, which can be found in the cell wall of *Aspergillus*. Liu et al. vaccinated immunocompetent mice with mannans derived from *C. albicans*, leading to increased survival rates after challenge with *A. fumigatus* conidia. Mortality was further decreased by the addition of bovine serum albumin (BSA) to the mannans [109].

Even though vaccine development in immunocompromised patients is difficult because of their weakened immune system, advances have been made to improve vaccination strategies in this patient cohort. However, T and B cell counts, as well as functionality, have to be at least partially restored in order to elicit a protective response. After allo-SCT, the reconstitution of the adaptive immune system takes several months [110]. Therefore, *Aspergillus* vaccination might not be effective in *Aspergillus* infections early after allo-SCT. It is still difficult and costly to develop vaccines against fungal pathogens, and in contrast to other microbes, no fungal vaccine has been licensed yet. Vaccines for other fungi, such as NDV-3A for *C. albicans*, which was used in a recent promising clinical trial, might lead to increased interest in the development of vaccines for *Aspergillus* [102,111].

4.2. Antibodies

Two decades ago, the humoral response was thought to play little to no role in the defense against fungi. More recent findings, however, show that this dogma needs to be revised. Humoral responses, in fact, are important for the host defense against fungal infection, including *Aspergillus* [112]. Patients with Good syndrome, a disease characterized by hypogammaglobulinemia, show increased incidences of fungal infections, including aspergillosis [113]. Anti-*Aspergillus* antibodies bind to swollen conidia and germ tubes, activating the classical pathway of the complement system. Complement activation leads to the killing of *Aspergillus* by neutrophils [114].

The efficacy of different kinds of antibodies against *Aspergillus* has been evaluated. One approach is to target polysaccharides found on the cell wall of fungi. The monoclonal antibody (mAb) 2G8 targets the cell wall polysaccharide laminarin, which consists of ß-glucan. It has demonstrated antifungal effects, including activity against *A. fumigatus* [115]. A different method is the usage of anti-idiotypic mAbs to yeast killer toxin, found in *Pichia anomala* and *Williopsis mrakii*, which displays antimicrobial effects. Administration of these mAbs to immunocompromised mice infected with *A. fumigatus* decreased fungal growth and increased survival [116]. Radioimmunotherapy has the potential to be another antibody-based immunotherapeutic strategy against *Aspergillus*. In this approach, an antibody directed against the fungus is tagged with radionuclides in order to deliver a lethal dose of radiation to the fungus [117].

The administration of antibodies might strengthen the ability of allo-SCT patients to prevent or clear IA in absence of a fully functional adaptive immune system. In contrast to adoptive T cell or CAR T cell transfer, in which autologous T cells have to be generated for each single patient over the period of weeks, one type of antibody would be instantly available for all affected patients, which might be a major advantage in acute infections. The research on the humoral response against *Aspergillus* and the implementation of immunotherapeutic strategies based on these findings is still in its early stages. However, the initial results generated are promising, and more data should be collected.

5. Summary and Outlook

The treatment of IA patients with standard antifungal drugs faces numerous challenges. No new class of antifungal drugs has been invented for over a decade, the number of fungal isolates resistant to azoles has been steadily increasing, and the side effects of conventional antifungal drugs are still considered to be severe. Immunotherapeutic approaches hold promise for improving antifungal therapy in order to decrease high mortality rates. In general, immunotherapy protocols treating *Aspergillus* infections are still exploratory, cost-intensive, might be accompanied by severe side effects, and involve complex as well as time-intensive genetic and cellular manipulations before use. Different immunotherapeutic strategies have been investigated for their efficacy, safety, and their potential to overcome these challenges. The most promising candidates should be evaluated in well-designed clinical trials. Up to this point, the low prevalence of IA has first resulted in the clinical evaluation of these exploratory methods in small patient cohorts with low statistical power; and second, the analysis of a treatment's efficacy has often been assessed in combined IFIs. Various IFIs are known to differ in their pathology and susceptibility to certain treatments. Thus, multicenter clinical trials for IA should be performed.

There are promising weapons against *Aspergillus* on the horizon. In the future, this fight might involve the use of new NK CAR technology, a tool that can be used as an allogeneic "off-the-shelf" product [118]. It might also include checkpoint inhibitors. These molecules disable inhibiting receptors on immune cells and therefore increase their activity. They have demonstrated their efficacy in cancer research and might attenuate the clinical progression of IA [119]. Another promising approach is the usage of neutrophil-dendritic cell hybrids (PMN-DCs), which are cells with the microbicide function of PMNs and the capacity of DCs to stimulate adaptive immunity [120]. In addition, as drug development is expensive, and only a few drug candidates reach market maturity, the repurposing of approved drugs for potential use in IA might be worthwhile. Drugs such as auranofin and ebselen have shown activity against *Aspergillus* in vitro. Both drugs block the thioredoxin reductase pathway, which is essential for cells to manipulate disulfide bonds. This pathway is different in humans compared to bacteria, as well as fungi, and therefore might be a suitable target [121,122]. Moreover, combining novel immunotherapeutic approaches with antifungals might yield positive synergistic effects. For example, echinocandins are drugs that uncover immunologically active epitopes in the fungal cell wall. Many immunotherapeutic strategies such as D-CARs or ß-glucan-specific antibodies target these epitopes, which might result in more efficient fungal clearance [119].

In conclusion, the fight against IA still relies heavily on conventional antifungal drugs. Immunotherapy has made a lot of progress in the last decade and might be used as an adjuvant therapy or even on its own in the future. In order to bring these new treatment strategies to the bedside, well-designed multicenter clinical trials are of the upmost importance.

Author Contributions: C.D.L., H.E., and J.L. wrote the manuscript. C.D.L designed the figures.

Acknowledgments: We thank Lukas Page for proofreading the manuscript.

References

1. Taccone, F.S.; Van den Abeele, A.M.; Bulpa, P.; Misset, B.; Meersseman, W.; Cardoso, T.; Paiva, J.A.; Blasco-Navalpotro, M.; De Laere, E.; Dimopoulos, G.; et al. Epidemiology of invasive aspergillosis in critically ill patients: Clinical presentation, underlying conditions, and outcomes. *Crit. Care* **2015**, *19*, 7. [CrossRef] [PubMed]
2. Filler, S.G.; Sheppard, D.C. Fungal invasion of normally non-phagocytic host cells. *PLoS Pathog.* **2006**, *2*, e129. [CrossRef] [PubMed]
3. White, P.L.; Posso, R.B.; Barnes, R.A. Analytical and Clinical Evaluation of the PathoNostics AsperGenius Assay for Detection of Invasive Aspergillosis and Resistance to Azole Antifungal Drugs Directly from Plasma Samples. *J. Clin. Microbiol.* **2017**, *55*, 2356–2366. [CrossRef] [PubMed]
4. Hohl, T.M. Immune responses to invasive aspergillosis: New understanding and therapeutic opportunities. *Curr. Opin. Infect. Dis.* **2017**, *30*, 364–371. [CrossRef] [PubMed]
5. Aimanianda, V.; Bayry, J.; Bozza, S.; Kniemeyer, O.; Perruccio, K.; Elluru, S.R.; Clavaud, C.; Paris, S.; Brakhage, A.A.; Kaveri, S.V.; et al. Surface hydrophobin prevents immune recognition of airborne fungal spores. *Nature* **2009**, *460*, 1117–1121. [CrossRef] [PubMed]
6. Bidula, S.; Schelenz, S. A Sweet Response to a Sour Situation: The Role of Soluble Pattern Recognition Receptors in the Innate Immune Response to Invasive Aspergillus fumigatus Infections. *PLoS Pathog.* **2016**, *12*, e1005637. [CrossRef]
7. Garth, J.M.; Reeder, K.M.; Godwin, M.S.; Mackel, J.J.; Dunaway, C.W.; Blackburn, J.P.; Steele, C. IL-33 Signaling Regulates Innate IL-17A and IL-22 Production via Suppression of Prostaglandin E_2 during Lung Fungal Infection. *J. Immunol.* **2017**. [CrossRef]
8. Espinosa, V.; Rivera, A. First line of defense: Innate cell-mediated control of pulmonary aspergillosis. *Front. Microbiol.* **2016**, *7*, 272. [CrossRef]
9. Khanna, N.; Stuehler, C.; Lünemann, A.; Wójtowicz, A.; Bochud, P.Y.; Leibundgut-Landmann, S. Host response to fungal infections—How immunology and host genetics could help to identify and treat patients at risk. *Swiss Med. Wkly.* **2016**, *146*. [CrossRef]
10. Heinz, W.J.; Vehreschild, J.J.; Buchheidt, D. Diagnostic workout to assess early response indicators in invasive pulmonary aspergillosis in adult patients with hematologic malignancies. *Mycoses* **2018**. [CrossRef]
11. Leroux, S.; Ullmann, A.J. Management and diagnostic guidelines for fungal diseases in infectious diseases and clinical microbiology: Critical appraisal. *Clin. Microbiol. Infect. Off. Publ. Eur. Soc. Clin. Microbiol. Infect. Dis.* **2013**, *19*, 1115–1121. [CrossRef]
12. Chowdhary, A.; Sharma, C.; Meis, J.F. Azole-Resistant Aspergillosis: Epidemiology, Molecular Mechanisms, and Treatment. *J. Infect. Dis.* **2017**, *216*, S436–S444. [CrossRef] [PubMed]
13. Hickey, M.J.; Kubes, P. Intravascular immunity: The host-pathogen encounter in blood vessels. *Nat. Rev. Immunol.* **2009**, *9*, 364–375. [CrossRef]
14. Shoham, S.; Levitz, S.M. The immune response to fungal infections. *Br. J. Haematol.* **2005**, *129*, 569–582. [CrossRef] [PubMed]
15. Hubel, K.; Carter, R.A.; Liles, W.C.; Dale, D.C.; Price, T.H.; Bowden, R.A.; Rowley, S.D.; Chauncey, T.R.; Bensinger, W.I.; Boeckh, M. Granulocyte transfusion therapy for infections in candidates and recipients of HPC transplantation: A comparative analysis of feasibility and outcome for community donors versus related donors. *Transfusion* **2002**, *42*, 1414–1421. [CrossRef] [PubMed]
16. Price, T.H.; Bowden, R.A.; Boeckh, M.; Bux, J.; Nelson, K.; Liles, W.C.; Dale, D.C. Phase I/II trial of neutrophil transfusions from donors stimulated with G-CSF and dexamethasone for treatment of patients with infections in hematopoietic stem cell transplantation. *Blood* **2000**, *95*, 3302–3309. [PubMed]

17. Seidel, M.G.; Peters, C.; Wacker, A.; Northoff, H.; Moog, R.; Boehme, A.; Silling, G.; Grimminger, W.; Einsele, H. Randomized phase III study of granulocyte transfusions in neutropenic patients. *Bone Marrow Transplant.* **2008**, *42*, 679–684. [CrossRef]
18. Mousset, S.; Hermann, S.; Klein, S.A.; Bialleck, H.; Duchscherer, M.; Bomke, B.; Wassmann, B.; Bohme, A.; Hoelzer, D.; Martin, H. Prophylactic and interventional granulocyte transfusions in patients with haematological malignancies and life-threatening infections during neutropenia. *Ann. Hematol.* **2005**, *84*, 734–741. [CrossRef]
19. Price, T.H.; Boeckh, M.; Harrison, R.W.; McCullough, J.; Ness, P.M.; Strauss, R.G.; Nichols, W.G.; Hamza, T.H.; Cushing, M.M.; King, K.E.; et al. Efficacy of transfusion with granulocytes from G-CSF/dexamethasone-treated donors in neutropenic patients with infection. *Blood* **2015**, *126*, 2153–2161. [CrossRef]
20. BitMansour, A.; Burns, S.M.; Traver, D.; Akashi, K.; Contag, C.H.; Weissman, I.L.; Brown, J.M. Myeloid progenitors protect against invasive aspergillosis and Pseudomonas aeruginosa infection following hematopoietic stem cell transplantation. *Blood* **2002**, *100*, 4660–4667. [CrossRef]
21. BitMansour, A.; Cao, T.M.; Chao, S.; Shashidhar, S.; Brown, J.M. Single infusion of myeloid progenitors reduces death from Aspergillus fumigatus following chemotherapy-induced neutropenia. *Blood* **2005**, *105*, 3535–3537. [CrossRef] [PubMed]
22. Patterson, T.F.; Thompson, G.R., 3rd; Denning, D.W.; Fishman, J.A.; Hadley, S.; Herbrecht, R.; Kontoyiannis, D.P.; Marr, K.A.; Morrison, V.A.; Nguyen, M.H.; et al. Practice Guidelines for the Diagnosis and Management of Aspergillosis: 2016 Update by the Infectious Diseases Society of America. *Clin. Infect. Dis.* **2016**, *63*, e1–e60. [CrossRef] [PubMed]
23. Ramirez-Ortiz, Z.G.; Means, T.K. The role of dendritic cells in the innate recognition of pathogenic fungi (A. fumigatus, C. neoformans and C. albicans). *Virulence* **2012**, *3*, 635–646. [CrossRef] [PubMed]
24. Thakur, R.; Anand, R.; Tiwari, S.; Singh, A.P.; Tiwary, B.N.; Shankar, J. Cytokines induce effector T-helper cells during invasive aspergillosis; what we have learned about T-helper cells? *Front. Microbiol.* **2015**, *6*, 429. [CrossRef] [PubMed]
25. Zelante, T.; Wong, A.Y.; Ping, T.J.; Chen, J.; Sumatoh, H.R.; Vigano, E.; Hong Bing, Y.; Lee, B.; Zolezzi, F.; Fric, J.; et al. CD103(+) Dendritic Cells Control Th17 Cell Function in the Lung. *Cell Rep.* **2015**, *12*, 1789–1801. [CrossRef] [PubMed]
26. Bozza, S.; Gaziano, R.; Lipford, G.B.; Montagnoli, C.; Bacci, A.; Di Francesco, P.; Kurup, V.P.; Wagner, H.; Romani, L. Vaccination of mice against invasive aspergillosis with recombinant Aspergillus proteins and CpG oligodeoxynucleotides as adjuvants. *Microbes Infect.* **2002**, *4*, 1281–1290. [CrossRef]
27. Bozza, S.; Perruccio, K.; Montagnoli, C.; Gaziano, R.; Bellocchio, S.; Burchielli, E.; Nkwanyuo, G.; Pitzurra, L.; Velardi, A.; Romani, L. A dendritic cell vaccine against invasive aspergillosis in allogeneic hematopoietic transplantation. *Blood* **2003**, *102*, 3807–3814. [CrossRef]
28. Shao, H.J.; Chen, L.; Su, Y.B. DNA fragment encoding human IL-1beta 163-171 peptide enhances the immune responses elicited in mice by DNA vaccine against foot-and-mouth disease. *Vet. Res. Commun.* **2005**, *29*, 35–46. [CrossRef]
29. Zhu, F.; Ramadan, G.; Davies, B.; Margolis, D.A.; Keever-Taylor, C.A. Stimulation by means of dendritic cells followed by Epstein-Barr virus-transformed B cells as antigen-presenting cells is more efficient than dendritic cells alone in inducing Aspergillus f16-specific cytotoxic T cell responses. *Clin. Exp. Immunol.* **2008**, *151*, 284–296. [CrossRef]
30. Roy, R.M.; Klein, B.S. Dendritic cells in antifungal immunity and vaccine design. *Cell Host Microbe* **2012**, *11*, 436–446. [CrossRef]
31. Schmidt, S.; Tramsen, L.; Perkhofer, S.; Lass-Florl, C.; Hanisch, M.; Roger, F.; Klingebiel, T.; Koehl, U.; Lehrnbecher, T. Rhizopus oryzae hyphae are damaged by human natural killer (NK) cells, but suppress NK cell mediated immunity. *Immunobiology* **2013**, *218*, 939–944. [CrossRef] [PubMed]
32. Schmidt, S.; Tramsen, L.; Lehrnbecher, T. Natural Killer Cells in Antifungal Immunity. *Front. Immunol.* **2017**, *8*, 1623. [CrossRef] [PubMed]
33. Ziegler, S.; Weiss, E.; Schmitt, A.L.; Schlegel, J.; Burgert, A.; Terpitz, U.; Sauer, M.; Moretta, L.; Sivori, S.; Leonhardt, I.; et al. CD56 Is a Pathogen Recognition Receptor on Human Natural Killer Cells. *Sci. Rep.* **2017**, *7*, 6138. [CrossRef] [PubMed]

34. Schmidt, S.; Tramsen, L.; Hanisch, M.; Latge, J.P.; Huenecke, S.; Koehl, U.; Lehrnbecher, T. Human natural killer cells exhibit direct activity against Aspergillus fumigatus hyphae, but not against resting conidia. *J. Infect. Dis.* **2011**, *203*, 430–435. [CrossRef] [PubMed]
35. Stuehler, C.; Kuenzli, E.; Jaeger, V.K.; Baettig, V.; Ferracin, F.; Rajacic, Z.; Kaiser, D.; Bernardini, C.; Forrer, P.; Weisser, M.; et al. Immune Reconstitution After Allogeneic Hematopoietic Stem Cell Transplantation and Association With Occurrence and Outcome of Invasive Aspergillosis. *J. Infect. Dis.* **2015**, *212*, 959–967. [CrossRef] [PubMed]
36. Park, S.J.; Hughes, M.A.; Burdick, M.; Strieter, R.M.; Mehrad, B. Early NK cell-derived IFN-{gamma} is essential to host defense in neutropenic invasive aspergillosis. *J. Immunol.* **2009**, *182*, 4306–4312. [CrossRef] [PubMed]
37. Benedetto, N.; Sabatini, P.; Sellitto, C.; Romano Carratelli, C. Interleukin-2 and increased natural killer activity in mice experimentally infected with Aspergillus niger. *Microbiologica* **1988**, *11*, 339–345.
38. Tonn, T.; Schwabe, D.; Klingemann, H.G.; Becker, S.; Esser, R.; Koehl, U.; Suttorp, M.; Seifried, E.; Ottmann, O.G.; Bug, G. Treatment of patients with advanced cancer with the natural killer cell line NK-92. *Cytotherapy* **2013**, *15*, 1563–1570. [CrossRef] [PubMed]
39. Arai, S.; Meagher, R.; Swearingen, M.; Myint, H.; Rich, E.; Martinson, J.; Klingemann, H. Infusion of the allogeneic cell line NK-92 in patients with advanced renal cell cancer or melanoma: A phase I trial. *Cytotherapy* **2008**, *10*, 625–632. [CrossRef] [PubMed]
40. Boyiadzis, M.; Agha, M.; Redner, R.L.; Sehgal, A.; Im, A.; Hou, J.Z.; Farah, R.; Dorritie, K.A.; Raptis, A.; Lim, S.H.; et al. Phase 1 clinical trial of adoptive immunotherapy using "off-the-shelf" activated natural killer cells in patients with refractory and relapsed acute myeloid leukemia. *Cytotherapy* **2017**, *19*, 1225–1232. [CrossRef] [PubMed]
41. Klingemann, H.; Grodman, C.; Cutler, E.; Duque, M.; Kadidlo, D.; Klein, A.K.; Sprague, K.A.; Miller, K.B.; Comenzo, R.L.; Kewalramani, T.; et al. Autologous stem cell transplant recipients tolerate haploidentical related-donor natural killer cell-enriched infusions. *Transfusion* **2013**, *53*, 412–418. [CrossRef] [PubMed]
42. Shah, N.; Li, L.; McCarty, J.; Kaur, I.; Yvon, E.; Shaim, H.; Muftuoglu, M.; Liu, E.; Orlowski, R.Z.; Cooper, L.; et al. Phase I study of cord blood-derived natural killer cells combined with autologous stem cell transplantation in multiple myeloma. *Br. J. Haematol.* **2017**, *177*, 457–466. [CrossRef] [PubMed]
43. Dewi, I.; van de Veerdonk, F.; Gresnigt, M. The Multifaceted Role of T-Helper Responses in Host Defense against Aspergillus fumigatus. *J. Fungi* **2017**. [CrossRef] [PubMed]
44. Perruccio, K.; Tosti, A.; Burchielli, E.; Topini, F.; Ruggeri, L.; Carotti, A.; Capanni, M.; Urbani, E.; Mancusi, A.; Aversa, F.; et al. Transferring functional immune responses to pathogens after haploidentical hematopoietic transplantation. *Blood* **2005**, *106*, 4397–4406. [CrossRef]
45. Papadopoulou, A.; Kaloyannidis, P.; Yannaki, E.; Cruz, C.R. Adoptive transfer of Aspergillus-specific T cells as a novel anti-fungal therapy for hematopoietic stem cell transplant recipients: Progress and challenges. *Crit. Rev. Oncol. Hematol.* **2016**, *98*, 62–72. [CrossRef]
46. Tramsen, L.; Koehl, U.; Tonn, T.; Latge, J.P.; Schuster, F.R.; Borkhardt, A.; Uharek, L.; Quaritsch, R.; Beck, O.; Seifried, E.; et al. Clinical-scale generation of human anti-Aspergillus T cells for adoptive immunotherapy. *Bone Marrow Transplant.* **2009**, *43*, 13–19. [CrossRef] [PubMed]
47. Tramsen, L.; Schmidt, S.; Boenig, H.; Latge, J.P.; Lass-Florl, C.; Roeger, F.; Seifried, E.; Klingebiel, T.; Lehrnbecher, T. Clinical-scale generation of multi-specific anti-fungal T cells targeting Candida, Aspergillus and mucormycetes. *Cytotherapy* **2013**, *15*, 344–351. [CrossRef]
48. Khanna, N.; Stuehler, C.; Conrad, B.; Lurati, S.; Krappmann, S.; Einsele, H.; Berges, C.; Topp, M.S. Generation of a multipathogen-specific T-cell product for adoptive immunotherapy based on activation-dependent expression of CD154. *Blood* **2011**, *118*, 1121–1131. [CrossRef]
49. Stuehler, C.; Nowakowska, J.; Bernardini, C.; Topp, M.S.; Battegay, M.; Passweg, J.; Khanna, N. Multispecific Aspergillus T cells selected by CD137 or CD154 induce protective immune responses against the most relevant mold infections. *J. Infect. Dis.* **2015**, *211*, 1251–1261. [CrossRef]
50. Bacher, P.; Jochheim-Richter, A.; Mockel-Tenbrink, N.; Kniemeyer, O.; Wingenfeld, E.; Alex, R.; Ortigao, A.; Karpova, D.; Lehrnbecher, T.; Ullmann, A.J.; et al. Clinical-scale isolation of the total Aspergillus fumigatus-reactive T-helper cell repertoire for adoptive transfer. *Cytotherapy* **2015**, *17*, 1396–1405. [CrossRef]

51. Tramsen, L.; Schmidt, S.; Roeger, F.; Schubert, R.; Salzmann-Manrique, E.; Latge, J.P.; Klingebiel, T.; Lehrnbecher, T. Immunosuppressive compounds exhibit particular effects on functional properties of human anti-Aspergillus Th1 cells. *Infect. Immun.* **2014**, *82*, 2649–2656. [CrossRef] [PubMed]
52. Tzannou, I.; Papadopoulou, A.; Naik, S.; Leung, K.; Martinez, C.A.; Ramos, C.A.; Carrum, G.; Sasa, G.; Lulla, P.; Watanabe, A.; et al. Off-the-Shelf Virus-Specific T Cells to Treat BK Virus, Human Herpesvirus 6, Cytomegalovirus, Epstein-Barr Virus, and Adenovirus Infections After Allogeneic Hematopoietic Stem-Cell Transplantation. *J. Clin. Oncol.* **2017**, *35*, 3547–3557. [CrossRef] [PubMed]
53. Iannitti, R.G.; Carvalho, A.; Romani, L. From memory to antifungal vaccine design. *Trends Immunol.* **2012**, *33*, 467–474. [CrossRef] [PubMed]
54. Cutler, J.E.; Deepe, G.S., Jr.; Klein, B.S. Advances in combating fungal diseases: Vaccines on the threshold. *Nat. Rev. Microbiol.* **2007**, *5*, 13–28. [CrossRef] [PubMed]
55. Sun, Z.; Zhu, P.; Li, L.; Wan, Z.; Zhao, Z.; Li, R. Adoptive immunity mediated by HLA-A*0201 restricted Asp f16 peptides-specific CD8+ T cells against Aspergillus fumigatus infection. *Eur. J. Clin. Microbiol. Infect. Dis. Off. Publ. Eur. Soc. Clin. Microbiol.* **2012**, *31*, 3089–3096. [CrossRef] [PubMed]
56. Maldini, C.R.; Ellis, G.I.; Riley, J.L. CAR T cells for infection, autoimmunity and allotransplantation. *Nat. Rev. Immunol.* **2018**, *18*, 605–616. [CrossRef] [PubMed]
57. Zheng, P.-P.; Kros, J.M.; Li, J. Approved CAR T cell therapies: Ice bucket challenges on glaring safety risks and long-term impacts. *Drug Discov. Today* **2018**, *23*, 1175–1182. [CrossRef]
58. Johnson, L.A.; June, C.H. Driving gene-engineered T cell immunotherapy of cancer. *Cell Res.* **2017**, *27*, 38–58. [CrossRef]
59. Dotti, G.; Gottschalk, S.; Savoldo, B.; Brenner, M.K. Design and development of therapies using chimeric antigen receptor-expressing T cells. *Immunol. Rev.* **2014**, *257*, 107–126. [CrossRef]
60. Kumaresan, P.R.; Silva, T.; Kontoyiannis, D.P. Methods of Controlling Invasive Fungal Infections Using CD8+ T Cells. *Front. Immunol.* **2018**, *8*, 1939. [CrossRef]
61. Bridgeman, J.S.; Hawkins, R.E.; Bagley, S.; Blaylock, M.; Holland, M.; Gilham, D.E. The optimal antigen response of chimeric antigen receptors harboring the CD3zeta transmembrane domain is dependent upon incorporation of the receptor into the endogenous TCR/CD3 complex. *J. Immunol.* **2010**, *184*, 6938–6949. [CrossRef] [PubMed]
62. Abken, H. Costimulation Engages the Gear in Driving CARs. *Immunity* **2016**, *44*, 214–216. [CrossRef] [PubMed]
63. Kumaresan, P.R.; Manuri, P.R.; Albert, N.D.; Maiti, S.; Singh, H.; Mi, T.; Roszik, J.; Rabinovich, B.; Olivares, S.; Krishnamurthy, J.; et al. Bioengineering T cells to target carbohydrate to treat opportunistic fungal infection. *Proc. Natl. Acad. Sci. USA* **2014**, *111*, 10660–10665. [CrossRef] [PubMed]
64. Singh, H.; Manuri, P.R.; Olivares, S.; Dara, N.; Dawson, M.J.; Huls, H.; Hackett, P.B.; Kohn, D.B.; Shpall, E.J.; Champlin, R.E.; et al. Redirecting specificity of T-cell populations for CD19 using the Sleeping Beauty system. *Cancer Res.* **2008**, *68*, 2961–2971. [CrossRef] [PubMed]
65. Wright, C.R.; Ward, A.C.; Russell, A.P. Granulocyte Colony-Stimulating Factor and Its Potential Application for Skeletal Muscle Repair and Regeneration. *Mediat. Inflamm.* **2017**, *2017*, 7517350. [CrossRef] [PubMed]
66. Clark, O.A.; Lyman, G.H.; Castro, A.A.; Clark, L.G.; Djulbegovic, B. Colony-stimulating factors for chemotherapy-induced febrile neutropenia: A meta-analysis of randomized controlled trials. *J. Clin. Oncol.* **2005**, *23*, 4198–4214. [CrossRef] [PubMed]
67. Sionov, E.; Mendlovic, S.; Segal, E. Experimental systemic murine aspergillosis: Treatment with polyene and caspofungin combination and G-CSF. *J. Antimicrob. Chemother.* **2005**, *56*, 594–597. [CrossRef]
68. Liles, W.C.; Huang, J.E.; van Burik, J.A.; Bowden, R.A.; Dale, D.C. Granulocyte colony-stimulating factor administered in vivo augments neutrophil-mediated activity against opportunistic fungal pathogens. *J. Infect. Dis.* **1997**, *175*, 1012–1015. [CrossRef]
69. Smith, T.J.; Khatcheressian, J.; Lyman, G.H.; Ozer, H.; Armitage, J.O.; Balducci, L.; Bennett, C.L.; Cantor, S.B.; Crawford, J.; Cross, S.J.; et al. 2006 update of recommendations for the use of white blood cell growth factors: An evidence-based clinical practice guideline. *J. Clin. Oncol.* **2006**, *24*, 3187–3205. [CrossRef]
70. Ringden, O.; Labopin, M.; Gorin, N.C.; Le Blanc, K.; Rocha, V.; Gluckman, E.; Reiffers, J.; Arcese, W.; Vossen, J.M.; Jouet, J.P.; et al. Treatment with granulocyte colony-stimulating factor after allogeneic bone marrow transplantation for acute leukemia increases the risk of graft-versus-host disease and death: A study

from the Acute Leukemia Working Party of the European Group for Blood and Marrow Transplantation. *J. Clin. Oncol.* **2004**, *22*, 416–423. [CrossRef]

71. Hume, D.A.; MacDonald, K.P. Therapeutic applications of macrophage colony-stimulating factor-1 (CSF-1) and antagonists of CSF-1 receptor (CSF-1R) signaling. *Blood* **2012**, *119*, 1810–1820. [CrossRef] [PubMed]
72. Nemunaitis, J.; Shannon-Dorcy, K.; Appelbaum, F.R.; Meyers, J.; Owens, A.; Day, R.; Ando, D.; O'Neill, C.; Buckner, D.; Singer, J. Long-term follow-up of patients with invasive fungal disease who received adjunctive therapy with recombinant human macrophage colony-stimulating factor. *Blood* **1993**, *82*, 1422–1427. [PubMed]
73. Kandalla, P.K.; Sarrazin, S.; Molawi, K.; Berruyer, C.; Redelberger, D.; Favel, A.; Bordi, C.; de Bentzmann, S.; Sieweke, M.H. M-CSF improves protection against bacterial and fungal infections after hematopoietic stem/progenitor cell transplantation. *J. Exp. Med.* **2016**, *213*, 2269–2279. [CrossRef] [PubMed]
74. Gonzalez, C.E.; Lyman, C.A.; Lee, S.; Del Guercio, C.; Roilides, E.; Bacher, J.; Gehrt, A.; Feuerstein, E.; Tsokos, M.; Walsh, T.J. Recombinant human macrophage colony-stimulating factor augments pulmonary host defences against Aspergillus fumigatus. *Cytokine* **2001**, *15*, 87–95. [CrossRef] [PubMed]
75. Shiomi, A.; Usui, T. Pivotal roles of GM-CSF in autoimmunity and inflammation. *Mediat. Inflamm.* **2015**, *2015*, 568543. [CrossRef] [PubMed]
76. Scriven, J.E.; Tenforde, M.W.; Levitz, S.M.; Jarvis, J.N. Modulating host immune responses to fight invasive fungal infections. *Curr. Opin. Microbiol.* **2017**, *40*, 95–103. [CrossRef] [PubMed]
77. Ruef, C.; Coleman, D.L. Granulocyte-macrophage colony-stimulating factor: Pleiotropic cytokine with potential clinical usefulness. *Rev. Infect. Dis.* **1990**, *12*, 41–62. [CrossRef]
78. Wan, L.; Zhang, Y.; Lai, Y.; Jiang, M.; Song, Y.; Zhou, J.; Zhang, Z.; Duan, X.; Fu, Y.; Liao, L.; et al. Effect of Granulocyte-Macrophage Colony-Stimulating Factor on Prevention and Treatment of Invasive Fungal Disease in Recipients of Allogeneic Stem-Cell Transplantation: A Prospective Multicenter Randomized Phase IV Trial. *J. Clin. Oncol.* **2015**, *33*, 3999–4006. [CrossRef]
79. Safdar, A.; Rodriguez, G.; Zuniga, J.; Al Akhrass, F.; Georgescu, G.; Pande, A. Granulocyte macrophage colony-stimulating factor in 66 patients with myeloid or lymphoid neoplasms and recipients of hematopoietic stem cell transplantation with invasive fungal disease. *Acta Haematol.* **2013**, *129*, 26–34. [CrossRef]
80. Brummer, E.; Maqbool, A.; Stevens, D.A. In vivo GM-CSF prevents dexamethasone suppression of killing of Aspergillus fumigatus conidia by bronchoalveolar macrophages. *J. Leukoc. Biol.* **2001**, *70*, 868–872.
81. Quezada, G.; Koshkina, N.V.; Zweidler-McKay, P.; Zhou, Z.; Kontoyiannis, D.P.; Kleinerman, E.S. Intranasal granulocyte-macrophage colony-stimulating factor reduces the Aspergillus burden in an immunosuppressed murine model of pulmonary aspergillosis. *Antimicrob. Agents Chemother.* **2008**, *52*, 716–718. [CrossRef] [PubMed]
82. Brummer, E.; Kamberi, M.; Stevens, D.A. Regulation by granulocyte-macrophage colony-stimulating factor and/or steroids given in vivo of proinflammatory cytokine and chemokine production by bronchoalveolar macrophages in response to Aspergillus conidia. *J. Infect. Dis.* **2003**, *187*, 705–709. [CrossRef] [PubMed]
83. Cenci, E.; Mencacci, A.; Fe d'Ostiani, C.; Del Sero, G.; Mosci, P.; Montagnoli, C.; Bacci, A.; Romani, L. Cytokine- and T helper-dependent lung mucosal immunity in mice with invasive pulmonary aspergillosis. *J. Infect. Dis.* **1998**, *178*, 1750–1760. [CrossRef] [PubMed]
84. Brieland, J.K.; Jackson, C.; Menzel, F.; Loebenberg, D.; Cacciapuoti, A.; Halpern, J.; Hurst, S.; Muchamuel, T.; Debets, R.; Kastelein, R.; et al. Cytokine networking in lungs of immunocompetent mice in response to inhaled Aspergillus fumigatus. *Infect. Immun.* **2001**, *69*, 1554–1560. [CrossRef] [PubMed]
85. Chai, L.Y.; van de Veerdonk, F.; Marijnissen, R.J.; Cheng, S.C.; Khoo, A.L.; Hectors, M.; Lagrou, K.; Vonk, A.G.; Maertens, J.; Joosten, L.A.; et al. Anti-Aspergillus human host defence relies on type 1 T helper (Th1), rather than type 17 T helper (Th17), cellular immunity. *Immunology* **2010**, *130*, 46–54. [CrossRef] [PubMed]
86. Estrada, C.; Desai, A.G.; Chirch, L.M.; Suh, H.; Seidman, R.; Darras, F.; Nord, E.P. Invasive aspergillosis in a renal transplant recipient successfully treated with interferon-gamma. *Case Rep. Transplant.* **2012**, *2012*, 493758. [CrossRef] [PubMed]
87. Mezidi, M.; Belafia, F.; Nougaret, S.; Pageaux, G.P.; Conseil, M.; Panaro, F.; Boniface, G.; Morquin, D.; Jaber, S.; Jung, B. Interferon gamma in association with immunosuppressive drugs withdrawal and antifungal combination as a rescue therapy for cerebral invasive Aspergillosis in a liver transplant recipient. *Minerva Anestesiol.* **2014**, *80*, 1359–1360. [PubMed]

88. Ellis, M.; Watson, R.; McNabb, A.; Lukic, M.L.; Nork, M. Massive intracerebral aspergillosis responding to combination high dose liposomal amphotericin B and cytokine therapy without surgery. *J. Med. Microbiol.* **2002**, *51*, 70–75. [CrossRef]
89. Kelleher, P.; Goodsall, A.; Mulgirigama, A.; Kunst, H.; Henderson, D.C.; Wilson, R.; Newman-Taylor, A.; Levin, M. Interferon-gamma therapy in two patients with progressive chronic pulmonary aspergillosis. *Eur. Respir. J.* **2006**, *27*, 1307–1310. [CrossRef]
90. The International Chronic Granulomatous Disease Cooperative Study Group. A controlled trial of interferon gamma to prevent infection in chronic granulomatous disease. *N. Engl. J. Med.* **1991**, *324*, 509–516. [CrossRef]
91. Armstrong-James, D.; Teo, I.A.; Shrivastava, S.; Petrou, M.A.; Taube, D.; Dorling, A.; Shaunak, S. Exogenous interferon-gamma immunotherapy for invasive fungal infections in kidney transplant patients. *Am. J. Transplant.* **2010**, *10*, 1796–1803. [CrossRef] [PubMed]
92. Delsing, C.E.; Gresnigt, M.S.; Leentjens, J.; Preijers, F.; Frager, F.A.; Kox, M.; Monneret, G.; Venet, F.; Bleeker-Rovers, C.P.; van de Veerdonk, F.L.; et al. Interferon-gamma as adjunctive immunotherapy for invasive fungal infections: A case series. *BMC Infect. Dis.* **2014**, *14*, 166. [CrossRef] [PubMed]
93. Bandera, A.; Trabattoni, D.; Ferrario, G.; Cesari, M.; Franzetti, F.; Clerici, M.; Gori, A. Interferon-gamma and granulocyte-macrophage colony stimulating factor therapy in three patients with pulmonary aspergillosis. *Infection* **2008**, *36*, 368–373. [CrossRef] [PubMed]
94. Gil-Lamaignere, C.; Winn, R.M.; Simitsopoulou, M.; Maloukou, A.; Walsh, T.J.; Roilides, E. Inteferon gamma and granulocyte-macrophage colony-stimulating factor augment the antifungal activity of human polymorphonuclear leukocytes against Scedosporium spp.: Comparison with Aspergillus spp. *Med. Mycol.* **2005**, *43*, 253–260. [CrossRef] [PubMed]
95. Gaviria, J.M.; van Burik, J.A.; Dale, D.C.; Root, R.K.; Liles, W.C. Comparison of interferon-gamma, granulocyte colony-stimulating factor, and granulocyte-macrophage colony-stimulating factor for priming leukocyte-mediated hyphal damage of opportunistic fungal pathogens. *J. Infect. Dis.* **1999**, *179*, 1038–1041. [CrossRef] [PubMed]
96. Safdar, A.; Rodriguez, G.; Ohmagari, N.; Kontoyiannis, D.P.; Rolston, K.V.; Raad, I.I.; Champlin, R.E. The safety of interferon-gamma-1b therapy for invasive fungal infections after hematopoietic stem cell transplantation. *Cancer* **2005**, *103*, 731–739. [CrossRef]
97. Sainz, J.; Perez, E.; Hassan, L.; Moratalla, A.; Romero, A.; Collado, M.D.; Jurado, M. Variable number of tandem repeats of TNF receptor type 2 promoter as genetic biomarker of susceptibility to develop invasive pulmonary aspergillosis. *Hum. Immunol.* **2007**, *68*, 41–50. [CrossRef]
98. Roilides, E.; Dimitriadou-Georgiadou, A.; Sein, T.; Kadiltsoglou, I.; Walsh, T.J. Tumor necrosis factor alpha enhances antifungal activities of polymorphonuclear and mononuclear phagocytes against Aspergillus fumigatus. *Infect. Immun.* **1998**, *66*, 5999–6003.
99. Nagai, H.; Guo, J.; Choi, H.; Kurup, V. Interferon-gamma and tumor necrosis factor-alpha protect mice from invasive aspergillosis. *J. Infect. Dis.* **1995**, *172*, 1554–1560. [CrossRef]
100. Mehrad, B.; Strieter, R.M.; Standiford, T.J. Role of TNF-alpha in pulmonary host defense in murine invasive aspergillosis. *J. Immunol.* **1999**, *162*, 1633–1640.
101. Roberts, N.J.; Zhou, S.; Diaz, L.A., Jr.; Holdhoff, M. Systemic use of tumor necrosis factor alpha as an anticancer agent. *Oncotarget* **2011**, *2*, 739–751. [CrossRef] [PubMed]
102. Pikman, R.; Ben-Ami, R. Immune modulators as adjuncts for the prevention and treatment of invasive fungal infections. *Immunotherapy* **2012**, *4*, 1869–1882. [CrossRef] [PubMed]
103. Cassone, A.; Casadevall, A. Recent progress in vaccines against fungal diseases. *Curr. Opin. Microbiol.* **2012**, *15*, 427–433. [CrossRef] [PubMed]
104. Ito, J.I.; Lyons, J.M. Vaccination of corticosteroid immunosuppressed mice against invasive pulmonary aspergillosis. *J. Infect. Dis.* **2002**, *186*, 869–871. [CrossRef] [PubMed]
105. Liu, M.; Capilla, J.; Johansen, M.E.; Alvarado, D.; Martinez, M.; Chen, V.; Clemons, K.V.; Stevens, D.A. Saccharomyces as a vaccine against systemic aspergillosis: 'the friend of man' a friend again? *J. Med. Microbiol.* **2011**, *60*, 1423–1432. [CrossRef] [PubMed]
106. Cenci, E.; Mencacci, A.; Bacci, A.; Bistoni, F.; Kurup, V.P.; Romani, L. T cell vaccination in mice with invasive pulmonary aspergillosis. *J. Immunol.* **2000**, *165*, 381–388. [CrossRef] [PubMed]

107. Ito, J.I.; Lyons, J.M.; Hong, T.B.; Tamae, D.; Liu, Y.-K.; Wilczynski, S.P.; Kalkum, M. Vaccinations with recombinant variants of Aspergillus fumigatus allergen Asp f 3 protect mice against invasive aspergillosis. *Infect. Immun.* **2006**, *74*, 5075–5084. [CrossRef]
108. Bozza, S.; Clavaud, C.; Giovannini, G.; Fontaine, T.; Beauvais, A.; Sarfati, J.; D'Angelo, C.; Perruccio, K.; Bonifazi, P.; Zagarella, S.; et al. Immune sensing of Aspergillus fumigatus proteins, glycolipids, and polysaccharides and the impact on Th immunity and vaccination. *J. Immunol.* **2009**, *183*, 2407–2414. [CrossRef]
109. Liu, M.; Machova, E.; Nescakova, Z.; Medovarska, I.; Clemons, K.V.; Martinez, M.; Chen, V.; Bystricky, S.; Stevens, D.A. Vaccination with mannan protects mice against systemic aspergillosis. *Med. Mycol.* **2012**, *50*, 818–828. [CrossRef]
110. Tomblyn, M.; Chiller, T.; Einsele, H.; Gress, R.; Sepkowitz, K.; Storek, J.; Wingard, J.R.; Young, J.A.; Boeckh, M.J. Guidelines for preventing infectious complications among hematopoietic cell transplantation recipients: A global perspective. *Biol. Blood Marrow Transplant.* **2009**, *15*, 1143–1238. [CrossRef]
111. Edwards, J.E., Jr.; Schwartz, M.M.; Schmidt, C.S.; Sobel, J.D.; Nyirjesy, P.; Schodel, F.; Marchus, E.; Lizakowski, M.; DeMontigny, E.A.; Hoeg, J.; et al. A Fungal Immunotherapeutic Vaccine (NDV-3A) for Treatment of Recurrent Vulvovaginal Candidiasis-A Phase 2 Randomized, Double-Blind, Placebo-Controlled Trial. *Clin. Infect. Dis.* **2018**, *66*, 1928–1936. [CrossRef] [PubMed]
112. Casadevall, A.; Pirofski, L.A. Immunoglobulins in defense, pathogenesis, and therapy of fungal diseases. *Cell Host Microbe* **2012**, *11*, 447–456. [CrossRef] [PubMed]
113. Malphettes, M.; Gerard, L.; Galicier, L.; Boutboul, D.; Asli, B.; Szalat, R.; Perlat, A.; Masseau, A.; Schleinitz, N.; Le Guenno, G.; et al. Good syndrome: An adult-onset immunodeficiency remarkable for its high incidence of invasive infections and autoimmune complications. *Clin. Infect. Dis.* **2015**, *61*, e13–e19. [CrossRef] [PubMed]
114. Braem, S.G.; Rooijakkers, S.H.; van Kessel, K.P.; de Cock, H.; Wosten, H.A.; van Strijp, J.A.; Haas, P.J. Effective Neutrophil Phagocytosis of Aspergillus fumigatus Is Mediated by Classical Pathway Complement Activation. *J. Innate Immun.* **2015**, *7*, 364–374. [CrossRef] [PubMed]
115. Torosantucci, A.; Chiani, P.; Bromuro, C.; De Bernardis, F.; Palma, A.S.; Liu, Y.; Mignogna, G.; Maras, B.; Colone, M.; Stringaro, A.; et al. Protection by anti-beta-glucan antibodies is associated with restricted beta-1,3 glucan binding specificity and inhibition of fungal growth and adherence. *PLoS ONE* **2009**, *4*, e5392. [CrossRef] [PubMed]
116. Cenci, E.; Mencacci, A.; Spreca, A.; Montagnoli, C.; Bacci, A.; Perruccio, K.; Velardi, A.; Magliani, W.; Conti, S.; Polonelli, L.; et al. Protection of killer antiidiotypic antibodies against early invasive aspergillosis in a murine model of allogeneic T-cell-depleted bone marrow transplantation. *Infect. Immun.* **2002**, *70*, 2375–2382. [CrossRef] [PubMed]
117. Nosanchuk, J.D.; Dadachova, E. Radioimmunotherapy of fungal diseases: The therapeutic potential of cytocidal radiation delivered by antibody targeting fungal cell surface antigens. *Front. Microbiol.* **2011**, *2*, 283. [CrossRef]
118. Rezvani, K.; Rouce, R.; Liu, E.; Shpall, E. Engineering Natural Killer Cells for Cancer Immunotherapy. *Mol. Ther. J. Am. Soc. Gene Ther.* **2017**, *25*, 1769–1781. [CrossRef]
119. Daver, N.; Kontoyiannis, D.P. Checkpoint inhibitors and aspergillosis in AML: The double hit hypothesis. *Lancet Oncol.* **2017**, *18*, 1571–1573. [CrossRef]
120. Fites, J.S.; Gui, M.; Kernien, J.F.; Negoro, P.; Dagher, Z.; Sykes, D.B.; Nett, J.E.; Mansour, M.K.; Klein, B.S. An unappreciated role for neutrophil-DC hybrids in immunity to invasive fungal infections. *PLoS Pathog.* **2018**, *14*, e1007073. [CrossRef]
121. Ngo, H.X.; Shrestha, S.K.; Garneau-Tsodikova, S. Identification of Ebsulfur Analogues with Broad-Spectrum Antifungal Activity. *ChemMedChem* **2016**, *11*, 1507–1516. [CrossRef] [PubMed]
122. Wiederhold, N.P.; Patterson, T.F.; Srinivasan, A.; Chaturvedi, A.K.; Fothergill, A.W.; Wormley, F.L.; Ramasubramanian, A.K.; Lopez-Ribot, J.L. Repurposing auranofin as an antifungal: In vitro activity against a variety of medically important fungi. *Virulence* **2017**, *8*, 138–142. [CrossRef] [PubMed]

14

Genome-Wide Comparative Analysis of *Aspergillus fumigatus* Strains: The Reference Genome as a Matter of Concern

Rocio Garcia-Rubio [1,†], Sara Monzon [2,†], Laura Alcazar-Fuoli [1], Isabel Cuesta [2] and Emilia Mellado [1,*]

1 Mycology Reference Laboratory, National Centre for Microbiology, Instituto de Salud Carlos III (ISCIII), Majadahonda, 28220 Madrid, Spain; rgarciar@isciii.es (R.G.-R.); lalcazar@isciii.es (L.A.-F.)
2 Bioinformatics Unit, Common Scientific Technical Units, ISCIII, Majadahonda, 28220 Madrid, Spain; smonzon@isciii.es (S.M.); isabel.cuesta@isciii.es (I.C.)
* Correspondence: emellado@isciii.es
† These authors contributed equally to this work.

Abstract: *Aspergillus fumigatus* is a ubiquitous saprophytic mold and a major pathogen in immunocompromised patients. The effectiveness of triazole compounds, the *A. fumigatus* first line treatment, is being threatened by a rapid and global emergence of azole resistance. Whole genome sequencing (WGS) has emerged as an invaluable tool for the analysis of genetic differences between *A. fumigatus* strains, their genetic background, and antifungal resistance development. Although WGS analyses can provide a valuable amount of novel information, there are some limitations that should be considered. These analyses, based on genome-wide comparative data and single nucleotide variant (SNV) calling, are dependent on the quality of sequencing, assembling, the variant calling criteria, as well as on the suitable selection of the reference genome, which must be genetically close to the genomes included in the analysis. In this study, 28 *A. fumigatus* genomes sequenced in-house and 73 available in public data bases have been analyzed. All genomes were distributed in four clusters and showed a variable number of SNVs depending on the genome used as reference (Af293 or A1163). Each reference genome belonged to a different cluster. The results highlighted the importance of choosing the most suitable *A. fumigatus* reference genome to avoid misleading conclusions.

Keywords: *Aspergillus fumigatus*; whole genome sequencing; reference genomes; azole resistance; *cyp51A*

---

1. Introduction

Aspergillus fumigatus is a saprophytic filamentous fungus and the principal causative agent of human aspergillosis [1,2]. There are many types of diseases caused by *A. fumigatus* and their symptoms vary according to the site of infection and host health condition. Predominantly, this species causes invasive infections, such as invasive pulmonary aspergillosis (IPA), with high mortality rates in immunocompromised or immunosuppressed patients [3–5]. Currently, the treatment options are limited to three classes of antifungal drugs (azoles, echinocandins and polyenes) and azoles are drugs of first line for treating *Aspergillus*-caused diseases. However, azole drug efficacy is threatened by the worldwide spreading of resistance [6].

Despite all the technological improvements developed in recent years, many basic aspects about the biology of this opportunistic pathogen remained largely unknown. Genomics and whole genome sequencing (WGS) have emerged as useful tools to greatly enhance knowledge and understanding of infectious diseases and clinical microbiology [7–10]. In this context, genome-wide sequencing using high throughput sequencing (HTS) together with alignment comparison analysis has been described as a good approach to identify single nucleotide variants (SNVs) or polymorphisms (SNPs) for the analysis of genetic differences between *A. fumigatus* strains [11]. The genetic diversity between isolates can be used to explain many different aspects such as the strain background lineage, strain specific virulence phenotypes, the potential factors involved in antifungal resistant development, and more commonly, determining the genetic strain relatedness in epidemiological surveillance and outbreak studies [12–14].

Although WGS studies provide a valuable amount of novel data, there are some considerations that should be taken into account. To date, most WGS analyses are based on identifying SNVs in a set of strains in comparison to a reference genome, and consequently the results will be completely dependent on the chosen reference. Therefore, the identified SNVs will have a different significance depending on how genetically close the reference genome will be from the strains included in the analysis. Classically, most advances have been focused on unravelling the genomics of two different *A. fumigatus* reference strains [15], Af293 (AAHF00000000.1) and A1163 (ABDB00000000.1), or their derivatives. First, the Af293 strain was fully sequenced in 2005 [16], and soon after, the A1163 strain was the second *A. fumigatus* genome sequenced by the J. Craig Venter Institute [17]. This strain was a derivative of another clinical isolate, the CBS144-89/CEA10. The first genome comparison between both strains showed that despite high synteny and identity in most of the regions of their genomes, there were some hundreds of genes unique from each strain and not present in the other [18]. This heterogeneity could potentially lead to confusion, so care must be taken in drawing conclusions on different aspects from a single genetic background [15]. A recent study carried out in our laboratory [19] showed that the Af293 reference genome belonged to a specific lineage of *A. fumigatus* strains which harbors five polymorphisms (F46Y, M172V, N248T, D255E, E427K) in *cyp51A* gene which codes for the azole target. Based on these phylogenetic studies from whole genome sequencing, the other classic reference genome, the A1163 strain, belonged to a different and distant phylogenetic lineage, which implies that both genomes are significantly different. Also, and apart from the relevance of choosing the most suitable reference genome, the quality of sequencing and assembling will be of great importance for getting reliable results.

In this work, we describe the in-house genome sequencing and comparative analysis of 28 *A. fumigatus* genomes, including the *A. fumigatus* genomes of six strains routinely used in *Aspergillus* basic research laboratories. All these genomes were distributed in four separate clusters, corresponding to very different lineages. In addition, 73 *A. fumigatus* genomes, including azole susceptible and resistant strains from a worldwide distribution, were included in the study. The whole sequence analysis of these 101 *A. fumigatus* genomes provided information that led to an increase in the knowledge of *A. fumigatus* genetic background and the development of azole resistance.

2. Materials and Methods

2.1. *Aspergillus fumigatus* Isolates

A total of 169 genomes were evaluated including in-house sequenced *Aspergillus fumigatus* isolates and genomes downloaded from NCBI Sequence Read Archive (SRA) public database (www.ncbi.nlm.nih.gov/sra). The genomic samples were selected following this criteria: (i) all genomes had to be sequenced with Illumina platform; and (ii) had to be paired-end. After quality control filtering (>85% mapping rate against Af293 reference genome and >95% of genome coverage at more than 10× depth of coverage), a total of 101 *A. fumigatus* strain genome sequences representing 8 different geographical locations were selected for further analysis. Among them, 28 *A. fumigatus* strains were from the Mycology Reference Laboratory Collection (Table 1). Most of them were clinical azole susceptible strains. Some of them had specific *cyp51A* modifications: 12 strains harbored three changes (F46Y, M172V, and E427K) and 3 strains had five (F46Y, M172V, N248T, D255E and E427K) [19]. Af293 was included in the latter group of five *cyp51A* modifications and sequenced again in-house (named as AF293). Another group of *A. fumigatus* azole susceptible strains were isolates that have been classically used as reference or control strains in most *Aspergillus* laboratories. This set of strains included the A1163 (also known as CEA10, CBS144.89, FGSC A1163 or AF10), AF237 (called CM237), ATCC204305, *akuB*^{KU80} (FGSC A1160) [20], and ATCC46645. Two azole resistant strains without modifications in *cyp51A* were also included and sequenced in this work (CM7510 and CM7555).

Table 1. *Aspergillus fumigatus* strains whole genome sequenced in our laboratory. The assigned lineage was based on the phylogenetic study.

Samples	Origin	*cyp51A* Modifications	AZL SC	Mating Type	Source	Lineage
AF293	SP	5SNPs	S	M1.2	CL	3
akuB^{KU80}	SP	WT	S	M1.1	CL	1.1
ATCC204305	SP	I242V	S	M1.1	CL	1.2
ATCC46645	SP	WT	S	M1.1	CL	2.1
CEA10	SP	WT	S	M1.1	CL	1.1
CM2141	SP	WT	S	M1.1	CL	2.2
CM237	SP	WT	S	M1.1	CL	1.1
CM2495	SP	3SNPs	S	M1.1	CL	4
CM2730	SP	3SNPs	S	M1.2	CL	4
CM2733	SP	3SNPs	S	M1.1	CL	4
CM3248	SP	N248K	S	M1.1	CL	1.1
CM3249	SP	3SNPs	S	M1.1	CL	4
CM3249b	SP	3SNPs	S	M1.1	CL	4
CM3262	SP	3SNPs	S	M1.1	CL	4
CM3720	SP	3SNPs	S	M1.1	CL	4
CM4602	SP	3SNPs	S	M1.2	CL	4
CM4946	SP	3SNPs	S	M1.2	CL	4
CM5419	SP	WT	S	M1.2	CL	2.2
CM5757	SP	WT	S	M1.2	CL	1.1
CM6126	SP	WT	S	M1.2	CL	1.1
CM6458	SP	WT	S	M1.2	CL	1.3
CM7510	SP	WT	R	M1.1	CL	1.1
CM7555	SP	WT	R	M1.2	CL	1.3
CM7560	SP	3SNPs	S	M1.1	CL	4
CM7570	SP	3SNPs	S	M1.1	CL	4
CM7632	SP	5SNPs	S	M1.1	CL	3
TP12	SP	5SNPs	S	M1.2	CL	3
TP32	SP	3SNPs	S	M1.1	CL	4

SP (Spain), SNPS (single nucleotide polymorphisms), 3SNPs *cyp51A* modifications (F46Y, M172V, E427K) and 5SNPs *cyp51A* modifications (F46Y, M172V, N248T, D255E, E427K), AZL susceptibility (azole susceptibility), S (susceptible), R (resistant), CL (clinical).

The remaining 73 strain genomes were obtained from public data bases and belonged to strains from the United Kingdom, the Netherlands, Portugal, Denmark, India, Japan and Canada [13,21,22] (NCBI SRA public database) (Table 2). Some of the isolates from The Netherlands and India came from clinical samples (n = 8) and others from environmental soil sources (n = 8). Strains from Japan, UK and Canada were all from clinical origin while the Portuguese strains had an unknown origin (Table 2).

Table 2. *Aspergillus fumigatus* genomes from public data bases included in this study. The assigned lineage is based on the phylogenetic study.

Samples	Origin	*cyp51A* Modifications	AZL SC	Mating Type	Source	Lineage	Ref.
08-12-12-13	NT	TR_{34}/L98H, S297T, F495I	R	M1.1	CL	2.2	[13]
08-19-02-10	NT	TR_{34}/L98H	R	M1.2	ENV	2.2	[13]
08-19-02-30	NT	WT	S	M1.1	ENV	1.3	[13]
08-19-02-46	NT	TR_{34}/L98H	R	M1.1	ENV	2.2	[13]
08-19-02-61	NT	TR_{34}/L98H	R	M1.1	ENV	2.2	[13]
08-31-08-91	NT	TR_{34}/L98H	R	M1.1	CL	2.2	[13]
08-36-03-25	NT	TR_{34}/L98H, S297T, F495I	R	Unclear	CL	2.2	[13]
09-7500806	UK	WT	S	M1.2	CL	1.3	[13]
10-01-02-27	NT	TR_{34}/L98H	R	M1.2	CL	2.2	[13]
12-7504462	UK	WT	S	M1.2	CL	1.3	[13]
12-7504652	UK	WT	S	M1.1	CL	2.1	[13]
12-7505054	UK	WT	S	M1.1	CL	2.1	[13]

Table 2. *Cont.*

Samples	Origin	*cyp51A* Modifications	AZL SC	Mating Type	Source	Lineage	Ref.
12-7505220	UK	TR_{34}/L98H	R	M1.1	CL	2.2	[13]
12-7505446	UK	TR_{34}/L98H	R	M1.2	CL	2.2	[13]
Af293	UK	5SNPs	S	M1.2	CL	3	[13]
AF41	UK	WT	S	M1.2	CL	1.1	[13]
Af65	UK	WT	S	M1.2	CL	2.1	[13]
AF72	UK	G54E	R	M1.2	CL	1.1	[13]
AF90	UK	M220V	R	M1.1	CL	1.1	[13]
Afu1042-09	IN	TR_{34}/L98H	R	M1.1	CL	2.2	[13]
Afu124-E11	IN	TR_{34}/L98H	R	M1.1	ENV	2.2	[13]
Afu166-E11	IN	TR_{34}/L98H	R	M1.1	ENV	2.2	[13]
Afu218-E11	IN	TR_{34}/L98H	R	M1.1	ENV	2.2	[13]
Afu257-E11	IN	TR_{34}/L98H	R	M1.1	ENV	2.2	[13]
Afu343-P-11	IN	TR_{34}/L98H	R	Unclear	CL	2.2	[13]
Afu591-12	IN	TR_{34}/L98H	R	M1.1	CL	2.2	[13]
Afu942-09	IN	TR_{34}/L98H	R	M1.1	CL	2.2	[13]
F12041	UK	G138C	R	M1.2	CL	2.1	[21] *
F12219	UK	G54R	R	M1.2	CL	1.1	[21] *
F12636	UK	G54E	R	M1.1	CL	2.1	[21] *
F13535	UK	G138C	R	M1.2	CL	2.1	[21] *
F13619	UK	H147Y, G448S	R	M1.1	CL	2.1	[21] *
F13952	UK	G138C	R	M1.2	CL	2.1	[21] *
F14403	UK	G54R	R	M1.1	CL	1.1	[21] *
F14513G	UK	G138C	R	M1.2	CL	2.1	[21] *
F14532	UK	M220T	R	M1.1	CL	2.1	[21] *
F14946G	UK	WT	S	M1.2	CL	1.1	[21] *
F15390	UK	M220T	R	M1.1	CL	2.1	[21] *
F15927	CN	3SNPs	S	M1.1	CL	4	[21] *
F16134	DN	M220K	R	M1.2	CL	1.1	[21] *
F16216	UK	TR_{34}/L98H	R	M1.2	CL	2.1	[21] *
F16311	UK	WT	S	M1.1	CL	1.1	[21] *
F17582	UK	WT	S	M1.2	CL	2.1	[21] *
F17729	UK	WT	S	M1.2	CL	1.1	[21] *
F17729W	UK	WT	S	M1.2	CL	1.1	[21] *
F17764	CN	WT	S	M1.1	CL	1.1	[21] *
F18085	UK	WT	S	M1.1	CL	1.1	[21] *
F5211G	UK	WT	S	M1.1	CL	2.1	[21] *
F7763	UK	5SNPs	S	M1.1	CL	3	[21] *
IFM55369	JP	WT	S	M1.1	CL	1.2	[22]
IFM58026	JP	N248K	S	M1.2	CL	1.1	[22]
IFM58029	JP	WT	S	M1.2	CL	1.2	[22]
IFM58401	JP	WT	S	M1.2	CL	1.1	[22]
IFM59056	JP	WT	S	M1.1	CL	1.1	[22]
IFM59073	JP	WT	S	M1.2	CL	1.2	[22]
IFM59359	JP	WT	S	Unclear	CL	1.2	[22]
IFM59361	JP	WT	S	M1.1	CL	1.3	[22]
IFM59365	JP	WT	S	M1.2	CL	1.1	[22]
IFM59777	JP	WT	S	M1.1	CL	1.2	[22]
IFM60514	JP	WT	S	M1.2	CL	1.1	[22]
IFM61118	JP	N248K	S	M1.1	CL	1.1	[22]
IFM61407	JP	WT	S	Unclear	CL	1.1	[22]
IFM61578	JP	P216L	S	M1.2	CL	1.1	[22]
IFM61610	JP	WT	S	M1.2	CL	1.1	[22]
IFM62516	JP	P329P	S	M1.1	CL	1.2	[22]
SL143435	PT	N248K	S	M1.2	UNK	1.1	*
SL143436	PT	WT	S	M1.2	UNK	1.1	*
SL143437	PT	WT	S	M1.1	UNK	1.3	*
SL143438	PT	N248K	S	M1.2	UNK	1.1	*
SL143439	PT	WT	S	M1.1	UNK	1.3	*
SL143440	PT	3SNPs	S	M1.1	UNK	4	*
SL143441	PT	WT	S	M1.1	UNK	1.1	*
SL146112	PT	N248K	S	M1.2	UNK	1.1	*

NT (the Netherlands), UK (the United Kingdom), IN (India), CN (Canada), JP (Japan), PT (Portugal). SNPs (single nucleotide polymorphisms), 3SNPs *cyp51A* modifications (F46Y, M172V, E427K) and 5SNPs *cyp51A* modifications (F46Y, M172V, N248T, D255E, E427K), AZL SC (azole susceptibility), S (susceptible), R (resistant), CL (clinical), ENV (environmental), UNK (unknown), * NCBI SRA.

2.2. *DNA Extraction and Aspergillus fumigatus Identification*

First, conidia from each selected strain were cultured in 3 mL of glucose-yeast extract-peptone (GYEP) broth (2% glucose, 0.3% yeast extract, 1% peptone; OXOID LTD, Basingstoke, Hampshire, England) and grown overnight at 37 °C, after which mycelium mats were harvested and DNA was extracted [23]. The *A. fumigatus* Spanish isolates included in this work were identified to the species level on the basis of PCR amplification and sequencing of the internal transcribed spacer (ITS) region and the partial amplification of the *β-tubulin* gene [24].

2.3. *DNA Quality and Quantity Assessment*

The DNA quality and quantity was assessed using a spectrophotometer (Thermo Scientific NanoDrop One Spectrophotometer, Waltham, MA, USA). Since genomic DNA (gDNA) must be clean and pure for preparing WGS libraries, when the 260/280 or 260/230 rates were lower than 1.8 or higher than 2.2, the DNA was rejected. The strain was extracted again from a new mycelium mat and its quality was assessed. Genomic DNA (gDNAs) were stored at −20 °C until further use.

2.4. *Screening of cyp51A Changes: PCR Amplification and Sequence Analysis*

The full coding sequences of *cyp51A* including its promoter, were amplified and sequenced using the PCR conditions described before [25]. To exclude the possibility that any change identified in the sequences was due to PCR-induced errors, each isolate was independently analyzed twice. Isolates were screened for the presence of tandem repeat insertions in the *cyp51A* promoter region, as well as for the presence of other *cyp51A* modifications. All the nucleotide sequences were analyzed using the DNASTAR Lasergene package (DNASTAR Inc., Madison, WI, USA).

2.5. *DNA Library Preparation and Illumina Whole-Genome Sequencing*

Genomic DNA was extracted as previously described. Genomic DNA were quantified afterwards using the QuantiFluor ® dsDNA System and the QuantiFluor ® ST Fluorometer (Promega, Madison, WI, USA) and their quality was determined with the Agilent 2100 Bioanalyzer (Agilent Technologies, Inc., Santa Clara, CA, USA). The preparation of fragmented gDNA libraries was performed using Nextera ® XT Library Prep Kit (Illumina Inc., San Diego, CA, USA), according to the manufacturer's protocols. The mean fragment length of the libraries ranged from 800 to 1800 bp. Sequencing was conducted in paired-end 2 × 150 bp on a NextSeq 500 system, according to the manufacturer's protocols (Illumina Inc., San Diego, CA, USA).

2.6. *Whole-Genome Sequencing Alignment*

The Illumina reads were trimmed using Trimmomatic (version 0.32) [26]. The sequencing adapters and sequences with low quality scores on 3′ ends (Phred score [Q], <20) were trimmed. Raw Illumina WGS reads were quality checked performing a quality control with FastQC (version 0.11.3; Babraham Institute). Data sets were analyzed against two different *A. fumigatus* reference genomes, the Af293 (GenBank accession number AAHF00000000.1) and the A1163 (GenBank accession number ABDB00000000.1) using WGS-outbreaker v1.0 (Instituto de Salud Carlos III, Madrid, Spain) (https://github.com/BU-ISCIII/WGS-Outbreaker) with default parameters. The pipeline comprised all steps needed for SNV analysis using whole genome sequencing data. Mapping against genome reference was performed with bwa mem (version 0.7.12-r1039) [27], duplicated reads removed using Picard (version 1.140) (http://broadinstitute.github.io/picard), and the bedtools coverage v2.26 program [28] was used to perform further quality controls. Hereafter, in order to identify genetic variations among strains, single nucleotide variant (SNV) detection (variant calling) and SNV matrix generation were performed using GATK version 3.8.0 [29] with best practices parameters. ENSEMBL variant effect predictor script (version 88) was used for variant annotation. The whole genome sequencing project has been deposited in NCBI SRA (project accession number SRP151231).

2.7. Phylogenetic Analysis and Single Nucleotide Variant Comparison

Final step of WGS-Outbreaker pipeline comprised Maximum-likelihood trees construction using RaxML software (version 8.2.9) [30] with GTRCAT model and 100 bootstrap replicates. Phylogenetic trees were visualized and annotated using ggtree R package [31]. SNV comparisons were performed using a custom R script, mapping all genomes to Af293 and A1163 reference genomes.

2.8. Analysis of Genetic Diversity

Genetic diversity was calculated using the Molecular Evolutionary Genetics Analysis software (MEGA, version 7) [32]. The *A. fumigatus* population was analyzed according to the formed groups (clusters and subclusters) from the previous phylogenic studies. In MEGA, evolutionary distances between sequences can be estimated by computing the number or proportion of nucleotide differences between sequences using the FASTA alignment against each reference genome [33]. Two different models have been used in this work, the p-distance model and another based on the number of differences; (i) the p-distance model calculates the distance as the proportion of different nucleotide sites compared. It is obtained by dividing the number of nucleotide differences (transitions and transversions) by the total number of nucleotides compared. As recommended [34], when the genetic distance was estimated, the complete-deletion option was used, since it normalizes the number of differences based on the number of valid sites compared, not taking into account the alignment gaps and missing data that sequences could contain. However, this model does not make any correction for multiple substitutions at the same site, substitution rate biases (for example, differences in the transitional and transversional rates), or differences in evolutionary rates among sites; (ii) The second model, based on the number of differences, estimates the genetic distances according to the number of sites at which the compared sequences differ (transitions and transversions). In this model, the complete-deletion option was also used.

2.9. Determining Modifications in Genes of Interest

In order to see if the population structure could be based on particular genomic modifications, some genes that have already been described as important in *A. fumigatus* biology were analyzed in depth in each of the *A. fumigatus* population clusters formed from the SNV comparisons. One of the genes was the *cyp51A* gene including its promoter (AFUA_4G06890 in Af293, and AFUB_063960 in A1163). This region was used to determine the azole resistant phenotype based on the resistance mechanism. Since both reference genomes, Af293 and A1163, have opposite mating types, the mating locus genes were included in the analysis: Mat1.1.1 (AFUB_042900), Mat1.2.1 (AFUA_3G06170), and Mat1.2.4 (AFUA_3G06160). The presence or absence of these loci was also tested in all genomes using srst2 software (version 0.1.8) [35]. Every gene of interest was analyzed independently in all genomes.

2.10. Visualization of Depth of Coverage

An exploratory approach using Circos (v 0.69.3) [36], a tool to represent visual data, was used to plot the depth of coverage of 20 whole-sequenced genomes selected to represent each cluster and subcluster in comparison to the Af293 reference genome. Mean coverage data in 10,000 length bins was calculated from bam files with bedtools (version 2.2.17) (http://bedtools.readthedocs.io/en/latest/).

2.11. Mating Type Analysis

A mapping approach was used in order to identify genes associated with each mating type. Since Af293 was Mat1.2 and A1163 was Mat1.1, all samples were mapped against both references using the workflow displayed in Figure S1: (i) samples that had been determined with srst2 as Mat1.2 and mapped against A1163 were selected, and unmapped reads were retained in this step; (ii) the unmapped reads were then mapped against Af293. Statistics of coverage and depth of coverage were calculated for all genes annotated in A1163 reference genome using the bam generated in this step; (iii) genes with at least 70% of coverage were selected; (iv) to discard genes that may be found due to the lack of presence in the A1163 assembly, the same procedure was performed for Mat1.1 samples; (v) finally, genes in common among all Mat1.2 samples minus one but not present in any Mat1.1 sample were exported as a result (Figure S1A). The reverse procedure was performed starting with Mat1.1 samples determining the genes only present in Mat1.1 samples (Figure S1B).

3. Results

3.1. Species Identification

The isolates were identified at the species level and also the azole resistance mechanism was analyzed by PCR amplification and sequencing of the *cyp51A* gene and its promoter as explained in Materials and Methods section. All the strains were identified as *A. fumigatus* sensu stricto. The azole susceptibility profile of most of the strains sequenced in the laboratory is described elsewhere [19]. For the remaining strains, the azole susceptibility profile was determined based on the known *cyp51A* modifications detected by WGS analysis. According to the azole resistance mechanism, the *A. fumigatus* strains included in this study harbored the following *cyp51A* modifications: (i) strains with *cyp51A* single point mutations (G54E/R, M220V/T/K, and G138C) or double point mutations (G448S together with H147Y) in the minority of cases (only one strain); or (ii) strains with tandem integrations and *cyp51A* modifications (TR34/L98H, TR34/L98H/S297T/F495I). Two azole resistant *cyp51A* wild type (WT) strains were also included. All these strain features (*cyp51A* modifications and azole susceptibility profile, as well as the geographical origin and mating type), were described in Tables 1 and 2. Afterwards, the DNAs were further analyzed using WGS.

3.2. Whole-Genome Sequencing Analysis

All genome sequences mapped to a range of 85–99% genome coverage with at least 10x of depth of coverage and a mapping rate > 94% against Af293 reference genome. Similarly, sequences were mapped to a range of 84–99% genome coverage with at least 10× of depth of coverage against A1163 reference with a mapping rate > 88% (Table S1). The Af293 and the A1163 strains were resequenced in our laboratory (and named hereafter AF293 and CEA10) and had a total of 313 and 1009 SNVs, respectively, compared to their respective reference genomes.

3.3. Phylogenetic Analysis

Phylogenetic analysis using SNV data of Spanish genomes (Table 1) clearly showed that our strains were divided into four clusters independently of the genome used as reference (Figure 1, with Af293 as reference genome and Figure 2, with A1163 as reference genome). In this previous analysis, the different wild type reference strains used, *akuB*^{KU80} and CEA10 as derivative strains of A1163, AF293, CM237, ATCC204305 and ATCC46645 were located in separated clusters (Figures 1 and 2). Those clusters were further confirmed when the remaining 73 *A. fumigatus* genomes available from other countries were included.

Therefore, based on phylogenetic analysis, the complete *A. fumigatus* population was divided into four well defined clusters (I, II, III, and IV). Two of them could be further subdivided into subclusters: cluster I split in 3 subclusters (I.1, I.2, I.3), and cluster II in 2 (II.1, II.2). Clusters III and IV remained undivided, because any subcluster was identified. Each subcluster was considered as an independent population group, and was used to compare itself against each reference genome (Table 3). The two reference genomes used were distributed in different clusters when compared against the other: A1163 in cluster I and Af293 in cluster III. The number of clusters and the tree topology was maintained regardless of the reference genome chosen.

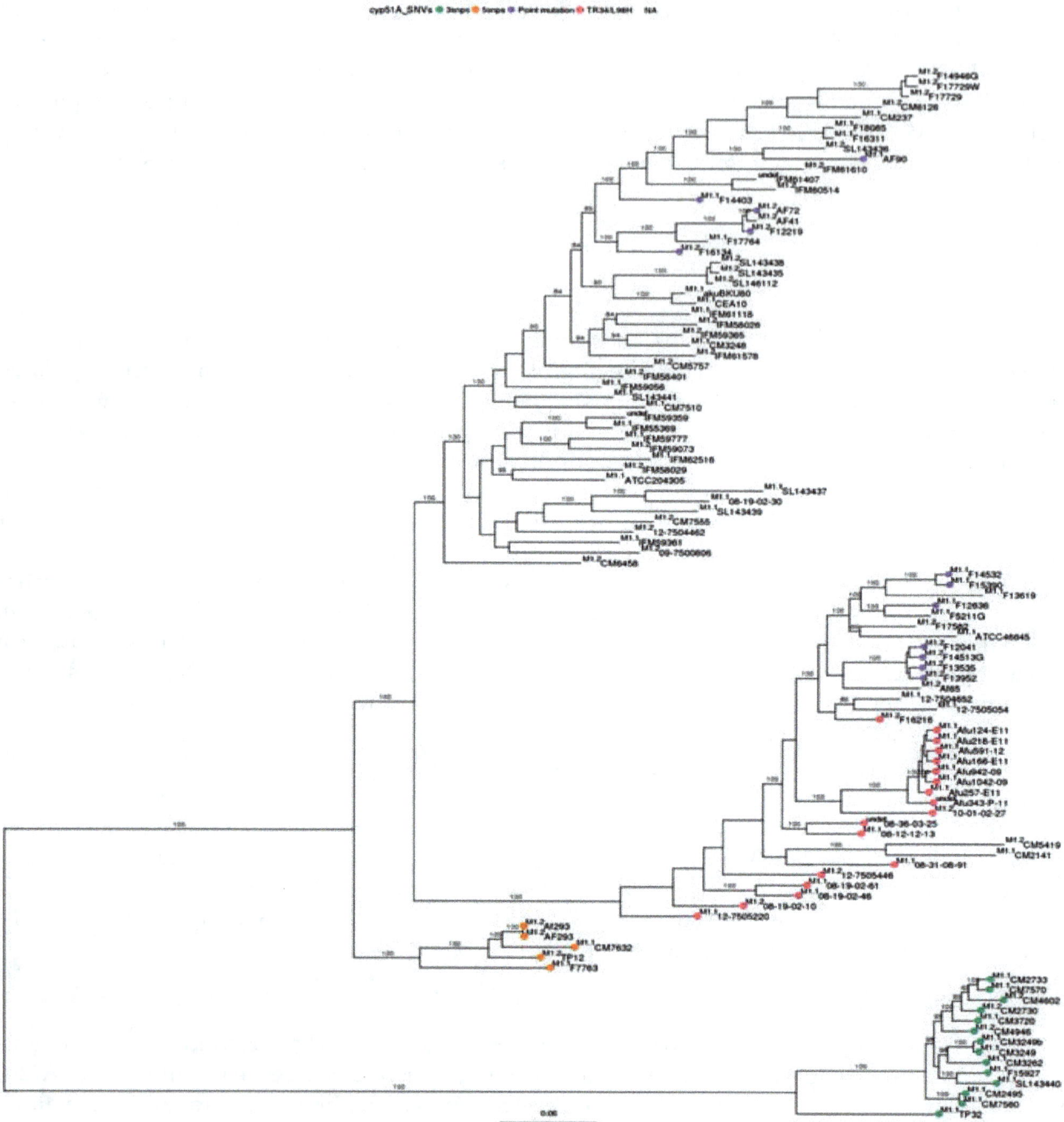

Figure 1. Whole genome phylogenetic analysis of 101 *Aspergillus fumigatus* genomes included in the study. Dendrogram was performed using Af293 as reference genome.

Table 3. Mean of single nucleotide variants (SNVs). Variants within clusters and subclusters compared to both reference genomes.

Phylogenetic Groups	SNVs vs. A1163 Reference Genome	SNVs vs. Af293 Reference Genome
Subcluster I.1	34,544	75,653
Subcluster I.2	40,124	65,121
Subcluster I.3	46,811	79,899
Subcluster II.1	81,478	98,423
Subcluster II.2	80,994	97,749
Cluster III	82,235	35,268
Cluster IV	158,154	159,742

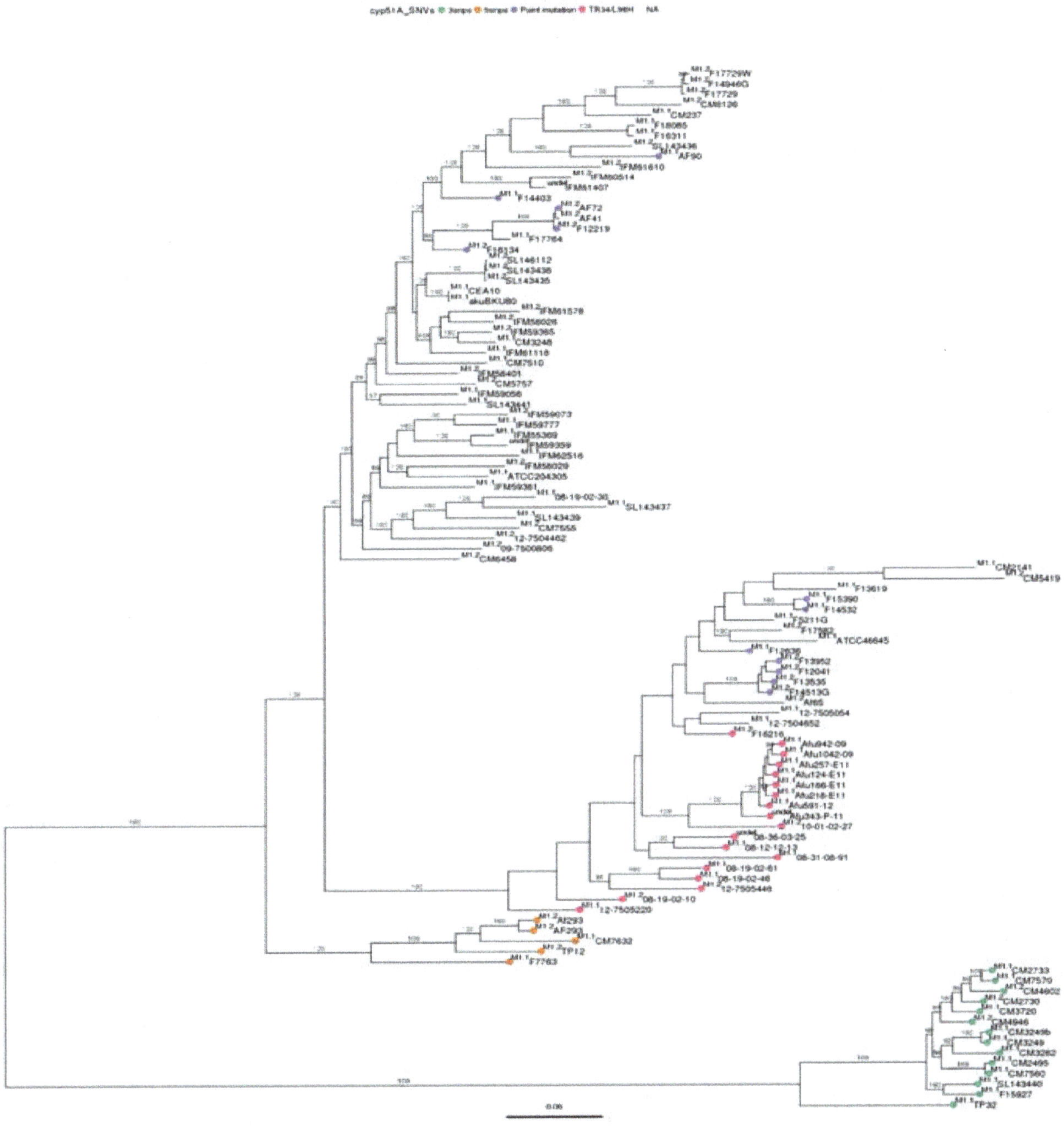

Figure 2. Whole genome phylogenetic analysis of 101 *Aspergillus fumigatus* genomes included in the study. Dendrogram was performed using A1163 as reference genome.

Based on *cyp51A* modifications, azole susceptible *cyp51A*-WT strains together with azole resistant *cyp51A* single point mutation strains were grouped together in cluster I. In cluster II, there were azole susceptible and resistant strains, with both *cyp51A* single point mutations and TR_{34}/L98H mechanisms. In cluster III, a set of strains with five *cyp51A* modifications (F46Y, M172V, N248T, D255E, E427K) grouped together. While in cluster IV strains with three *cyp51A* modifications (F46Y, M172V, E427K) also grouped together [19]. The Netherlands, Portugal and Canada genomes were distributed in two clusters. The United Kingdom genomes were distributed in three, while Japanese genomes (*cyp51A*-WT) were only in cluster I and Indian genomes (*cyp51A*-TR_{34}) in cluster II. Except for the tightly clustered isolates from India in cluster II.2, there was no relationship between the geographical origin of the isolates and the cluster where they grouped.

3.4. Single Nucleotide Variant Analysis against Both References

To explore the genomic differences between the clusters formed from phylogenetic studies, total SNVs between populations were determined. There were a total of 93,609 and 71,844 SNV positions identified against the reference genomes, Af293 and A1163, respectively. No noticeable differences were found in the SNV ranges when all strains were mapped against Af293 (313–165,788) or A1163 (1043–163,367). However, the number of specific SNVs identified in each strain was notably different depending on the genome that was used as reference (Table 4). In fact, some particular SNVs previously detected in our laboratory by PCR (L98H, F46Y, M172V, N248T, D255E, E427K) were specifically searched for in both reference whole genomes. The L98H variant was found in all genomes that harbored this mutation since none of the reference genomes had this change in its own genome. However, the remaining 5 SNVs (F46Y, M172V, N248T, D255E, E427K) were only detected when the reference genome chosen was the A1163 genome, as Af293 specifically harbored these 5 same polymorphisms.

Table 4. Single nucleotide variant differences compared to both reference genomes. Variants of each *A. fumigatus* genome included in this study.

Samples	A1163	Af293	Samples	A1163	Af293	Samples	A1163	Af293
08-12-12-13	80,791	91,956	CM2495	151,089	148,524	F17582	79,598	97,024
08-19-02-10	75,401	89,762	CM2730	157,505	159,177	F17729	44,054	79,106
08-19-02-30	42,487	87,831	CM2733	154,361	160,494	F17729W	43,663	78,416
08-19-02-46	78,449	96,243	CM3248	22,834	74,568	F17764	25,812	70,013
08-19-02-61	80,244	96,416	CM3249	157,242	159,900	F18085	51,241	78,553
08-31-08-91	88,972	98,911	CM3249b	154,510	157,780	F5211G	82,091	99,726
08-36-03-25	83,921	102,006	CM3262	161,695	160,926	F7763	84,764	55,332
09-7500806	45,286	74,134	CM3720	156,600	158,781	IFM55369	42,849	64,003
10-01-02-27	72,487	93,299	CM4602	155,381	161,767	IFM58026	22,186	68,777
12-7504462	48,927	75,301	CM4946	158,692	161,082	IFM58029	36,521	63,106
12-7504652	80,203	93,323	CM5419	89,354	99,771	IFM58401	26,669	63,489
12-7505054	86,952	101,471	CM5757	36,027	74,420	IFM59056	30,841	61,481
12-7505220	75,479	100,229	CM6126	55,871	86,902	IFM59073	43,230	68,775
12-7505446	86,194	100,736	CM6458	42,482	71,670	IFM59359	39,309	67,118
Af293	83,486	313	CM7510	33,559	79,283	IFM59361	42,795	73,228
AF293	78,045	659	CM7555	51,657	77,679	IFM59365	21,830	74,248
AF41	34,879	72,914	CM7560	158,657	153,769	IFM59777	40,117	65,300
Af65	90,143	103,614	CM7570	160,908	162,292	IFM60514	39,629	75,765
AF72	35,271	73,632	CM7632	81,519	25,490	IFM61118	21,905	70,230
AF90	40,262	73,395	F12041	78,812	93,712	IFM61407	32,025	76,034
Afu1042-09	80,346	96,348	F12219	35,440	73,872	IFM61578	26,201	67,946
Afu124-E11	81,115	97,509	F12636	80,359	98,501	IFM61610	41,690	74,102
Afu166-E11	80,948	97,350	F13535	78,741	93,777	IFM62516	41,229	67,364
Afu218-E11	80,571	96,955	F13619	85,412	107,985	SL143435	22,037	81,031
Afu257-E11	80,499	97,008	F13952	78,466	93,926	SL143436	52,604	84,188
Afu343-P11	73,797	101,305	F14403	27,476	74,454	SL143437	61,289	91,394
Afu591-12	80,781	97,039	F14513G	78,647	94,213	SL143438	22,676	81,649
Afu942-09	80,827	97,149	F14532	79,931	102,436	SL143439	39,562	87,955
akuB^{KU80}	1043	78,152	F14946G	44,442	79,719	SL143440	162,993	165,788
ATCC 204305	37,614	60,180	F15390	79,743	101,967	SL143441	38,498	72,994
ATCC 46645	84,994	103,941	F15927	161,157	164,076	SL146112	21,782	81,137
CEA10	1009	75,854	F16134	19,660	77,718	TP12	83,363	24,982
CM2141	88,704	107,238	F16216	78,073	90,736	TP32	163,367	162,032
CM237	48,402	83,874	F16311	51,387	78,630	F17582	79,598	97,024

Although the tree topology was maintained regardless of the reference genome chosen, the number of SNVs within clusters changed significantly when comparing each reference against each cluster, showing that both reference genomes were genetically very different (Table 3). The number of SNVs of clusters II and IV were similar against both references, while remarkable differences in SNVs were present in clusters I (closer to A1163) and III (closer to Af293) (Table 3). Considering subclusters, the number of SNVs in subclusters I.1, I.2 and I.3 were almost half when the reference genome was the

A1163, than the SNVs obtained using Af293 as reference genome. Another remarkable result was the small number of SNVs found in cluster III when compared to Af293 genome. The SNV differences found against both references were slighter but also considerable in cluster II, higher when compared to A1163. Cluster IV had the greatest number of SNVs, independent of the reference genome used.

Moreover, in order to explore any genomic differences between clusters and subclusters, some features of the SNVs found in each population were determined (Table 5). This table shows that all populations had a similar amount of SNVs, excluding cluster IV, which had much more variants, specifically missense and synonymous, compared to the other clusters.

Table 5. Types of SNVs and features. Variants found within each cluster compared to both genomes.

Variants	A1163 Reference Genome				Af293 Reference Genome			
	I	II	III	IV	I	II	III	IV
Frameshift variants	256	512	477	828	446	587	133	819
Inframe deletions	149	278	264	511	246	330	94	527
Inframe insertions	191	369	291	561	325	447	91	556
Intergenic variants	6405	11,107	12,819	6730	13,428	16,394	3,785	8792
Intron variants	1568	3668	3418	9066	3120	4322	960	8670
Missense variants	4342	10,251	10,008	23,107	8766	11,973	2562	22,746
Protein altering	8	19	12	18	16	22	4	21
Start lost	9	16	23	57	21	24	6	57
Stop gained	95	230	264	298	141	218	43	288
Stop lost	13	27	32	61	25	33	9	61
Stop retained	10	22	21	52	17	24	5	52
Synonymous variants	3675	9026	9005	26,080	8189	11,058	2365	25,418

3.5. Genetic Diversity

Evolutionary distances were estimated by computing the mean proportion or number of nucleotide differences between each subcluster and each reference genome using two different models provided by MEGA: the p-model and the number of differences model.

The pairwise distance matrices referred to the distance between each genome and the others in pairs and was calculated and expressed in proportion and number of differences (Tables S2–S5). The matrices obtained from the mean distance between groups in which each subcluster was compared to each other, were indicated also as the proportion and number of differences of all these comparisons (Tables S6 and S7). Cluster IV was identified as the most distant cluster, according to phylogenetic results, with 123,259, 118,271 and 114,815 differences in SNVs against cluster I, II and III, respectively. Moreover, while cluster III was more similar to cluster II with 36,031 differences, cluster I was closer to cluster II than to III with 38,197 and 50,040 differences, respectively. These data were calculated using Af293 genome as reference. Data using A1163 were not shown since no significant differences were found.

Homogeneity within a group or cluster could be inferred through the analysis of the mean distance within groups (Tables S8 and S9). Cluster IV was the most homogeneous since the number of differences was lower than in the remaining groups, followed by subcluster II.1, independently of the genome that was chosen as reference.

3.6. Genome-Wide Visualization of Depth of Coverage

The depth of coverage from a selected group of whole-sequenced genomes was plotted in a Circos image to make an exploratory analysis, and to visualize similarities and differences in genome structure (Figure 3). None of the 20 *A. fumigatus* genomes included in this study displayed chromosomal or copy number variations. However, small deletions were observed in multiple chromosomes: regions smaller than 100 kbp seemed to be deleted in chromosomes 3, 4, 5, 6, 7 and 8. Also, what seemed to be large-scale deletions (bigger than 300 kbp) were detected in the edges of chromosomes 1 and 7 in genomes of cluster I and II. It is noteworthy that there was a huge red region in chromosome 4 present in all genomes marked as an expected deletion, even in the two different Af293 genomes downloaded and sequenced in-house although the reference genome used was the same Af293 strain genome.

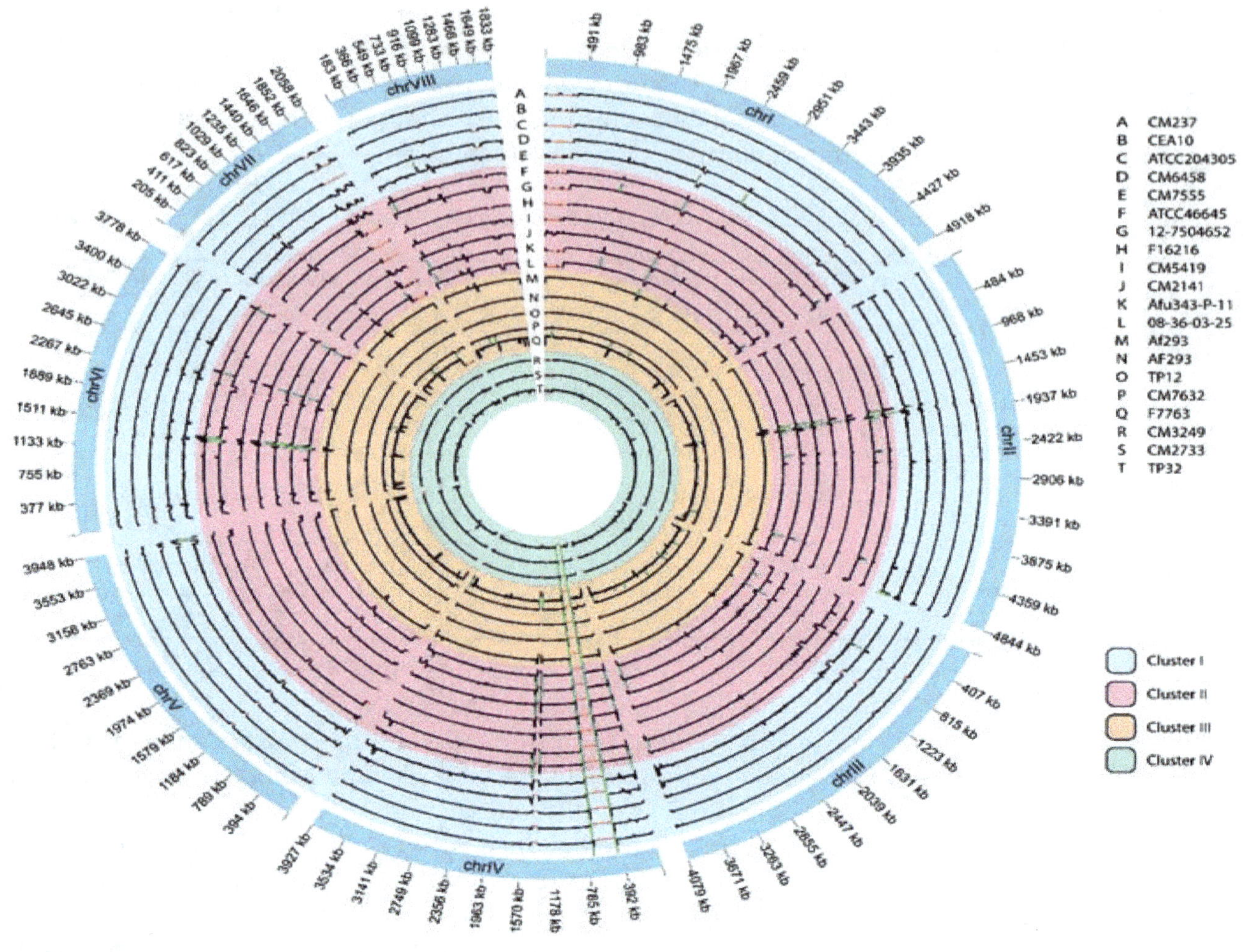

Figure 3. Circos representation of whole-genome depth of coverage of 20 *A. fumigatus* genomes, averaged over 10,000-bp bins. Red marks showed null coverage, black marks a range of coverage between 1–500, and green marks showed a coverage higher than 500. Color legend shows the selected genomes of each cluster: I (blue), II (pink), III (orange) and IV (green).

3.7. Genome Comparisons Based on Their Mating Type

There were no differences in the strain genetic background between genomes harboring the mating type 1 or 2. In fact, strain genomes of both mating types were present in all clusters. In order to detect if there was any differential presence or absence of certain genes based on their particular mating type, all genomes were divided according to their mating type and mapped to both reference genomes (Af293, Mat1.2 and A1163, Mat1.1). No differences in the presence of genes were found in Mat1.1 strain genomes other than those encoded by the Mat1.2 locus itself (Mat1.2.1 and Mat1.2.4). The same situation was found within strains with Mat1.2 genomes; there were no differences in genes other than the gene Mat1.1.1 itself encoded by the Mat1.1 locus.

4. Discussion

Different typing techniques have demonstrated remarkable genomic diversity among strains of *A. fumigatus* [13,37]. *Aspergillus fumigatus* is found in multiple environmental niches which contribute to its genotypic and phenotypic heterogeneity among isolates [38]. Therefore, understanding the association between genomic diversity and different biological and phenotypic features, such as the spectrum of pathogenicity and antifungal resistance, among others, is a challenge for multiple *Aspergillus* laboratories. In this context, WGS is emerging as a promising tool for strain characterization [18,39]. Since WGS considers the entire genetic material of every isolate, it provides the highest discriminatory power that any technique can reach, allowing for the differentiation of closely related strains [39]. In addition, WGS could emerge as a useful tool for gene detection and other sequence-based investigations [9]. This source of an unprecedented amount of novel and comparative data could aid in the development of a huge database which would contain information about the biological differences between *A. fumigatus* strains, such as their origin, diversity and population structure. Previous WGS studies with a suitable depth of coverage had shown variation in genome structure with small-scale insertions and deletions, and recombination events among *A. fumigatus* isolates [40]. However, due to the complexity of biological systems, some difficulties need to be overcome in order to correlate complex biological traits with genomic features.

To date, most of the WGS studies are based on genome-scale comparisons in which the number of SNVs of each strain are obtained comparing its genome to a previously selected reference genome. In this work, we have made all comparison independently using two *A. fumigatus* reference genomes, Af293 and A1163. The differential grouping of the *A. fumigatus* population in four clusters is driven by the different SNVs found. In fact, the number of SNVs in each cluster and subcluster differed depending on the reference genome used to determine the number of variants. Particularly, the small number of SNVs found in cluster III when it was compared to Af293 reference genome is due to the fact that the genomes included in this cluster were more similar to Af293 and had twice the SNVs obtained with A1163 as a reference. Because cluster III was the smallest, formed by only five genomes, the WGS analysis would be improved by the addition of more genomes when available. In addition, it is important to highlight that the specific five SNVs in *cyp51A* present in all genomes belonging to cluster III (F46Y, M172V, N248T, D255E, and E427K) would have not been detected when Af293 genome was used as reference since those changes are also found in its genome. Other important changes could have been missed during the analysis depending on which genome was used as a reference, highlighting the importance of choosing an appropriate reference genome for each case.

The highest number of SNVs was found in cluster IV, which means that was the furthest and most different population compared to both references (Table 3). In fact, this result was in agreement with those computed using MEGA. Cluster IV was the most distant (in number of differences as well as in proportion) from all the subclusters (Tables S6 and S7). When the differences within subclusters were analyzed (Tables S8 and S9), this cluster had the greatest homogeneity. In conclusion, cluster IV is the most different *A. fumigatus* population compared to the others but also the most homogeneously composed. The results obtained by MEGA to study the evolutionary distances among genomes were in line with the results obtained from WGS phylogenetic studies, since the evolutionary distances supported the formed clusters and subclusters (Figures 1 and 2, Tables S6 and S7).

Regarding the Circos visual representation of the depth of coverage (Figure 3), it is noteworthy that the described large-scale deletions were detected in the edges of chromosomes 1 and 7, so these possible deletion events could be confined to telomeric or subtelomeric regions. Notably, all cluster III genomes did not have these deletions, as well as the reference genome used, which belonged to this same cluster. Remarkably, a huge deletion in chromosome 4 was present in all genomes. This might be due to a misassembly or to sequencing errors since two different Af293 genomes (downloaded and sequenced in-house) were included in the analysis and also had this deletion in spite of being the same strain that the genome used as reference. Similar results have been found by other authors although no comments were made about it, probably because it was difficult to realize without sequencing in-house the Af293 [13]. Areas with higher depth of coverage might be a consequence of possible duplication events, pseudogene presence or artefacts. However, since these regions appeared specifically in chromosomes 2, 4 and 6 in most of the genomes of cluster II, it would be worthy to explore them further. A specific mapping approach should be developed to analyze all these regions and to determine if there are real duplications and also if they represent a hallmark for cluster characterization. Further research is in progress to clarify which genes are in these differential regions and which are their biological processes or functions in which they are involved.

Experimental investigations on *A. fumigatus* biology and virulence have historically used only a few particular strains, of which Af293 and A1163 are the most used. More than in any other comparisons, the genetic background must be highly considered in the genomes used as references, since it can be responsible for the variability in many biological aspects between isolates and thus responsible for different phenotypes. The first genome comparison study between Af293 and A1163 was accomplished in 2007, showing that both genomes were highly syntenic in most regions, having core genes highly conserved and with levels of identity of 99.8% at the genome level [18]. These results were confirmed later by Fedorova et al. [17]. Specifically, the Af293 genome contained 143 [17] to 208 unique genes [18], while the A1163, 218 [17] to 320 [18]. In both cases, more than 60% of the strain-specific genes were related to cellular metabolism, secondary metabolism, signaling and transcriptional regulation [17,18]. These sequence divergences could explain the phenotypic differences described by other authors who reported a high heterogeneity among these two isolates regarding abiotic stimuli physiological responses, levels of growth, and virulence [15,38,41], as well as in immunogenic responses [42]. The variability in the total amount of unique genes in each genome could be due to sequencing errors or, less probably, to new mutations generated during the repeated subculture [13]. These results are in agreement with our study, in which the Af293 and the A1163 reference genomes belonged to different phylogenetic clusters which means that there are considerable differences between both genomes. Therefore, the appropriate election of the most suitable reference genome in each context will ultimately result in a more appropriate comparison and lead to solid conclusions.

Apart from the differences already discussed between Af293 and A1163, comparative analyses of the mating loci showed that both strains belonged to opposite mating types [40,43]. Mating type genes are not true idiomorphs, as they occupy adjacent positions on the chromosome. Mat1.1 strains have only one gene in this locus that encodes a transcriptional factor with an alpha box domain (AFUB_042900, Mat1.1.), while Mat1.2 strains contain a truncated copy of the high mobility group (HMG) box (Afu3g06170, Mat1.2.1) and another gene (Afu3g06160, Mat1.2.4) needed for heterokaryon formation as part of the mating process [44–46]. In this study we also checked if there were gene differences (presence or absence) other than those responsible for the mating type (Mat1.1, Mat1.2.1 and Mat1.2.4) among both groups of *A. fumigatus* genomes using an innovative approach (Figure S1). No gene absences were found in Mat1.1 strain genomes other than those encoded by the Mat1.2 locus itself (Mat1.2.1 and Mat1.2.4). Some previous works have reported differential gene presence between strains that coincidentally had different mating types [17,18]. However, the differences found must be due to their own different genetic background and not because of their opposite mating type.

One of the main concerns of invasive aspergillosis treatment is the global emergence of azole resistance. Regarding azole resistance mechanisms, Cyp51A protein is the target of these drugs and the *cyp51A* gene is a hotspot for mutations that confer azole resistance. The most common *cyp51A* modifications could be grouped into two categories: *A. fumigatus* strains that harbor *cyp51A* single point mutations (G54, G138, M220, or G448) [47–50], and isolates with specific point mutations in *cyp51A* gene together with various size tandem repeat (TR) integrations in the promoter of the gene (TR34/L98H, TR34/L98H/S297T/F495I, TR46/Y121F/T289A, or TR53) [24,51–53]. Moreover, all these *cyp51A* modifications have been described to evolve from two different azole resistance acquisition routes: the first set of strains come from the clinical setting as a consequence of the in-host drug adaptation after azole exposure in the patient [54], while the second set of isolates with TR insertions are hypothesized to develop from the azole exposure in the environmental setting [13,37,55–58]. Thanks to the high amount of isolates harboring different azole resistance mechanisms included in the study, a clear tendency in terms of grouping can be observed. In agreement with previous studies [13,37,55,56,58–60], all genomes included in our work that harbor a TR integration with single point mutations in *cyp51A* gene were grouped in cluster II, while isolates with punctual modifications in this gene were spread across clusters I and II. The same happened with *cyp51A*-WT strains that were distributed across those clusters. Therefore, our study supported the idea that isolates with punctual modifications in *cyp51A* (G54, G138, M220, or G448) and also *cyp51A*-WT strains have a greater genetic diversity than TR azole resistant isolates (TR34/L98H, TR34/L98H/S297T/F495I), which reinforces the previously suggested idea that TR resistance mechanisms have developed from a reduced set of clonally related strains with shorter genetic distances among them [59,60]. In this study, only genomes from strains which harbor the TR34/L98H resistance mechanism (with or without the S297T and F495I modifications) have been included. It would be most interesting to include isolates harboring TR46/Y121F/T289A, and TR53 azole resistance mechanisms. Furthermore, it is noteworthy that cluster III and IV were formed specifically by particular isolates that harbor 3 or 5 *cyp51A* modifications (F46Y, M172V, E427K and F46Y, M172V, N248T, D255E, E427K, respectively). This result was in agreement with previous studies developed in our group [19]. Further characterization of clado-specific genes would enhance our understanding of antifungal resistance mechanisms and help to unravel the environmental route resistance development.

Despite all these known azole resistance mechanisms, there is an increasing number of *A. fumigatus* azole resistant isolates for which the underlying mechanism remains unknown [61,62] or which are independent of *cyp51A* modifications [63]. The availability of *A. fumigatus* genomes to compare closely related strains but with differences in their azole susceptibility phenotype will increase the chance of finding genetic differences that could explain the phenotypic variations.

In conclusion, a great amount of novel and useful information can be derived from WGS studies. Here we particularly demonstrated that the selection of strains and reference genomes is crucial for comparative analysis at genomic and phenotypic level. Further compilation of *A. fumigatus* data generated by WGS studies could greatly enhance the understanding of molecular mechanisms involved in antifungal drug resistance and its development, as well as in many other biological functions that remain unknown. As the number of *A. fumigatus* genomes have increasingly been publically available, researchers will be able to increase the possibilities for data analysis which will ultimately allow them to come up with possible conclusions about an infinite number of hypotheses.

Supplementary Materials
Figure S1: Workflow for obtaining genes present in all Mat1.1 samples but not present in Mat1.2 (A); and on the contrary (B). Table S1: Mapping rate and coverage at 10× of 101 *A. fumigatus* strains against both reference genomes. Table S2: MEGA genetic distance estimations: pairwise distance matrix calculating the proportion of differences (p-model) and using Af293 as reference genome. Table S3: MEGA genetic distance estimations: pairwise distance matrix calculating the number of differences and using Af293 as reference genome. Table S4: MEGA genetic distance estimations: pairwise distance matrix calculating the proportion of differences (p-model) and using A1163 as reference genome. Table S5: MEGA genetic distance estimations: pairwise distance matrix calculating the number of differences and using A1163 as reference genome. Table S6: MEGA genetic distance estimations: mean distances within subclusters calculating the proportion and number of differences and using Af293 as reference genome. Table S7: MEGA genetic distance estimations: mean distances within subclusters calculating the proportion and number of differences and using A1163 as reference genome. Table S8: MEGA genetic distance estimations: matrix of the mean distances between subclusters calculating the proportion and number of differences and using Af293 as reference genome. Table S9: MEGA genetic distance estimations: matrix of the mean distances between subclusters calculating the proportion and number of differences and using A1163 as reference genome.

Author Contributions: Conceptualization, E.M.; Data curation, S.M. and I.C.; Formal analysis, R.G.-R. and S.M.; Funding acquisition, E.M.; Investigation, R.G.-R. and S.M.; Project administration, E.M.; Resources, E.M.; Software, S.M. and I.C.; Supervision, E.M.; Validation, I.C. and E.M.; Visualization, R.G.-R. and S.M.; Writing-original draft,

References

1. Kontoyiannis, D.P.; Marr, K.A.; Park, B.J.; Alexander, B.D.; Anaissie, E.J.; Walsh, T.J.; Ito, J.; Andes, D.R.; Baddley, J.W.; Brown, J.M.; et al. Prospective surveillance for invasive fungal infections in hematopoietic stem cell transplant recipients, 2001–2006: Overview of the Transplant-Associated Infection Surveillance Network (TRANSNET) Database. *Clin. Infect. Dis.* **2010**, *50*, 1091–1100. [CrossRef] [PubMed]
2. Pappas, P.G.; Alexander, B.D.; Andes, D.R.; Hadley, S.; Kauffman, C.A.; Freifeld, A.; Anaissie, E.J.; Brumble, L.M.; Herwaldt, L.; Ito, J.; et al. Invasive fungal infections among organ transplant recipients: Results of the Transplant-Associated Infection Surveillance Network (TRANSNET). *Clin. Infect. Dis.* **2010**, *50*, 1101–1111. [CrossRef] [PubMed]
3. Denning, D.W. Invasive aspergillosis. *Clin. Infect. Dis.* **1998**, *26*, 781–805. [CrossRef] [PubMed]
4. Latgé, J.P. *Aspergillus fumigatus* and aspergillosis. *Clin. Microbiol. Rev.* **1999**, *12*, 310–350. [PubMed]
5. Kosmidis, C.; Denning, D.W. The clinical spectrum of pulmonary aspergillosis. *Thorax* **2015**, *70*, 270–277. [CrossRef] [PubMed]
6. Verweij, P.E.; Chowdhary, A.; Melchers, W.J.G.; Meis, J.F. Azole Resistance in *Aspergillus fumigatus*: Can We Retain the Clinical Use of Mold-Active Antifungal Azoles? *Clin. Infect. Dis.* **2016**, *62*, 362–368. [CrossRef] [PubMed]
7. Köser, C.U.; Ellington, M.J.; Peacock, S.J. Whole-genome sequencing to control antimicrobial resistance. *Trends Genet.* **2014**, *30*, 401–407. [CrossRef] [PubMed]
8. Peacock, S. Bring microbial sequencing to hospitals. *Nature* **2014**, *509*, 557–559. [CrossRef] [PubMed]
9. Kwong, J.C.; McCallum, N.; Sintchenko, V.; Howden, B.P. Whole genome sequencing in clinical and public health microbiology. *Pathology* **2015**, *47*, 199–210. [CrossRef] [PubMed]
10. Zoll, J.; Snelders, E.; Verweij, P.E.; Melchers, W.J.G. Next-Generation Sequencing in the Mycology Lab. *Curr. Fungal Infect. Rep.* **2016**, *10*, 37–42. [CrossRef] [PubMed]
11. Araujo, R. Towards the genotyping of fungi: Methods, benefits and challenges. *Curr. Fungal Infect. Rep.* **2014**, *8*, 203–210. [CrossRef]
12. Hagiwara, D.; Takahashi, H.; Watanabe, A.; Takahashi-Nakaguchi, A.; Kawamoto, S.; Kamei, K.; Gonoi, T. Whole-genome comparison of *Aspergillus fumigatus* strains serially isolated from patients with aspergillosis. *J. Clin. Microbiol.* **2014**, *52*, 4202–4209. [CrossRef] [PubMed]
13. Abdolrasouli, A.; Rhodes, J.; Beale, M.A.; Hagen, F.; Rogers, T.R.; Chowdhary, A.; Meis, J.F.; Armstrong-James, D.; Fisher, M.C. Genomic context of azole resistance mutations in *Aspergillus fumigatus* determined using whole-genome sequencing. *MBio* **2015**, *6*, e00536-15. [CrossRef] [PubMed]
14. Wei, X.; Chen, P.; Gao, R.; Li, Y.; Zhang, A.; Liu, F.; Lu, L. Screening and characterization of a non-cyp51A mutation in an *Aspergillus fumigatus* cox10 strain conferring azole resistance. *Antimicrob. Agents Chemother.* **2017**, *61*, e02101-16. [CrossRef] [PubMed]
15. Keller, N. Heterogeneity Confounds Establishment of "a" Model Microbial Strain. *mBio* **2017**, *8*, e00135-17. [CrossRef] [PubMed]
16. Nierman, W.C.; Pain, A.; Anderson, M.J.; Wortman, J.R.; Kim, H.S.; Arroyo, J.; Berriman, M.; Abe, K.; Archer, D.B.; Bermejo, C.; et al. Genomic sequence of the pathogenic and allergenic filamentous fungus *Aspergillus fumigatus*. *Nature* **2005**, *438*, 1151–1156. [CrossRef] [PubMed]
17. Fedorova, N.D.; Khaldi, N.; Joardar, V.S.; Maiti, R.; Amedeo, P.; Anderson, M.J.; Crabtree, J.; Silva, J.C.; Badger, J.H.; Albarraq, A.; et al. Genomic islands in the pathogenic filamentous fungus *Aspergillus fumigatus*. *PLoS Genet.* **2008**, *4*, e1000046. [CrossRef] [PubMed]
18. Rokas, A.; Payne, G.; Fedorova, N.D.; Baker, S.E.; Machida, M.; Yu, J.; Georgianna, D.R.; Dean, R.A.; Bhatnagar, D.; Cleveland, T.E.; et al. What can comparative genomics tell us about species concepts in the genus Aspergillus? *Stud. Mycol.* **2007**, *59*, 11–17. [CrossRef] [PubMed]
19. Garcia-Rubio, R.; Alcazar-Fuoli, L.; Monteiro, M.C.; Monzon, S.; Cuesta, I.; Pelaez, T.; Mellado, E. Insight into the significance of *Aspergillus fumigatus* cyp51A polymorphisms. *Antimicrob. Agents Chemother.* **2018**, *62*, e00241-18. [CrossRef] [PubMed]
20. Da Silva Ferreira, M.E.; Kress, M.R.V.Z.; Savoldi, M.; Goldman, M.H.S.; Härtl, A.; Heinekamp, T.; Brakhage, A.A.; Goldman, G.H. The akuBKU80 mutant deficient for nonhomologous end joining is a powerful tool for analyzing pathogenicity in *Aspergillus fumigatus*. *Eukaryot. Cell* **2006**, *5*, 207–211. [CrossRef] [PubMed]

21. Howard, S.J.; Cerar, D.; Anderson, M.J.; Albarrag, A.; Fisher, M.C.; Pasqualotto, A.C.; Laverdiere, M.; Arendrup, M.C.; Perlin, D.S.; Denning, D.W. Frequency and evolution of Azole resistance in *Aspergillus fumigatus* associated with treatment failure. *Emerg. Infect. Dis.* **2009**, *15*, 1068–1076. [CrossRef] [PubMed]
22. Takahashi-Nakaguchi, A.; Muraosa, Y.; Hagiwara, D.; Sakai, K.; Toyotome, T.; Watanabe, A.; Kawamoto, S.; Kamei, K.; Gonoi, T.; Takahashi, H. Genome sequence comparison of *Aspergillus fumigatus* strains isolated from patients with pulmonary aspergilloma and chronic necrotizing pulmonary aspergillosis. *Med. Mycol.* **2015**, *53*, 353–360. [CrossRef] [PubMed]
23. Tang, C.M.; Cohen, J.; Holden, D.W. An *Aspergillus fumigatus* alkaline protease mutant constructed by gene disruption is deficient in extracellular elastase activity. *Mol. Microbiol.* **1992**, *6*, 1663–1671. [CrossRef] [PubMed]
24. Alcazar-Fuoli, L.; Mellado, E.; Alastruey-Izquierdo, A.; Cuenca-Estrella, M.; Rodriguez-Tudela, J.L. Aspergillus section Fumigati: Antifungal susceptibility patterns and sequence-based identification. *Antimicrob. Agents Chemother.* **2008**, *52*, 1244–1251. [CrossRef] [PubMed]
25. Mellado, E.; Garcia-Effron, G.; Alcazar-Fuoli, L.; Melchers, W.J.; Verweij, P.E.; Cuenca-Estrella, M.; Rodriguez-Tudela, J.L. A new *Aspergillus fumigatus* resistance mechanism conferring in vitro cross-resistance to azole antifungals involves a combination of cyp51A alterations. *Antimicrob. Agents Chemother.* **2007**, *51*, 1897–1904. [CrossRef] [PubMed]
26. Bolger, A.M.; Lohse, M.; Usadel, B. Trimmomatic: A flexible trimmer for Illumina sequence data. *Bioinformatics* **2014**, *30*, 2114–2120. [CrossRef] [PubMed]
27. Langmead, B.; Salzberg, S.L. Fast gapped-read alignment with Bowtie2. *Nat. Methods* **2012**, *9*, 357–359. [CrossRef] [PubMed]
28. Quinlan, A.R.; Hall, I.M. BEDTools: A flexible suite of utilities for comparing genomic features. *Bioinformatics* **2010**, *26*, 841–842. [CrossRef] [PubMed]
29. McKenna, A.; Hanna, M.; Banks, E.; Sivachenko, A.; Cibulskis, K.; Kernytsky, A.; Garimella, K.; Altshuler, D.; Gabriel, S.; Daly, M.; et al. The Genome Analysis toolkit: A MapReduce framework for analyzing nextgeneration DNA sequencing data. *Genome Res.* **2010**, *20*, 1297–1303. [CrossRef] [PubMed]
30. Stamatakis, A. RAxML version 8: A tool for phylogenetic analysis and post-analysis of large phylogenies. *Bioinformatics* **2014**, *30*, 1312–1313. [CrossRef] [PubMed]
31. Yu, G.; Smith, D.K.; Zhu, H.; Guan, Y.; Lam, T.T.-Y. ggtree: An R package for visualization and annotation of phylogenetic trees with their covariates and other associated data. *Methods Ecol. Evol.* **2017**, *8*, 28–36. [CrossRef]
32. Kumar, S.; Stecher, G.; Tamura, K. MEGA7: Molecular Evolutionary Genetics Analysis version 7.0. *Mol. Biol. Evol.* **2016**, *33*, 1870–1874. [CrossRef] [PubMed]
33. Pearson, W.R.; Lipman, D.J. Improved tools for biological sequence comparison. *Proc. Natl. Acad. Sci. USA* **1988**, *85*, 2444–2448. [CrossRef] [PubMed]
34. Nei, M.; Kumar, S. *Molecular Evolution and Phylogenetics*; Oxford University Press: New York, NY, USA, 2000; ISBN 9780195135855.
35. Inouye, M.; Dashnow, H.; Raven, L.A.; Schultz, M.B.; Pope, B.J.; Tomita, T.; Zobel, J.; Holt, K.E. SRST2: Rapid genomic surveillance for public health and hospital microbiology labs. *Genome Med.* **2014**, *6*, 90. [CrossRef] [PubMed]
36. Krzywinski, M.; Schein, J.; Birol, I.; Connors, J.; Gascoyne, R.; Horsman, D.; Jones, S.J.; Marra, M.A. Circos: An information aesthetic for comparative genomics. *Genome Res.* **2009**, *19*, 1639–1645. [CrossRef] [PubMed]
37. Ashu, E.E.; Hagen, F.; Chowdhary, A.; Meis, J.F.; Xu, J. Global population genetic analysis of *Aspergillus fumigatus*. *mSphere* **2017**, *2*, e00019-17. [CrossRef] [PubMed]
38. Kowalski, C.H.; Beattie, S.R.; Fuller, K.K.; McGurk, E.A.; Tang, Y.-W.; Hohl, T.M.; Obar, J.J.; Cramer, R.A., Jr. Heterogeneity among isolates reveals that fitness in low oxygen correlates with *Aspergillus fumigatus* virulence. *mBio* **2016**, *7*, e01515-16. [CrossRef] [PubMed]
39. Popovich, K.J.; Snitkin, E.S. Whole Genome Sequencing—Implications for Infection Prevention and Outbreak Investigations. *Curr. Infect. Dis. Rep.* **2017**, *19*, 15. [CrossRef] [PubMed]
40. Wortman, J.R.; Fedorova, N.; Crabtree, J.; Joardar, V.; Maiti, R.; Haas, B.J.; Amedeo, P.; Lee, E.; Angiuoli, S.V.; Jiang, B.; et al. Whole genome comparison of the *A. fumigatus* family. *Med. Mycol.* **2006**, *44* (Suppl. 1), S3–S7. [CrossRef]
41. Fuller, K.K.; Cramer, R.A.; Zegans, M.E.; Dunlap, J.C.; Loros, J.J. *Aspergillus fumigatus* photobiology illuminates the marked heterogeneity between isolates. *mBio* **2016**, *7*, e01517-16. [CrossRef] [PubMed]

42. Rizzetto, L.; Giovannini, G.; Bromley, M.; Bowyer, P.; Romani, L.; Cavalieri, D. Strain dependent variation of immune responses to *A. fumigatus*: Definition of pathogenic species. *PLoS ONE* **2013**, *8*, e56651. [CrossRef] [PubMed]
43. Losada, L.; Sugui, J.A.; Eckhaus, M.A.; Chang, Y.C.; Mounaud, S.; Figat, A.; Joardar, V.; Pakala, S.B.; Pakala, S.; Venepally, P. Genetic Analysis Using an Isogenic Mating Pair of *Aspergillus fumigatus* Identifies Azole Resistance Genes and Lack of MAT Locus's Role in Virulence. *PLoS Pathog.* **2015**, *11*, e1004834. [CrossRef] [PubMed]
44. Dyer, P.S.; O'Gorman, C.M. Sexual development and cryptic sexuality in fungi: Insights from Aspergillus species. *FEMS Microbiol. Rev.* **2012**, *36*, 165–192. [CrossRef] [PubMed]
45. Dyer, P.S.; Inderbitzin, P.; Debuchy, R. Mating-type structure, function, regulation and evolution in the Pezizomycotina. In *Growth, Differentiation and Sexuality. The Mycota (A Comprehensive Treatise on Fungi as Experimental Systems for Basic and Applied Research)*; Wendland, J., Ed.; Springer International Publishing: Basel, Switzerland, 2016; Volume I, pp. 351–385. ISBN 978-3-319-25844-7.
46. Yu, Y.; Amich, J.; Will, C.; Eagle, C.E.; Dyer, P.S.; Krappmann, S. The novel *Aspergillus fumigatus* MAT1-2-4 mating-type gene is required for mating and cleistothecia formation. *Fungal Genet. Biol.* **2017**, *108*, 1–12. [CrossRef] [PubMed]
47. Diaz-Guerra, T.M.; Mellado, E.; Cuenca-Estrella, M.; Rodriguez-Tudela, J.L. A point mutation in the 14alpha-sterol demethylase gene cyp51A contributes to itraconazole resistance in *Aspergillus fumigatus*. *Antimicrob. Agents Chemother.* **2003**, *47*, 1120–1124. [CrossRef] [PubMed]
48. Mellado, E.; Garcia-Effron, G.; Alcazar-Fuoli, L.; Cuenca-Estrella, M.; Rodriguez-Tudela, J.L. Substitutions at methionine 220 in the 14-alpha sterol demethylase (Cyp51A) of *Aspergillus fumigatus* are responsible for resistance in vitro to azole antifungal drugs. *Antimicrob. Agents Chemother.* **2004**, *48*, 2747–2750. [CrossRef] [PubMed]
49. Howard, S.J.; Webster, I.; Moore, C.B.; Gardiner, R.E.; Park, S.; Perlin, D.S.; Denning, D.W. Multi-azole resistance in *Aspergillus fumigatus*. *Int. J. Antimicrob. Agents* **2006**, *28*, 450–453. [CrossRef] [PubMed]
50. Bellete, B.; Raberin, H.; Morel, J.; Flori, P.; Hafid, J.; Manhsung, R.T. Acquired resistance to voriconazole and itraconazole in a patient with pulmonary aspergilloma. *Med. Mycol.* **2010**, *48*, 197–200. [CrossRef] [PubMed]
51. Hodiamont, C.J.; Dolman, K.M.; Ten Berge, I.J.; Melchers, W.J.; Verweij, P.E.; Pajkrt, D. Multiple-azole-resistant *Aspergillus fumigatus* osteomyelitis in a patient with chronic granulomatous disease successfully treated with long-term oral posaconazole and surgery. *Med. Mycol.* **2009**, *47*, 217–220. [CrossRef] [PubMed]
52. Vermeulen, E.; Maertens, J.; Schoemans, H.; Lagrou, K. Azole-resistant *Aspergillus fumigatus* due to TR46/Y121F/T289A mutation emerging in Belgium, July 2012. *Eur. Surveill.* **2012**, *17*, 20326.
53. Chen, Y.; Li, Z.; Han, X.; Tian, S.; Zhao, J.; Chen, F.; Su, X.; Zhao, J.; Zou, Z.; Gong, Y.; et al. Elevated MIC values to imidazole drugs among *Aspergillus fumigatus* isolates with TR34/L98H/S297T/F495I mutation. *Antimicrob. Agents Chemother.* **2018**, *62*, e01549-17. [CrossRef] [PubMed]
54. Burgel, P.R.; Baixench, M.T.; Amsellem, M.; Audureau, E.; Chapron, J.; Kanaan, R.; Honoré, I.; Dupouy-Camet, J.; Dusser, D.; Klaassen, C.H.; et al. High prevalence of azole-resistant *Aspergillus fumigatus* in adults with cystic fibrosis exposed to itraconazole. *Antimicrob. Agents Chemother.* **2012**, *56*, 869–874. [CrossRef] [PubMed]
55. Chowdhary, A.; Kathuria, S.; Xu, J.; Sharma, C.; Sundar, G.; Singh, P.K.; Gaur, S.N.; Hagen, F.; Klaassen, C.H.; Meis, J.F. Clonal expansion and emergence of environmental multiple-triazole-resistant *Aspergillus fumigatus* strains carrying the TR34/L98H mutations in the *cyp51A* gene in India. *PLoS ONE* **2012**, *7*, e52871. [CrossRef] [PubMed]
56. Chang, H.; Ashu, E.; Sharma, C.; Kathuria, S.; Chowdhary, A.; Xu, J. Diversity and origins of Indian multi-triazole resistant strains of *Aspergillus fumigatus*. *Mycoses* **2016**, *59*, 450–466. [CrossRef] [PubMed]
57. Garcia-Rubio, R.; Cuenca-Estrella, M.; Mellado, E. Triazole Resistance in Aspergillus Species: An Emerging Problem. *Drugs* **2017**, *77*, 599–613. [CrossRef] [PubMed]
58. Wang, H.C.; Huang, J.C.; Lin, Y.H.; Chen, Y.H.; Hsieh, M.I.; Choi, P.C.; Lo, H.J.; Liu, W.L.; Hsu, C.S.; Shih, H.I.; et al. Prevalence, mechanisms and genetic relatedness of the human pathogenic fungus *Aspergillus fumigatus* exhibiting resistance to medical azoles in the environment of Taiwan. *Environ. Microbiol.* **2017**, *20*, 270–280. [CrossRef] [PubMed]
59. Snelders, E.; Rijs, A.J.; Kema, G.H.; Melchers, W.J.; Verweij, P.E. Possible environmental origin of resistance of *Aspergillus fumigatus* to medical triazoles. *Appl. Environ. Microbiol.* **2009**, *75*, 4053–4057. [CrossRef] [PubMed]

60. Camps, S.M.T.; Rijs, A.J.M.M.; Klaassen, C.H.W.; Meis, J.F.; O'Gorman, C.M.; Dyer, P.S.; Melchers, W.J.G.; Verweij, P.E. Molecular epidemiology of *Aspergillus fumigatus* isolates harboring the TR34/L98H azole resistance mechanism. *J. Clin. Microbiol.* **2012**, *50*, 2674–2680. [CrossRef] [PubMed]
61. Chowdhary, A.; Sharma, C.; Hagen, F.; Meis, J.F. Exploring azole antifungal drug resistance in *Aspergillus fumigatus* with special reference to resistance mechanisms. *Future Microbiol.* **2014**, *9*, 697–711. [CrossRef] [PubMed]
62. Moye-Rowley, W.S. Multiple mechanisms contribute to the development of clinically significant azole resistance in *Aspergillus fumigatus*. *Front. Microbiol.* **2015**, *6*, 70. [CrossRef] [PubMed]
63. Fraczek, M.G.; Bromley, M.; Buied, A.; Moore, C.B.; Rajendran, R.; Rautemaa, R.; Ramage, G.; Denning, D.W.; Bowyer, P. The cdr1B efflux transporter is associated with non-cyp51 a mediated itraconazole resistance in *Aspergillus fumigatus*. *J. Antimicrob. Chemother.* **2013**, *68*, 1486–1496. [CrossRef] [PubMed]

Permissions

All chapters in this book were first published by MDPI; hereby published with permission under the Creative Commons Attribution License or equivalent. Every chapter published in this book has been scrutinized by our experts. Their significance has been extensively debated. The topics covered herein carry significant findings which will fuel the growth of the discipline. They may even be implemented as practical applications or may be referred to as a beginning point for another development.

The contributors of this book come from diverse backgrounds, making this book a truly international effort. This book will bring forth new frontiers with its revolutionizing research information and detailed analysis of the nascent developments around the world.

We would like to thank all the contributing authors for lending their expertise to make the book truly unique. They have played a crucial role in the development of this book. Without their invaluable contributions this book wouldn't have been possible. They have made vital efforts to compile up to date information on the varied aspects of this subject to make this book a valuable addition to the collection of many professionals and students.

This book was conceptualized with the vision of imparting up-to-date information and advanced data in this field. To ensure the same, a matchless editorial board was set up. Every individual on the board went through rigorous rounds of assessment to prove their worth. After which they invested a large part of their time researching and compiling the most relevant data for our readers.

The editorial board has been involved in producing this book since its inception. They have spent rigorous hours researching and exploring the diverse topics which have resulted in the successful publishing of this book. They have passed on their knowledge of decades through this book. To expedite this challenging task, the publisher supported the team at every step. A small team of assistant editors was also appointed to further simplify the editing procedure and attain best results for the readers.

Apart from the editorial board, the designing team has also invested a significant amount of their time in understanding the subject and creating the most relevant covers. They scrutinized every image to scout for the most suitable representation of the subject and create an appropriate cover for the book.

The publishing team has been an ardent support to the editorial, designing and production team. Their endless efforts to recruit the best for this project, has resulted in the accomplishment of this book. They are a veteran in the field of academics and their pool of knowledge is as vast as their experience in printing. Their expertise and guidance has proved useful at every step. Their uncompromising quality standards have made this book an exceptional effort. Their encouragement from time to time has been an inspiration for everyone.

The publisher and the editorial board hope that this book will prove to be a valuable piece of knowledge for researchers, students, practitioners and scholars across the globe.

List of Contributors

Tafese B. Tufa
Asella Teaching and Referral Hospital, College of Health Sciences, Arsi University, Asella, Ethiopia
Hirsch Institute of Tropical Medicine (HITM), Heinrich-Heine University, Asella, Ethiopia

David W. Denning
The National Aspergillosis Centre, Wythenshawe Hospital, Manchester M23 9LT, UK
The University of Manchester and Manchester Academic Health Science Centre, Manchester M13 9PL, UK

Jan Springer, Hermann Einsele and Juergen Loeer
Department for Internal Medicine II, University Hospital of Wuerzburg, 97080 Wuerzburg, Germany

Grit Walther
National Reference Center for Invasive Fungal Infections (NRZMyk), Leibniz Institute for Natural Product Research and Infection Biology, Hans Knöll Institute, 07745 Jena, Germany

Volker Rickerts
Robert Koch Institute Berlin, 13353 Berlin, Germany

Axel Hamprecht
Institute for Medical Microbiology, Immunology and Hygiene, University Hospital of Cologne, University of Cologne, 50935 Cologne, Germany
Institute for Medical Microbiology and Virology, Carl von Ossietzky University of Oldenburg, 26129 Oldenburg, Germany

Birgit Willinger
Division of Clinical Microbiology, Institute of Hygiene and Medical Microbiology of the University, Vienna University Hospital, 1090 Vienna, Austria

Daniel Teschner
Department of Hematology, Medical Oncology, and Pneumology, University Medical Center of the Johannes Gutenberg University, 55122 Mainz, Germany

Oliver Kurzai
National Reference Center for Invasive Fungal Infections (NRZMyk), Leibniz Institute for Natural Product Research and Infection Biology, Hans Knöll Institute, 07745 Jena, Germany
Institute for Hygiene and Microbiology, University Wuerzburg, 97080 Wuerzburg, Germany

Marta Stanzani
Institute of Hematology "Lorenzo e Ariosto Seràgnoli", Department of Hematology and Clinical Oncology, S. Orsola-Malpighi Hospital, University of Bologna, 40138 Bologna, Italy

Russell E. Lewis
Clinic of Infectious Diseases, Department of Medical and Surgical Sciences, S. Orsola-Malpighi Hospital, University of Bologna, 40138 Bologna, Italy

Sarah Dellière, Romain Guery and Claire Aguilar
Medical School, Paris-Descartes University, APHP, Necker-Enfants Malades Hospital, Infectious Disease Center Necker-Pasteur, IHU Imagine, 75015 Paris, France

Sophie Candon and Lucienne Chatenoud
Medical School, Paris-Descartes University, INSERM U1151-CNRS UMR 8253APHP, Necker-Enfants Malades Hospital, APHP, Clinical Immunology, 75015 Paris, France

Blandine Rammaert
Medical School, Poitiers University, Poitiers, France; Poitiers University Hospital, Infectious Disease Unit, Poitiers, France; INSERM U1070, 86022 Poitiers, France

Fanny Lanternier and Olivier Lortholary
Medical School, Paris-Descartes University, APHP, Necker-Enfants Malades Hospital, Infectious Disease Center Necker-Pasteur, IHU Imagine, 75015 Paris, France
Pasteur Institute, Molecular Mycology Unit, National Reference Center for Invasive Fungal Disease and Antifungals, CNRS UMR 2000, 75015 Paris, France

Sevtap Arikan-Akdagli
Department of Medical Microbiology, Mycology Laboratory, Hacettepe University Medical School, TR-06100 Ankara, Turkey

Mahmoud Ghannoum
Center for Medical Mycology, Department of Dermatology, University Hospitals Cleveland Medical Center, Case Western Reserve University, Cleveland, OH 44106, USA

Jacques F. Meis
Department of Medical Microbiology and Infectious Diseases, Canisius Wilhelmina Hospital (CWZ), 6532 Nijmegen, The Netherlands
Centre of Expertise in Mycology Radboudumc/CWZ, 6532 Nijmegen, The Netherlands

Liang Huo, Ping Zhang, Chenxi Li, Kashif Rahim, Xiaoran Hao, Biyun Xiang and Xudong Zhu
Beijing Key Laboratory of Genetic Engineering Drug and Biotechnology, Institute of Biochemistry and Molecular Biology, College of Life Sciences, Beijing Normal University (CLS-BNU), Beijing 100875, China

João N. de Almeida Jr.
Central Laboratory Division, Hospital das Clínicas da Faculdade de Medicina da Universidade de São Paulo, CEP 05403-000 São Paulo, Brazil

Paula M. Peçanha-Pietrobom and Arnaldo L. Colombo
Department of Medicine, Division of Infectious Diseases, Escola Paulista de Medicina, Universidade Federal de São Paulo, CEP 04039-032 São Paulo, Brazil

Thomas J. Walsh
Departments of Medicine, Pediatrics, and Microbiology & immunology, Weill Cornell Medicine of Cornell University and New York Presbyterian Hospital, New York, NY 10065, USA

Tempe Chen
Pediatric Infectious Diseases, Department of Pediatrics, Miller Children's Hospital and University of California Irvine, Long Beach, CA 90806, USA

Priya Madhavan
School of Medicine, Faculty of Health and Medical Sciences, Taylor's University Malaysia, Subang Jaya, 47500 Selangor, Malaysia

Emmanuel Roilides
Infectious Diseases Section, 3rd Department of Pediatrics, Faculty of Medicine, Aristotle University School of Health Sciences and Hippokration General Hospital, 54642 Thessaloniki, Greece

Mafalda Cavalheiro, Pedro Pais, Mónica Galocha and Miguel C. Teixeira
Department of Bioengineering, Instituto Superior Técnico, Universidade de Lisboa, 1049-001 Lisbon, Portugal
Biological Sciences Research Group, iBB—Institute for Bioengineering and Biosciences, Instituto Superior Técnico, Universidade de Lisboa, 1049-001 Lisboa, Portugal

Jorge Amich
Manchester Fungal Infection Group (MFIG), Faculty of Biology, Medicine and Health, University of Manchester, Manchester M13 9NT, UK

Rocío Vicentefranqueira, Laura Marín, Clara Inés Sánchez, Fernando Leal and José Antonio Calera
Instituto de Biología Funcional y Genómica (IBFG-CSIC), Departamento de Microbiología y Genética, Universidad de Salamanca, 37007 Salamanca, Spain

Thomas F. Patterson and J. Peter Donnelly
Division of Infectious Diseases, San Antonio Center for Medical Mycology, The University of Texas Health Science Center at San Antonio and the South Texas Veterans Health Care System, 7703 Floyd Curl Drive-MSC 7881, San Antonio, TX 78229-3900, USA

Pei Pei Chong, Voon Kin Chin, Voon Chen Yong and Chung Yeng Looi
School of Biosciences, Faculty of Health and Medical Sciences, Taylor's University Malaysia, Subang Jaya, 47500 Selangor, Malaysia

Won Fen Wong
Department of Medical Microbiology, Faculty of Medicine, University Malaya, 50603 Kuala Lumpur, Malaysia

Aspasia Katragkou
Department of Pediatrics, Division of Pediatric Infectious Diseases, Nationwide Children's Hospital and The Ohio State University School of Medicine, Columbus, OH 43205, USA

Christine M. Salvatore
Department of Pediatrics, Division of Pediatric Infectious Diseases,Weill Cornell Medicine of Cornell University and New York Presbyterian Hospital, New York, NY 10065, USA

Chris D. Lauruschkat, Hermann Einsele and Juergen Loeffler
Department of Internal Medicine II, University Hospital Wuerzburg, WÜ4i, Building C11, 7080 Wuerzburg, Germany

Rocio Garcia-Rubio, Laura Alcazar-Fuoli and Emilia Mellado
Mycology Reference Laboratory, National Centre for Microbiology, Instituto de Salud Carlos III (ISCIII), Majadahonda, 28220 Madrid, Spain

Sara Monzon and Isabel Cuesta
Bioinformatics Unit, Common Scientific Technical Units, ISCIII, Majadahonda, 28220 Madrid, Spain

Index

L

M

N

O

P

R

S

T

V